D1740223

NEW INSIGHTS IN
GYNECOLOGY & OBSTETRICS

RESEARCH AND PRACTICE

NEW INSIGHTS IN
GYNECOLOGY & OBSTETRICS
RESEARCH AND PRACTICE

Edited by

B. Ottesen and A. Tabor

Hvidovre University Hospital
Hvidovre, Denmark

The Proceedings of the XV FIGO World Congress
of Gynecology and Obstetrics

Copenhagen, August 1997

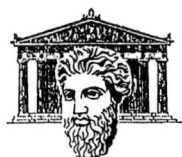

The Parthenon Publishing Group
International Publishers in Medicine, Science & Technology

NEW YORK   LONDON

Published in the USA by
The Parthenon Publishing Group Inc.
One Blue Hill Plaza, PO Box 1564,
Pearl River, New York 10965, USA

Published in the UK and Europe by
The Parthenon Publishing Group Ltd.
Casterton Hall, Carnforth,
Lancs. LA6 2LA, UK

Library of Congress Cataloging-in-Publication Data
FIGO World Congress of Gynecology and Obstetrics (15th : 1997 : Copenhagen, Denmark)
New insights in gynecology and obstetrics : research and practice / the proceedings of the XV FIGO
World Congress of Gynecology and Obstetrics, Copenhagen, Denmark, August 1997 : edited by
B. Ottesen and A. Tabor.
p. cm.
Includes bibliographical references and index.
ISBN 1-85070-966-1
1. Gynecology—Congresses. 2. Obstetrics—Congresses.
I. Ottesen, B. II. Tabor, A. III Title.
[DNLM: 1. Gynecology congresses. 2. Obstetrics congresses. 3. Women's Health congresses.
WP 100 F473n 1998]
RG31.F54 1997
618—dc21
DNLM/DLC
for Library of Congress   98-15899
                                                                                              CIP

British Library Cataloguing-in-Publication Data
New insights in gynecology and obstetrics: research and practice: the proceedings of the XV FIGO
World Congress of Gynecology and Obstetrics Copenhagen, Denmark, August 1997
1. Gynecology 2. Obstetrics
I. Ottesen, B. II. Tabor, A. III. International Federation of Gynecology and Obstetrics
618

ISBN 1-85070-966-1

First published 1998

Typeset by AMA Graphics Ltd., Preston, UK
Printed and bound by Butler & Tanner Ltd., Frome and London, UK

Contents

List of principal contributors

M. M. Anceschi
2nd Institute of Obstetrics and Gynecology
University of Rome 'La Sapienza'
Policlinico Umberto I
Viale Regina Elena 324
00161 Rome
Italy

S. Arulkumaran
Department of Obstetrics and Gynecology
National University Hospital
Lower Kent Ridge Road
Singapore 119074
Singapore

H. Ba'aqeel
Department of Obstetrics and Gynecology
King Abdulaziz University Hospital
Jeddah 21452
Saudi Arabia

D. T. Baird
Department of Obstetrics and Gynaecology
University of Edinburgh
Centre for Reproductive Biology
37 Chalmers Street
Edinburgh EH3 9EW
UK

E. Barrett-Connor
Department of Family and Preventive
    Medicine
University of California, San Diego
9500 Gilman Drive
La Jolla
California 92093-0607
USA

J. M. Belizán
CREP-Centro Rosarino de Estudios Perinatales
San Luis 2493
Rosario
RA 2000
Argentina

V. Beral
Imperial Cancer Research Fund
Cancer Epidemiology Unit
Gibson Building
Radcliffe Infirmary
Oxford OX2 6HE
UK

J. S. Berek
UCLA School of Medicine
CHS 24-127
10833 LeConte Avenue
Los Angeles
CA 90095-1740
USA

P. Bergsjø
Kvinneklinikum
Haukeland University Hospital
N-5021 Bergen
Norway

K. W. M. Bloemenkamp
Department of Obstetrics, Gynecology
    and Reproductive Medicine
Leiden University Hospital, Building 1-H3-P
PO Box 9600
2300 RC Leiden
The Netherlands

M. A. Bruhat
Polyclinique Gynécologie Obstétrique
    Médecine de la Reproduction
CHU - Université d'Auvergne
13 Boulevard Charles-De-Gaulle
63000 Clermont-Ferrand
France

R. J. Cook
Faculty of Law
University of Toronto
84 Queen's Park
Toronto
Canada M5S 2C5

E. V. Cosmi
2nd Institute of Obstetrics and Gynecology
University of Rome 'La Sapienza'
Policlinico Umberto I
Viale Regina Elena 324
00161 Rome
Italy

W. T. Creasman
Department of Obstetrics and Gynecology
Medical University of South Carolina
171 Ashley Avenue
Charleston
South Carolina 29425-2233
USA

A. E. Dastur
Nowrosjee Wadia Maternity Hospital
23 Nepean Sea Road
Colaba
Bombay 400 036
India

S. Daya
Department of Obstetrics and Gynecology
McMaster University
1200 Main Street West
Hamilton, Ontario
Canada L8N 3Z5

E. Diczfalusy
Karolinska Hospital
Rönningewägen 21
S-144 61 Rönninge
Sweden

C. Ellertson
The Population Council
1 Dag Hammaskjold Plaza
New York
NY 10017
USA

C. Garcia-Moreno
Women, Health and Development
World Health Organization
1211 Geneva 27
Switzerland

A. Glasier
University of Edinburgh
18 Dean Terrace
Edinburgh EH4 1NL
UK

C. B. Hammond
Post Office Box 3853
Duke University Medical Center
Durham
North Carolina 27710
USA

L. A. J. Heinemann
Center for Epidemilogy and Health Research
  Berlin
Schoenerlinder Strasse 11
D-16341 Zepernick
Germany

A. D. Hewson
48 Denison Street
Hamilton
New South Wales 2303
Australia

R. E. Leake
Department of Biochemistry
University of Glasgow
Glasgow G12 8QQ
UK

E. Lynge
Danish Cancer Society
Division for Cancer Epidemiology
Strandboulevarden 49
Box 839
DK-2100 Copenhagen
Denmark

G. P. Mandruzzato
Instituto per l'Infanzia
Divisione di Obstetricia e Ginecologia
Via dell'Istria 65/1
34100 Trieste
Italy

G. C. Montruccoli
Toniolo Clinic
Via Toscana n 34
I-40141 Bologna
Italy

A. F. P. L. d'Oliveira
Rua Apinagés 854 – Sumaré
Sao Paulo
CEP 05017-000
SP
Brazil

B. Ottesen
Hvidovre University Hospital
Kettegaards Alle 30
DK 2650 Hvidovre
Denmark

Z. Papp
I Department of Obstetrics and Gynecology
Semmelweis University Medical School
Baross Ut. 27
1088 Budapest
Hungary

O. M. Petrucco
Women's & Children's Hospital
1st Floor Queen Victoria Building
72 King William Road
North Adelaide, SA 5006
Australia

H. J. Philippe
College National des Gynecologues et
    Obstetricians Français
C.H. Léon Touhaldjan
F 78303 Poissy Cedex
France

B. Schei
The Centre for Research in Women's Health
790 Bay Street
Room 749
Toronto
Ontario
Canada M5G 1N8

D. Schopper
Medicins sans Frontières
Rue du lac 12
Case Postale 6090
CH-1211 Geneve 6
Switzerland

J. J. Sciarra
Department of Obstetrics and Gynecology
Northwestern University Medical School
333 East Superior 490
Chicago
IL 60611
USA

V. Seltzer
American College of Obstetricians and
    Gynecologists
Long Island Jewish Medical Center
270-05 76th Avenue
Lakeville Road
New Hyde Park
NY 11040
USA

J. L. Simpson
Department of Obstetrics and Gynecology
Baylor College of Medicine
6550 Fannin Street
Suite 729A
Houston
TX 77030
USA

S. O. Skouby
Department of Obstetrics and Gynecology
Frederiksberg Hospital
Copenhagen
Denmark

I. Szabó
Department of Obstetrics and Gynecology
Medical University of Pecs
Edesanyak u. 17
H-7624 Pecs
Hungary

A. Tabor
Hvidovre University Hospital
Kettegaards Alle 30
DK 2650 Hvidovre
Denmark

P. F. A. Van Look
Human Reproduction Special Programme
World Health Organization
1211 Geneva 27
Switzerland

A. Van Steirteghem
Center for Reproductive Medicine
Medical School and University Hospital
Vrije Universiteit Brussel - VUB
Laarbeeklaan 101
B-1090 Brussels
Belgium

M. J. do A. Vasconcellos
Department of Obstetrics and Gynecology
Rio de Janeiro University
Rua Esteves Junior 64, Apt. 501
BR-22231-160 Rio de Janeiro
Brazil

H. C. Visscher
5721 Lakeshore Avenue
N. Holland
MI 49424
USA

N. Wake
Department of Reproductive Physiology &
 Endocrinology
Medical Institute of Bioregulation
Kyushu University
4546 Tsurumihara Beppu
Oita 874
Japan

J. N. Wasserheit
Division of STD Prevention
National Center for HIV, STD, TB Prevention
Center for Disease Control and Prevention
1600 Clifton Road (Mailstop E02)
Atlanta, Georgia 30333
USA

C. Watts
Health Policy Unit
London School of Hygiene and Tropical
 Medicine
Keppel St
London WC1E 7HT
UK

In search of human dignity: gender equity, reproductive health and healthy aging

E. Diczfalusy

Birth of three worlds

'Time present and time past
Are both perhaps present in time future
And time future contained in time past.'
T. S. Eliot, 1935

What an incredible privilege, responsibility and challenge it is to deliver the De Watteville Memorial Lecture at the last FIGO Congress of the century and even of the millennium! The occasion fills me with humility, plenty of emotion, and also with a kind of philosophical spirit since this is the place and time to reflect over our common past and common future. *Quo vadimus?* Where are we heading?

This is also my opportunity to try – in a humble way – to differentiate between the universal and the unique, since I have witnessed so much in the history of the 20th century that was fundamentally unique and that has dramatically changed our perception of the world. Indeed, all of us here are revolutionaries: the revolutionaries of changing perceptions. Therefore, this is the time to reflect over our common past and present and to attempt to formulate a common vision of that common future, since only those with some knowledge of the past can have a vision of the future.

'*Es bueno vivir mucho para ver mucho*' (It is good to live long in order to see much)[1], says Sancho Panza in *Don Quixote,* and those who live longest, may, indeed, see most. I have certainly seen a great deal during a long life; I have seen the major part of the history of the 20th century and

I have seen much more of the world than all my ancestors together. When I was born, the world population was less than 2 billion; next year it will surpass 6 billion people. Hence – in my lifetime – I have seen the birth of another two worlds, equal in numbers, needs, aspirations, hopes and dreams. I also see on the horizon the birth of a third new world of tomorrow that will lead to a new global reality, an entirely different world of 8 billion fellow men and women in approximately two decades and of 10 billion people in 50 years' time[2,3].

Those who live longest have seen much; who knows, sometimes perhaps they have seen even too much? As Schopenhauer remarked almost 150 years ago: 'The man who sees two or three generations is like someone who sits in a conjurer's booth at a fair, and sees the tricks two or three times. They are meant to be seen only once'[4]. I have seen three generations in action, exercising the two powerful instruments that occasionally shape human history: the arrogance of power and the arrogance of ignorance.

Is history only a nightmare?

'Contempt for human nature is an error of human reason.'
Luc de Clapiers deVauvenargues, 1746

'History is a nightmare from which I am trying to awake', said James Joyce in his *Lestrygonians.* Many of us may be tempted to agree with him, at least on certain occasions. But, on other occasions, we may feel that the issue is much more complicated. In his reflections above about the advantages of a long life, Sancho Panza also remarks: '*el que larga vida vive mucho mal ha de pasar*' (those who live long also pass through much evil)[1], and I have certainly witnessed a fair amount of it. I have seen the devastating consequences of two world wars, the dangerous flirtation with apocalypse by the 'superpowers' of the time, the rise and fall of 'millennial' empires and the endless chain of so-called 'limited' or 'local' armed conflicts in all corners of the world. I have also seen the enthusiastic acceptance and embrace by many millions of people of pseudointellectual political 'ideologies', exposing many fellow men and women to terror, cruelty, moral horrors and an incredible amount of unnecessary human suffering. In fact, it is estimated that, during the 20th century, almost 200 million human beings were systematically killed by human beings on the orders of human beings.

Like others before me, I have also found it extremely difficult to quantitate human suffering at the level of millions. Two hundred may still be a meaningful figure; one may think of 200 patients with cervical cancer or HIV; one may even remember the individual faces, the case histories and the pathological anatomy of individual suffering. But what about 200 million people? That figure becomes very distant, abstract and 'faceless' statistical information. And still, by the end of the day, such 'faceless' information will be of paramount importance in shaping both national and international health policy and the research agenda of tomorrow, and may, thus, eventually contribute to the improvement of the human condition. Therefore, this review is going to place heavy emphasis on descriptive statistics.

In all fairness, however, it was not only terror, barbarism and cruelty that I observed around me in the world of the 20th century; I have also witnessed an incredible amount of progress. In fact, I have witnessed more progress in science and technology than all scientists of all preceding generations put together, since the dawn of history. This should not be too surprising, since 'The crude size of science in terms of manpower or in publications tends to double within a period of 10–15 years. Indeed, more than 90% of all scientists that have ever lived are alive now'[5]. As Friedrich Engels phrased it: 'Science progresses in proportion to the mass of knowledge that is left to it by preceding generations, that is under the most ordinary circumstances in geometrical proportion'[6]. From this, it also follows that, when I graduated from Medical School in Szeged, Hungary, in 1944, the 'crude size' of medical science and technology was probably 5–10% of that of today, if not less. What an incredible privilege it was to witness the world-wide progress in medical sciences in general, and in obstetrics and gynecology in particular, during half a century, and to realize again and again with Shakespeare, that 'what is past is prologue'. And what a particular privilege it was not only to witness this process, but also to be part of it. History is much more than just a nightmare.

Seven revolutions

'I believe in two-faced truth, in the Either, the Or and the Holy Both.'

Palinurus, 1944

Sometimes I feel that the 20th century will go down in history as the century of paradoxes. Some of these are attributable to increasing numbers of people, others not. One may argue that never before our time were so many people killed, not only brutally, but systematically in cold blood, or that so many victims were helped, also systematically and humanely. Claude Bernard told us that 'The generalisation alone constitutes science'[7], but the de Goncourt brothers, Edmond and Jules, assure us that – in fact – in this existence 'nothing is repeated and everything is unparalleled'[8]. Is everyone right and everyone wrong? Other paradoxes appear to be even more characteristic: we live in a time of great events, big global concerns and rather simplistic philosophies proposed to confront those big concerns. We live in a world which is more integrated and at the same time more fragmented than ever before.

However, many of the apparent paradoxes may be inherent in the human condition and already Aristotle emphasized that 'The knowledge of opposites is one'. Indeed – to me – fundamental truths are characterized by the fact that the opposite proposition is also a fundamental truth. Upon further reflection, one wonders whether perhaps all preceding centuries also were centuries of paradoxes, reflecting simply our basic human condition?

There were, however, some unique major events in the history of the 20th century: fundamental changes, real revolutions, and this review will consider several of them. The word revolution has many meanings and can correctly describe the movement of certain celestial bodies just as well as the complete overthrow of a government, but – according to the *Oxford English Dictionary* – the term can also be used to describe a 'great change in affairs or things', with fundamental changes in general perception and public attitude, as it is used in the present article.

Table 1 indicates seven major revolutions of my time; I have witnessed them to evolve, I was part of them and my perception of the world was – and still is – deeply influenced by them. Others may, of course, prefer a different 'menu' of their favorite revolutions; like so many things in life, revolutions are also a matter of taste.

I have briefly touched upon the demographic and scientific revolutions. I consider the revolution of global identity to be a characteristic of 'our time', the second half of the 20th century, that brought to humankind a holistic view of the world and resulted in the establishment of a wide variety of international organizations, *inter alia* the United Nations (UN), with its numerous

Table 1 Seven revolutions

Demographic
Scientific
Global identity
Environmental
Contraceptive
Reproductive health
Gender equity

specialized agencies, such as the World Health Organization (WHO), the United Nations Environmental Program (UNEP), the High Commissioner for Refugees (UNHCR), the United Nations Food and Agricultural Organization (FAO), the United Nations Population Program (UNFPA) and the World Bank (International Bank for Reconstruction and Development, IBRD), just to mention a few. Another dimension of our global identity is represented by the hundreds, if not thousands, of international professional organizations, the International Federation of Gynecology and Obstetrics (FIGO) being one of the most important and most successful examples of them.

During its – so far – short existence of half a century, the UN sailed through the straits of several international crises between the Scylla and Charybdis of human nature in general, and devastating politics in particular, and has frequently been exposed to heavy criticisms, maybe sometimes rightly so, sometimes not. As I see it in retrospect, the main problem with the UN is that it is so young, that humankind doesn't really know, as yet, how to utilize it in an optimal manner to solve those problems it is capable of solving. We are still heavily involved in a learning process in which time and experience will be our great teachers. However, whatever may or may not happen, I am firmly convinced that the concept of the UN has come to stay with humankind during the centuries to come, just as the fundamental – and, indeed, revolutionary – concept of global identity. It was Hegel who remarked, some 160 years ago, that 'It is easier to discover a deficiency in individuals, in states and Providence than to see their import and value'[9], and one wonders really whether we are always fair in our appraisal of the United Nations and of its specialized agencies.

The environmental revolution is also a relatively recent departure in the history of humankind. In my youth, the problem simply didn't exist, at least not in our perception. For us, the 'carrying capacity' of the world was infinitely large, and its resources inexhaustible. Surely, there were many problems around, but world-wide population and its environmental impact were certainly not among them. Indeed, it is not easy to explain to our grandchildren today that it was self-evident to us that the environment ('Mother Nature') will always provide all our material needs and will effectively dispose of any amount of waste generated by us. To put all this in proper perspective, we may remind ourselves of Aldous Huxley's *Brave New World Revisited*[10], a continuation of the vision of the *Brave New World*[11]. Huxley remarks 'In the *Brave New World* of my fable, the problem of human numbers in their relation to natural resources had been effectively solved. An optimum figure for world population had been calculated and numbers were maintained at this figure (a little under 2 billions, if I remember rightly) generation after generation.'

The big eye-opener for many governments was certainly the United Nations Conference on Environment and Development[12], which also convinced many of us that the environmental issue – like the population issue – will assume a dominant role and top priority on the international agenda of the 21st century.

The last three revolutions of Table 1, the contraceptive revolution and the revolutions in reproductive health and gender equity, represent three coherent dimensions of the greatest social revolution of our century, the universal search for human dignity, and will constitute the main subject of this article together with the very first and most decisive one, the demographic revolution, with its most recent and most acute aspect, the issue of aging populations.

Demographic revolution

'Humankind is growing rapidly and aging rapidly.'
E. Diczfalusy, 1995

Growth of world population

Humankind entered the 20th century with a global population of 1650 million people and will leave it behind with a population of 6158 million people[3]. The estimates and medium variant projections of the world population between 1950 and 2050 are indicated in Table 2. The growth rate of the world population peaked

in 1990 with an annual increment of 88 million people; in 1960 it was 53 million and by the year 2050 it is expected to be again around 50 million. The United Nations medium-fertility extension projects a global population of 11.2 billion for the year 2100[2].

The figures of Table 2 can be complemented with a shorter-term regional projection for the next 30 years. Of the projected total increase of some 2.7 billion people, approximately 1.6 billion are expected to be in Asia, 800 million in Africa, 235 million in Latin America and 80 million in North America, whereas the European population is expected to decrease from 726 to 718 million[3].

What about the long-term regional distribution of the world population in the more distant future? Such projections – as emphasized by the UN – are most uncertain, since they involve too many major assumptions about future fertility and mortality rates. Still, such projections – with all their inherent limitations – must constitute part of our vision of our destiny. In these times, we must learn to live with uncertainty and to plan for an uncertain future accordingly. With all these caveats, Table 3 presents the UN

Table 2 Estimates and projections of the world population[3]

Year	Population (billions)
1950	2.5
1970	3.7
1990	5.3
2010	7.0
2030	8.7
2050	9.8

Table 3 Percentage distribution of the world population[2]

Area	Year		
	1950	2050	2150
Africa	8.8	22.6	26.8
China	22.1	15.2	12.0
India	14.2	17.0	16.9
Other Asia	18.4	23.7	24.3
North America	6.6	3.3	2.7
Europe	15.6	4.9	3.7

projections of the percentage distribution of the global population during a 200-year period between 1950 and 2150. The data of Table 3 suggest a future demographic predominance by Africa and Asia, and a long day's march of Europe towards demographic irrelevance.

Life expectancy at birth

As indicated by the data of Table 4, during the past half century, life expectancy at birth increased by some 20 years for women and by more than 18 years for men. Table 4 also projects that, during the next 50 years, it will further increase with an additional 11.5 years for women and 10.7 years for men. It also appears from the data of Table 4 that, between 1950 and 2050, the gender difference in world-wide life expectancy at birth is expected to increase from 2.7 to 4.9 years.

There are, of course, major regional differences behind the global averages of Table 4, as illustrated by the data for the year 2000 (Table 5). Life expectancy at birth in Africa will remain lowest for some time to come, and the gender difference will be highest in Europe. It is projected that, by the year 2050, life expectancy at birth in Europe will be 83.3 years for women and 77.1 years for men, with a gender difference of 6.2 years[3]. The long-term assumption of the UN for the year 2150 suggests a 'final' world-wide life expectancy at birth of 84.7 years for both sexes[2].

Life expectancy at 60 years and over

Most of the increase in life expectancy in the first half of the 20th century resulted from reduced mortality among young age groups. In the past few decades, there have also been substantial reductions in mortality among the elderly, resulting in significant increases in life expectancy at higher ages in many countries, as illustrated by some examples from selected countries given in Table 6[13].

Since the increase in women's life expectancy considerably exceeds that of men[13,14], in several countries the gender difference among the

elderly has reached proportions never observed before[15]. Relevant data from selected countries are presented in Table 7.

Table 4 Life expectancy at birth (years) in the world[3]

Year	Females	Males	Difference
1950	47.8	45.1	2.7
2000	67.8	63.7	4.1
2050	79.3	74.4	4.9

Table 5 Life expectancy at birth (years) in the year 2000[3]

Region	Female	Male	Difference
Africa	55.7	52.7	3.0
Asia	67.7	64.9	2.8
Latin America	72.4	67.1	5.3
North America	80.2	73.5	6.7
Europe	77.3	69.3	8.0

Table 6 Life expectancy (years) at the age of 65 years as assessed in 1950–1954 and 1985–1990[13]

Country	1950–1954		1985–1990	
	Women	Men	Women	Men
Japan	13.5	11.4	20.2	16.2
France	14.4	12.1	19.9	15.3
Italy	13.3	13.0	18.5	14.6
Sweden	14.6	13.8	19.0	15.0
United Kingdom	14.6	11.8	17.7	13.8
Australia	14.9	12.2	18.8	14.7
United States	15.4	13.0	19.0	15.0

Table 7 Gender difference and the elderly (women per 100 men aged 60 years and over)[15]

Country	Ratio
Russian Federation	224
Ukraine	205
Korea, People's Republic of	182
Germany	159
Korea, Republic of	151
United States	138
Japan	127
Thailand	125
China	107
India	102

Median age

Recent UN estimates and projections[3] of the median age of humankind are rather illuminating and provide a great deal of food for thought (Table 8). At the time of the FIGO Congress in Buenos Aires in 1964, the median age of Asia was 20 years and that of Europe was 31 years. In about 20 years' time from now, the median age of Asia will be the same as that of Europe in 1964, whereas the median age of Europe will be twice as much as that of Africa, and will exceed 42 years. Humankind is growing rapidly and aging rapidly.

Dependent populations

Another important demographic parameter is the relationship between the dependent population (usually those aged 15 years and below and those aged 65 and over) and the population expected to cater for them (the so-called dependency ratio). Estimates and projections of the dependent population of the world between 1950 and 2050 are presented in Table 9.

The data of Table 9 seem to require few, if any, comments; although, between 1950 and 2050, the proportion of the total dependent

Table 8 Estimates and projections of median age (years)[3]

Region	Year			
	1965	2000	2020	2040
Africa	17.7	18.2	21.1	26.2
Asia	20.1	25.9	30.9	35.9
Latin America	18.6	24.9	30.5	35.8
North America	27.9	35.6	38.2	40.2
Europe	30.9	37.4	42.2	44.3

Table 9 Dependent population of the world: estimates and projections[3]

Year	Population (%)		
	< 15 years	> 65 years	Total
1950	34.5	5.1	39.6
2000	30.5	6.8	37.3
2050	20.8	14.7	35.5

population will slightly decrease, the crucial change is projected to be a drastic decrease in the proportion of children and an equally drastic increase in the proportion of the elderly. Humankind is growing rapidly and aging rapidly.

What about the age structure beyond 2050? The UN long-range, medium-fertility extension projects rather dramatic changes. By the year 2150, humankind will have aged considerably. The median age will have risen to 42 years from 24 years in 1990. In 2150, only 18% of the global population will be under age 15, and 24% will be aged 65 and over. The proportion of the 'old old' (those aged 80 years and over) is projected to increase nine-fold, from 1% in 1990 to 9% in 2150[2].

Contraceptive revolution

'Progress is
The law of life;
man is not man as yet.'

Robert Browning, 1835

Contraception: historical perspective

The world became technically (but not yet emotionally) ripe for the contraceptive revolution around 1960 when the development of modern methods enabled humankind to move contraception 'out of the bathroom'. The first oral contraceptive was approved by the US Food and Drug Administration in 1959[16], and the first 'modern' intrauterine device, the Margulies spiral, was introduced in 1960, followed by the Lippes loop 2 years later[17]. 'One of the greatest pains to human nature is the pain of a new idea', remarked Walter Bagehot in the 19th century[18], and we may concur. The idea of contraception as a new lifestyle of large populations was certainly both disturbing and painful to several sections of our multifaceted and complex society a century after Bagehot.

By chance, the breakthroughs in contraceptive technology coincided with a world-wide 'demographic awakening', with a notion that 1960 was the critical year (as if not every year would be a critical year); world population reached the 3-billion level, giving rise to a heated international debate about our common future on an Earth with 'standing room only'. However, the demographic development also raised genuine concerns among policy-makers – at least in some developing countries – as to the likely impact of rapid population growth on the standard and quality of life of their populations.

The credit should undoubtedly go to the Government of India for establishing in 1952, for the first time in history, a national family planning program. In retrospect, the foresight and courage of the Government of India of that time should be applauded, not only when viewed against the hostile international atmosphere of the 1950s, but also because the Indian national family planning program was established at a time when modern methods of contraception (steroidal contraceptives, intra-uterine devices) were not yet available.

The example of India was followed by other governments, first slowly and somewhat hesitantly and then in an accelerated manner. In the early 1960s, only seven governments provided family planning programs, mainly, if not entirely, because of demographic concerns. By the early 1980s, some 120 developing country governments supported such programs: 55 of them for the demographic rationale, but 65 for the reproductive health and human rights rationale[19]. Today, the number of governments directly or indirectly supporting family planning programs is close to 150. Hence, the contraceptive revolution was indeed a major revolution, since it generated a new intellectual atmosphere world-wide and spearheaded the onset of two other – very powerful – revolutions, those in reproductive health and gender equity, which will be the subjects of the next two sections.

Contraceptive prevalence

'What is amusing now had to be taken in desperate earnest once', said Virginia Woolf in her book *A Room of One's Own* (1929), and many of us who witnessed the highly emotional and sometimes pseudoscientific debates of the 1960s and 1970s about the continued existence of modern contraceptive technologies (the bitter Depoprovera controversy being just one of the examples) would certainly concur. In retrospect, we may feel today that it was simply the irresistible logic of technological progress, a sheer historical necessity, that, between 1960 and 1990, contraceptive prevalence rapidly increased in all developing countries from 9 to 51%; it increased from 13 to 70% in East Asia, from 14 to 60% in Latin America, from 7 to 40% in South Asia and from 5 to 17% in Africa[20]. That this could so easily happen was, in fact, most unexpected in the 1960s and 1970s.

More recent estimates indicate that around 1990 – with the exception of Africa – contraceptive prevalence in developing regions was about 58%, and that the number of contraceptive users world-wide exceeded half a billion (Table 10).

Viewed globally, by the year 2000, tubectomy will remain the quantitatively most important method (207 million users) followed by the use of intrauterine devices (125 million) and steroidal contraceptives: oral, injectable or implantable (96 million). The number of vasectomies is estimated at 47 million and that of condom users at 35 million, whereas some 57 million couples are expected to rely on traditional methods[21]. 'When an idea meets the necessity of the epoch', wrote Jean Monnet in his *Mémoires* (1978), 'it ceases to belong to those who invented it'. Modern contraceptives do not belong any longer to their inventors, but to humankind. They improve the quality of life of more than half a billion couples: is not this an ideal outcome of an ideal revolution? Whether

Table 10 Contraception around 1990[3]

Region	Couples (millions)	Users (%)
World	900	57
Africa	97	18
Asia	545	58
(Eastern Asia)	236	79
Latin America	67	58
Developed regions	189	72

it still can be considered as a revolution, or just a normal way of modern life, is open to discussion.

Revolution in reproductive health

'A human life is worth nothing, but nothing is worth a human life.'

André Malraux, 1937

Estimates of reproductive ill health

The World Health Organization estimates[22–24] that 120 million people around the world still have unmet family planning needs; 120–130 million women have been subjected to genital mutilation; there are some 60–80 million infertile couples; and at least 20 million adults are living with HIV/AIDS and 2 million women with invasive cervical cancer.

Annually, there are more than 330 million new cases of sexually transmitted diseases (STDs), 20 million unsafe abortions and 20 million cases of severe maternal morbidity. Of a global grand total of 50–52 million deaths each year, there are more than 12 million deaths under the age of 5 years, more than 7 million perinatal deaths and 600 000 maternal deaths, and some 25 million infants are born with low birth weight.

Hence, the most important dimensions of reproductive health are family planning, maternal and newborn health, prevention of unwanted pregnancy, STDs including HIV/AIDS, malnutrition, anemia, infertility, reproductive tract infections and malignancies and, perhaps the most critical issue for our common future, adolescent reproductive health, the key to a better reproductive health in the 21st century.

I feel that the credit should go to WHO for initiating an irreversible process[25], and to the UN Conference in Cairo, 1994[26] for adopting the WHO initiative and for recognizing the universal character of the problem, and subsequently for initiating one of the major intellectual revolutions of our time, the revolution in reproductive health.

Dimensions of reproductive health

Because of obvious limitations of scope and space, only a few aspects of the problem, and only in a very sketchy manner, will be considered here.

HIV/AIDS The HIV pandemic began in the late 1970s; around 20 million adults are currently infected in the world and their number will be around 26 million by the turn of the century. It is estimated that some 5 million infected adults have developed AIDS since the beginning of the pandemic. In 1996, the highest prevalence rate (per 100 000 population) was in the African region (5144), followed by South East Asia (694), the Americas (565), Europe (136), the Eastern Mediterranean (90) and Western Pacific (31/100 000) regions[24].

Approximately 2% of the annual 52 million deaths around the world are AIDS-related deaths; their world-wide distribution in 1996 is shown in Table 11.

Sexually transmitted diseases The World Health Organization estimates that, among the some 333 million new cases of STDs (other than HIV infection) that occurred in 1995, there were some 89 million chlamydial infections, 62 million cases of gonorrhea, 12 million syphilis and 170 million trichomonas infections. Chlamydia and gonorrhea, as well as syphilis, can be associated with a high prevalence of infertility; they can also be passed on to infants during pregnancy and childbirth, and might cause abortion,

Table 11 AIDS-related deaths in 1996 (adult population aged 15–49 years)[24]

WHO region	Deaths
Africa	780 000
Americas	150 000
South East Asia	140 000
Europe	22 000
Eastern Mediterranean	11 000
Western Pacific	4 000
Total	1 107 000

stillbirth and severe eye-infection and pneumonia in the newborn. Moreover, there is strong evidence indicating that STDs greatly increase the risk of sexual transmission of HIV infection, particularly when accompanied by genital ulcers[23].

Abortion Although abortion statistics are notoriously uncertain, the best estimates suggest that, of a yearly world-wide total of 200 million pregnancies, some 40–60 million are interrupted[27]. From a public health point of view, the fundamental issue is not whether abortion is legal or illegal, but whether it is safe or unsafe, and WHO estimates that some 20 million unsafe abortions carried out in 1990 resulted in 67 000 deaths[28].

The global situation with respect to legislation on abortion is indicated in Table 12[29]. Abortion is available upon request in 41 countries, representing approximately 44% of the global population. It would also appear that, in general terms, abortion laws in developing countries are more restrictive than in developed countries. Only 8% of the former accept economic and social reasons, and less than 5% make abortion available upon request. Corresponding percentages in developed countries are 81% and 56%, respectively[29].

Low birth weight and malnutrition The most powerful single predictor of death in the first months of life is low birth weight, which is, *inter alia* a function of intrauterine malnutrition. The association of intrauterine growth retardation with decreased cognitive development and school performance is well established. There is increasing evidence, however, that it also

Table 12 Abortion laws around the world[29]

Indication	Number of countries
To save the life of a woman	173
To preserve her physical health	119
To preserve her mental health	95
Rape or incest	81
Fetal impairment	78
Economic or social	56
Upon request	41

increases the risk in adult life of hypertensive heart disease, myocardial infarction and non-insulin-dependent diabetes[30].

The World Health Organization estimates that, around 1988–1990, some 600 million people – mostly women and children – were deficient in one or several micronutrients, such as iodine, vitamin A and iron. It is also estimated that between 2 and 7% of pregnant women in the developing world are severely anemic with a risk of maternal mortality at least five times that of those without anemia[23].

Maternal mortality The World Health Organization estimates that each year there are some 600 000 maternal deaths world-wide[31]. In 1990, maternal mortality rates in developing countries exhibited wide variation between 6/100 000 live births (Hong Kong) and 2000/100 000 (Mali). Very high rates were reported also from Bangladesh (600), Nigeria (800), Ghana (1000) and Somalia (1100/100 000 live births)[31].

These enormous differences in mortality rates are attributable to the absence of quality services in many developing countries; in general, fewer than 60% of pregnant women in developing countries have antenatal care, and only about 55% of women deliver with the help of trained persons. The effective skills of those 'trained' persons are frequently unknown[23].

Child, infant, neonatal and perinatal mortality
World-wide child mortality was 134/1000 live births in 1970 and 82/1000 by 1995, when it was 8.5/1000 live births in the developed world, 91/1000 in all developing countries and 156/1000 in the least developed countries[23]. Of a global total of 50 million deaths in 1960, 19 million were of children under 5 years of age; of the 52 million deaths in 1996, only 11 million were of children[24].

Infant, neonatal and perinatal mortality rates also considerably decreased during the past few decades. Recent perinatal and neonatal mortality rates in the various regions of the world are given in Table 13[23,32], and recent infant mortality rates in selected developing countries are indicated in Table 14[24].

Table 13 Perinatal and neonatal mortality around 1995[32]

Region	Mortality	
	Perinatal (per 1000 births)	Neonatal (per 1000 live births)
Africa	75	42
Asia	53	41
Oceania	44	24
Latin America	39	25
Europe	13	8
North America	9	6

Table 14 Infant mortality rates (per 1000 live births) in selected developing countries in 1996[24]

Country	Rate
Singapore	5
Malaysia	11
Thailand	30
Indonesia	48
China	70
India	72
Liberia	153
Sierra Leone	169

Perinatal and neonatal mortality rates reflect not only standards of obstetric and pediatric care, but also those of a country's educational, social and public health systems. Indeed, such figures reveal more about the public health situation of any country than any other statistical information. Show me the neonatal mortality rates of a country, and I will tell you the rest.

Reproductive tract malignancies World-wide mortality from reproductive tract malignancies rapidly approaches 1 million people; in 1993, some 358 000 women died from malignant neoplasms of the breast, 235 000 from those of the uterine cervix and 123 000 from ovarian cancer, in addition to 182 000 men who died from prostatic cancer[22].

Genital mutilation The World Health Organization estimates that there are, at present, 120 million, perhaps even 130 million, girls and women who have undergone some form of genital mutilation[33]. Genital mutilation is an unsafe and unjustifiable traditional practice – mainly in several African countries – that is based on misconceptions and myths. In essence, it is the violation of fundamental human rights and of the basic principle of gender equity. Recently (9 April 1997) the heads of three UN agencies, WHO, the United Nations Children's Fund (UNICEF) and UNFPA, appealed to the international community and world leaders to support efforts aimed at eliminating this harmful procedure. The joint plan of these agencies, which will be carried out in close collaboration with governments, aims at completely eliminating this practice within two or three generations.

Reproductive health and poverty 'The greatest of evils and the worst of crimes is poverty', said G. B. Shaw 90 years ago in the preface to his play, *Major Barbara*, and even the classically 'emotion-free' language of WHO softens when it refers to the poverty of our world: 'Poverty is the most widespread, pervasive and intractable disease in the world today'[25]. Indeed, perusal of the data of Table 15 may give rise to somewhat similar reflections, when one tries to correlate the most important indicators of reproductive health with estimates of gross national product (GNP).

Reproductive health and human dignity How important, then, is reproductive health? It should appear from this very brief review that it is extremely important. Indeed, it is so important that seven of the ten goals set by WHO for the period 1996–2001 are directly relevant to it[34]. Reproductive health is the core and quintessence of general health, and health in general is the quintessence of all human development. It is not only a fundamental human right for all; it is also a social and economic imperative[26].

Revolution of gender equity

'L'extension des privilèges des femmes est le principe général de tous progrès sociaux.'

Charles Fourier, 1808

Charles Fourier could be considered – and indeed with some justification – as the 'father'

Table 15 Reproductive health and poverty[23]

Indicator	Developed world		Developing world	
	Developed market economies	Economies in transition	Developing countries (other than LDCs)	Least developed countries (LDCs)
Gross national product (US$ per capita)*	23 262	1992	1043	200
Literacy rate for women	98	98	64	38
Under-5 mortality rate (per 1000 live births)	9	29	75	156
Maternal mortality (per 100 000 live births)	13	60	350	1050
Institutional delivery (% live births)	98	95	41	20
Unsafe abortion	1	22	15	26

*Data from 1993

of the revolution in gender equity, judged from the 190-year-old statement taken from his book *Théorie des Quatre Mouvements et des Destinées Générales* published in Lyon in 1808 and reproduced in the motto above. 'Increasing women's rights is the general principle of all social progress', he wrote in 1808. Is it not up-to-date today? It could well be part of a recent 'official' UN declaration, since humankind is still far from achieving gender equity with respect to some basic human needs, in areas as diverse as nutrition, education, health services, human rights, money income and personal security. Was it Friedrich Nietzsche who said that some of us are born posthumously?

It is, of course, not difficult to find different examples of gender discrimination in our greatly varying cultures around the globe today, be it prenatal sex selection, differential healthcare and nutrition of male and female infants, or the less subtle examples of infanticide and genital mutilation. Other examples are related to violence against women, ranging from battery, sexual abuse and rape to forced prostitution and human trafficking, a multibillion-dollar 'international business activity' of our times.

The United Nations Development Program (UNDP) provides another dimension of gender disparity, by pointing out that, whereas women constitute 70% of the world's poor and 60% of its illiterate, they occupy only 10% of all parliamentary seats and 6% of the world's cabinet positions[35].

Furthermore, in 1990, the UN Commission on the Status of Women recommended the 'principle of 30% threshold' of decision-making positions to be held by women. In parliamentary or cabinet representation, only Denmark, Finland, the Netherlands, Norway, Seychelles and Sweden have crossed this threshold so far and – as far as I know – Sweden is the only country with a 50% representation by women both in the Cabinet and in the Parliament.

The UN International Conference on Population and Development in Cairo, 1994 emphasized that 'The elimination of social and economic discrimination against women is a prerequisite for reducing poverty, promoting economic growth and achieving sound population policies'[26]. Indeed, the urgent improvement of the political, socioeconomic and health status of women in general, and of elderly women in particular, will certainly have a most prominent place on the international agenda of the early 21st century. To achieve gender equity without destabilizing the social infrastructure of certain specific cultural settings will be the challenge for the next generation in their endeavor to successfully complete the process of global revolution in gender equity by gradually eliminating millennial prejudices.

I am profoundly convinced that, like the contraceptive revolution and the revolution in reproductive health, the revolution in gender equity is also a fundamentally irreversible process that will accompany humankind on its journey of thousands of miles and perhaps thousands of years towards our ultimate goal at the end of the journey: human dignity for all.

Healthy aging, or the demographic revolution revisited

'And the first Morning of Creation wrote
What the last Dawn of Reckoning shall read.'
Edward Fitzgerald, 1859
Rubáiyat of Omar Khayyam

New demographic reality

Rapid aging is both a consequence and a fundamental constituent of the demographic revolution. One of the most characteristic features of our time is the dramatic increase in life expectancy both at birth (Tables 4 and 5) and at the age of 65 (Table 6), with a widening gender difference (Table 7), resulting in a new reality of our time: the world-wide emergence of increasing rates of aging population that accompany accelerated fertility decline.

Between 1970 and 2025, the proportion of elderly is expected to increase from 12.1 to 20.1% in North America and from 13.7 to 22.4% in Europe. However, because of the numbers involved, the most impressive increase will take place in Asia, with its elderly population more than doubling. Between 1990 and 2025, the elderly population of Indonesia is expected to increase by 414%, that of Thailand by 337%, and those of India and China by 242% and 220%, respectively. Moreover, by the year 2025, the proportion of population aged 80 years and over will be 1.8% in Latin America and Asia, 4.6% in North America and 6.4% in Europe[13].

The UN long-range projections point out that, of the past increase in world population size between 1950 and 1990, 30% occurred among children and 7% among the elderly. Between 1990 and 2050, 7% of the increase is projected to take place among children and 23% among the elderly. And between 2050 and 2150, 90% of world population increase is projected to occur among the elderly[2].

Today, it is generally recognized that we are dealing with an almost universal and irreversible phenomenon, deeply rooted within the perspective of the demographic transition. What is not understood equally well is that an aging humankind is a fundamentally new feature in the world's history, and that people and their governments have not had time enough to consider the likely consequences and to react to this new demographic reality, although it will profoundly affect every aspect of life, our social institutions and ethical values.

Another classical paradox of our time, in addition to those mentioned in the 'Seven revolutions' section above, is our attitude to longevity. As individuals, all of us hope to live a very long and healthy life; however, as a society, we refuse to see the rather obvious consequences of this new reality and to make the necessary – and, in part, fundamental – socioeconomic and political adjustments to meet one of the greatest challenges of the 21st century[36].

Gender inequality in aging

Between 1950 and 2000, the gender differences in world-wide life expectancy will increase from 2.7 to 4.1 years (Table 4), and the difference will be further augmented by a gender difference in life expectancy at the age of 65. The consequences of this can best be assessed by considering the difference in numbers, rather than in averages. In 1990, 2654 million male and 2514 million female human beings lived on our planet: 140 million more males than females. However, among those aged 65 and over, there were 141 million males and 187 million females, or a female excess of 46 million, and among those aged 70 years and over, there were 44 million males and 70 million females[3].

Health dimension

The various aspects of the health dimension of aging have been addressed in detail in recent reviews[36,37]. The classical areas of concern in relation to the elderly include, *inter alia* cardiovascular and cerebrovascular disease, malignant neoplasms, chronic respiratory disease, neuropsychiatric disease and a variety of age-related metabolic alterations, such as osteoporosis, sense organ and musculoskeletal changes, diabetes, other endocrine and nutritional diseases and oral ill health. The most important causes of mortality in the elderly population (in decreasing order) are cardiovascular diseases, malignant neoplasms and respiratory tract diseases, and the most important causes of morbidity parallel those of mortality.

Although aging need not be associated with disability, disability rates are higher after age 60 both for women and men, and highest among those aged 75 and over. Among the problems leading to increased isolation of the elderly are incontinence (urinary and fecal), impaired hearing and vision, reduced mobility, falls and their consequences and fear of falls, and oral ill health.

One of the most reliable indicators of human deprivation is the lack of access to health services. In a recent study by the World Bank, comprising 12 selected countries with a total population of almost 3 billion people, more than half a billion of them had no access to health services[38]. It is easy to predict how many of them would be elderly women living under the poverty line.

Social dimension

There are a large number of studies on the various economic and social aspects of rapid population aging. Many of them were supported by UNFPA on local-level policy development to deal with the consequences of population aging; some of those were recently reviewed[36]. These studies impel the greater recognition of the health and social situation of elderly women as a major concern. These studies also suggest that there is almost infinite scope for socioeconomic research related to the rapid aging of populations and its effect on society.

In the most extensive studies published from China[39], the greatest misery was experienced by the oldest women who live in the small towns. They are mainly widows without any retirement pension and who do not have a share in any household income.

It would not seem to be unfair to generalize from the Chinese example and to conclude that, for the time being, in most developing countries, the majority of those surviving to old age face a longer life of economic deprivation with little, if any, social support. For them, the process of aging could be a personal crisis of day-to-day survival. Because of the increasing gender gap in life expectancy, the majority of the elderly will increasingly be women, experiencing greater burdens than men in terms of disability and morbidity, including the most pervasive of all human diseases: poverty.

Ethical dimension

As emphasized above, the problem of aging populations is fundamentally new, and people and their governments have not as yet had sufficient time, vision, determination and perhaps even courage to consider the significant political, cultural and social readjustments required to meet the challenge of this new demographic reality. As a predictable consequence, we are already witnessing a crisis in our contemporary ethics; all one has to do is to have a glance at our daily newspapers debating the scope and extent of hospitalization of the very old for major surgical interventions and its financial implications.

Indeed, any serious discussion of future social and health policy for the elderly immediately opens a virtually endless frontier of ethical inquiry into our – frequently conflicting – premises. For instance, take the 'present versus the future' premise: what constitutes an ethically justifiable allocation of scant resources among and between generations? There is a widening gap (economic, social, emotional and perhaps even moral) between generations in many developed and also developing countries, and intergenerational solidarity is under serious debate[40]. Furthermore, in many developing countries, the majority of the younger generation will simply lack the material resources to provide adequate support to the older generation. This then raises the issue of the relationship between family and government obligations in providing care for the elderly, the classical 'individual versus community' premise.

The above two premises lead then to even more complex ones, like the premise of 'equity'; because of insufficient economic resources, should there be limits of health-care for the elderly and, if so, who should decide over life and death? What should be the role of the health establishment in general, and of the medical profession in particular, in such a 'Brave New World'? Who will be in charge of the 'sanctity of life' premise in such a society? Are we going to legalize, and how, euthanasia? And who is going to safeguard the rights of the poor, disabled or demented elderly in such a society? What did Chamfort say? '*Il faut recommencer la société humaine*'. Maybe the time has come for a fresh start for a human and humane world society?

A less dramatic, but equally critical, premise is that of 'sustainability'; in a world where the elderly will soon constitute 25% of the population, will they be able to productively contribute to the maintenance of a very expensive social fabric, or will they be forced to spend almost one-third of their entire lifetime in passive retirement? And how will they be permitted to participate fairly and effectively in determining their own fate and welfare?

As the second millennium approaches its end, we perceive more and more, to use Shelley's phrase, 'the gigantic shadows which futurity casts upon the present'. At the same time, however, we also recognize that never before has humankind had so many resources, so much knowledge, such powerful technologies and adequate international mechanisms to mobilize our global resources in order to confront the challenges of futurity.

Scientific revolution, or has humankind a future?

'Oh Man, strive on, strive on, have faith; and trust!'
Imre Madách, *The Tragedy of Man,* 1860

Prophets of 'gloom and doom'

Our times represent golden opportunities for the 'prophets of gloom and doom'; all they have to do is to tell us – and they are more than willing to oblige – that the 'carrying capacity' of the Earth cannot provide a living for some 10 billion people (among them 25% elderly), and that our social structures are unlikely to change in the couple of centuries to come in order to confront these powerful new challenges. They may even remind us that it is not very likely that the political leaders of tomorrow will represent a much higher morality than those of the past few millennia (by the way, why not?), or that the 10 billion fellow men and women of tomorrow will have entirely different ambitions and a higher morality than past generations. Their favorite argument is, of course, that human progress is mainly, if not entirely, scientific and technological, but that the dark aspects of 'human nature' – be they aggression, barbarity, senseless cruelty, terror, the moral corruption of power and naked cynicism – have hardly changed, and constitute the greatest obstacle to human happiness today.

Maybe so: I may even agree that the worst enemy of humankind is still mankind. However, the prophets of gloom and doom seem to ignore the fundamentals of evolutionary biology, the enormous adaptive ability of the human race and the fact that 'human nature' is not destiny; indeed, it can change and will change with time and circumstances. They also disregard what Bertrand Russell so strongly emphasized, that 'in a biological sense, Man, the latest of species, is still an infant', and, therefore, 'No limit can be set to what he may achieve in the future'[41]. Yes, humankind is still an infant, even if a rapidly aging one.

From mankind to humankind

The prophets of 'gloom and doom' also fail to see that our generation is the first since the dawn of history which could acquire a global vision and could provide to those stricken by famine, or other natural catastrophes, help and efficient assistance in any corner of the Earth. Sure enough, there still are major obstacles on humankind's 'golden road to Samarkand', the most important ones – in my view – being the growth and aging of populations; environmental degradation; poor health of populations; persistent poverty; and – the worst of all – intraspecies aggression.

However, to assume that this is and will always be our lot, and that nothing can be done to substantially improve the human condition world-wide, is an extremely nihilistic view, and I am convinced that few, if any, obstetricians and gynecologists are intellectually prepared to accept such a philosophy based on the randomness, absurdity and futility of life. After all, is it not self-evident that the intellectual resources of *Homo sapiens* are far in excess of those required for sheer survival?

Is it not also true that the unparalleled success of the human race as a biological species is largely attributable to the unique capacity of the human brain, which has made possible abstract thinking, the alpha and omega of human development? If so, is it really so unrealistic to predict that during the next millennium the youngest species on Earth, *Homo sapiens*, will gradually master those problems interfering with its march on the 'golden road' towards the 'Samarkand of human happiness'? At the end of that road is the 'Empire of human dignity', in a place where every single human being has sufficient food, potable water, shelter, appropriate sanitation and health services, a healthy, clean environment, education, employment and personal security. Is this merely 'a hope beyond the shadow of a dream'[42]? No! All this may happen if we let it happen.

After all, in essence, these are simply fundamental human rights[43]! I agree with Dr Karan Singh, that 'If our knowledge is used with wisdom, compassion and understanding, we can abolish poverty, illiteracy, malnutrition, hunger and unemployment from the face of this planet'[44]. He thinks that this can be achieved within the next 15–20 years; I believe it may take a couple of centuries, but it can be done and it will be done!

Seven approaches to reality?

In his frequently quoted poem, 'Burnt Norton'[45], T. S. Eliot says that '. . . human kind cannot bear very much reality'. Maybe this is the reason why we try to employ so many approaches to reality; in a recent paper, I have indicated seven such approaches, the scientific, religious, ethical, cultural, economical, ecological and, last but not least, the political. When those approaches converge, they create an intellectual environment that catalyzes an amazingly rapid progress[46].

All seven approaches can enrich human existence; however, one of them proved to be much more powerful in improving the human condition than all the others. That approach is represented by the scientific revolution, the most important revolution of our time. As C. P. Snow remarked in the early 1960s, 'The scientific revolution is the only method by which most people can gain the primal things (years of life, freedom from hunger, survival for children)'[47]. Indeed, it is only science in general and medical science in particular that will provide the 10 billion fellow men and women of the next century with a healthy life, including better reproductive health and healthy aging!

FIGO and the third millennium

Humankind is 'still an infant'[41] and so is FIGO. Hence, to paraphrase Bertrand Russell, no limit can be set to what FIGO can achieve in the future! In retrospect, it is obvious now that Hubert de Watteville's vision was indeed correct when he perceived a new, major role for this Federation in shaping a brighter future for humankind. Almost exactly 2000 years ago,

Horace (*Odes*, III, xxx, 1) exclaimed: '*Exegi monumentum aere perennius*'; this is translated by the *Oxford Dictionary of Quotations* as 'My work is done, the memorial more enduring than brass'. Hubert de Watteville could have said the same, with at least as much justification; indeed, I am profoundly convinced that the significance of FIGO for improving the health of every woman world-wide will further increase during the coming centuries, if not millennia.

Why? Because FIGO is the embodiment of the fundamental philosophy formulated by Lucius Apuleius, some 1800 years ago: '*Singillatim mortales, cunctim perpetui*'. As individual obstetricians, gynecologists and scientists, all members of the Federation are mortal beings but, together, they represent perpetuity. And, at the threshold of the third millennium, FIGO does indeed represent both universality and perpetuity in its important mission to conquer suffering and incessantly improve the human condition!

Therefore, in its continued endeavor, FIGO can look forward to a great future: a future immeasurably longer than its past, inspired by the breadth of vision of Hubert de Watteville, the endless achievements of the ceaseless scientific revolution and the infinite wisdom of hope – a robust hope in the final success of the human race in its struggle to eventually establish on this Earth the 'empire of human dignity'.

References

1. Cervantes de Saavedra, M. (1976). *El ingenioso hidalgo Don Quixote de la Mancha, 1620*, II, Ch. XXXII. (Valencia: Edicion IV Centenario, Castilla)
2. United Nations (1992). *Long-range World Population Projections. Two Centuries of Population Growth 1950–2150*. (New York: United Nations)
3. United Nations (1995). *World Population Prospects. The 1994 Revision*. (New York: United Nations)
4. Schopenhauer, A. (1851). On the doctrine of the suffering of the world. *Parerga und Paralipomena*
5. de Solla Price, D. J. (1963). *Little Science, Big Science*. (New York: Columbia UP)
6. Engels, F. In Karpov, M. M. (1963). *Osnovyyie Zakonomernosti Razvitiya Estestvoznaniya*, Rostov State University, 1963. Quoted by Ebison, M. (ed.) (1977) *Scientific Quotations: the Harvest of a Quiet Eye*, p.54. (New York: Crane, Russak and Co.)
7. Bernard, C. (1962). *Principes de Médecine Expérimentale, 1865*. Oeuvre posthume publiée pour la première fois en 1947 par le Dr. Léon Delhoume. (Paris: Masson et Cie)
8. de Goncourt, E. and de Goncourt, J. (Goncourt brothers) (1867). *Journal*
9. Hegel, G. W. F. (1948). *Vorlesungen über die Philosophie der Geschichte 1832*. Introduction. (Berlin: Duncker und Humblot)
10. Huxley, A. L. (1958). *Brave New World Revisited*. (New York: Harper & Row)
11. Huxley, A. L. (1932). *Brave New World*. (London)
12. United Nations (1993). *Conference on Environment and Development, Rio de Janeiro, 3–14 June*. (New York: United Nations) United Nations publication, Sales No. E93.I.8 and corrigenda
13. World Health Organization (1995). Epidemiology and prevention of cardiovascular disease in elderly people. *WHO Technical Report Series*, No. 853. (Geneva: World Health Organization)
14. United Nations (1995). *World Economic and Social Survey 1995. Current Trends and Policies in the World Economy*. (New York: United Nations)
15. United Nations (1995). *The World's Women 1995*. Trends and statistics. ST/ESA/STAT/SER.K/12. (New York: United Nations)
16. Diczfalusy, E. (1989). Keynote address. The history of steroidal contraception: what is past and what is present? In Michal, F. (ed.) *Safety Requirements for Contraceptive Steroids*, pp. 1–18. (Cambridge: Cambridge University Press)
17. Guttmacher, A. F. (1965). Intrauterine contraceptive devices (the 8th Oliver Bird Lecture). *J. Reprod. Fertil.*, **10**, 115–28
18. Bagehot, W. (1965). In Stevas, N. A. F. St. J. (ed.) *Physics and Politics in Collected Works of Walter Bagehot (1826–1877)*. (London: Economist)

19. Johnson, S. P. (1987). *World Population and the United Nations. Challenge and Response.* (Cambridge: Cambridge University Press)

20. United Nations (1989). *Levels and Trends of Contraceptive Use, as Assessed in 1988.* (New York: United Nations)

21. Shah, J. H. (1994). The advance of the contraceptive revolution. *World Health Stat. Q.,* **47**, 9–15

22. World Health Organization (1995). *The World Health Report 1995. Bridging the Gaps.* (Geneva: World Health Organization)

23. World Health Organization (1996). *The World Health Report 1996. Fighting Disease Fostering Development.* (Geneva: World Health Organization)

24. World Health Organization (1997). *The World Health Report 1997. Conquering Suffering. Enriching Humanity.* (Geneva: World Health Organization)

25. World Health Organization (1994). *Health, Population and Development:* WHO Position Paper for the *International Conference on Population and Development,* Cairo, 1994. WHO/FHE/94. (Geneva: World Health Organization)

26. United Nations (1994). *Report of the International Conference on Population and Development.* (Cairo 1994) A/CONF:171/13. (New York: United Nations)

27. Henshaw, S. K. (1990). Induced abortion: a world review, 1990. *Fam. Plann. Persp.,* **22**, 76–89

28. World Health Organization (1994). *Maternal and Child Health and Family Planning: the Health Situation of Women, Children and Families and Programme Experiences.* An overview based upon materials and analysis prepared for the *7th Expert Committee on Maternal and Child Health.* FHE/MCH/94.1. (Geneva: World Health Organization)

29. United Nations Population Fund (UNFPA) (1995). *The State of World Population 1995,* p.43. (New York: UNFPA)

30. Barker, D. J. P. (1992). *Foetal and Infant Origins of Adult Disease.* (London: Br. Med. J. Publishers)

31. World Health Organization – UNICEF (1996). *Revised 1990 Estimates of Maternal Mortality.* A new approach by WHO and UNICEF. WHO/FRH/MSH/96.11 and UNICEF/PLN/96.1. (Geneva: World Health Organization)

32. World Health Organization (1996). *Perinatal Mortality.* A listing of available information. WHO/FRH/MSM/96.7. (Geneva: World Health Organization)

33. World Health Organization (1996). *Female Genital Mutilation.* Report of a *WHO Technical Working Group,* Geneva, 17–19 July 1995. WHO/FRH/WHD/96.10. (Geneva: World Health Organization)

34. World Health Organization (1994). Ninth General Programme of Work covering the period of 1996–2001. *Health for All Series,* No.11. (Geneva: World Health Organization)

35. United Nations Development Programme (UNDP) (1995). *Human Development Report 1995.* (Oxford: Oxford University Press)

36. Diczfalusy, E. and Benagiano, G. (1997). Women and the third and fourth age. *Int. J. Gynaecol. Obstet.,* **58**, 177–88

37. Diczfalusy, E. (1996). The third age, the third world and the third millennium. *Contraception,* **53**, 1–7

38. World Bank (1995). *World Development Report 1995. Workers in an Integrating World.* (Oxford: Oxford University Press)

39. Chesnais, J.-C. and Wang, S. (1990). Population aging, retirement policy and living conditions of the elderly in China. *Population,* **2**, 3–28

40. Bengtson, V. L. (1994). Ageing and the problem of generations: prospects for a new generation contract. In United Nations (ed.) *Ageing and the Family.* Doc. ST/ESA/SER.R/124, pp. 178–185. (New York: United Nations)

41. Russell, B. (1961). *Has Man a Future?* (London: George Allen & Unwin)

42. Keats, J. (1818). Endymion, line 857. In Allotts, M. *The poems of John Keats,* 1970, London

43. United Nations (1990). *Declaration on International Economic Cooperation, in Particular the Revitalization of Economic Growth and Development of the Developing Countries.* (New York: UNDP)

44. Singh, K. (1993). Closing address, *IPPF Family Planning Congress,* New Delhi, October 1992. In Senanayake, P. and Kleinman, R. L. (eds.) *Family Planning: Meeting Challenges, Promoting Choices.* (Carnforth, UK: Parthenon Publishing)

45. Eliot, T. S. (1935). Burnt Norton (Four Quartets). In (1987) *The Complete Poems and Plays of T. S. Eliot,* p. 172. (London: Guild Publishing)

46. Diczfalusy, E. (1995). Reproductive health: a rendezvous with human dignity. *Contraception,* **52**, 1–12

47. Snow, C. P. (1963). *The Two Cultures: a Second Look.* (London: Cambridge University Press)

What happens to the health of women in crisis situations?

2

D. Schopper

Introduction

This paper attempts to highlight some of the crucial health issues women face in times of crisis. This does not refer to the small or big crisis any woman may face during her personal, individual life story, but refers to major breakdowns of the social and economic environment as a consequence of external conflict and war, and the consequences this has for the health of women.

In the early 1960s, wars of national liberation and the first conflicts in the newly independent states of Asia and Africa began to provoke important movements of refugees. This was the first time that the United Nations (UN) organizations, and in particular the United Nations High Commissioner for Refugees (UNHCR), had to turn their attention to a new situation of south–south movements of populations and large-scale exodus caused by war and insecurity. For the last three decades, the majority of the people fleeing war, famine and repression have been from developing countries, seeking refuge in neighboring countries. At the end of the 1970s, the hardening of the East–West confrontation and the multiplication of low-intensity conflicts caused major refugee movements in Afghanistan, Southeast Asia, Central America and the Horn of Africa. Since the end of the cold war, the greatest concentrations of refugees have been found around countries in conflict such as Burma, Tajikistan, Azerbaijan, Georgia, ex-Yugoslavia, Chechenya, Afghanistan, Liberia, Somalia, Sudan, Burundi, Rwanda . . . the list is long. The exodus of the Kurds from Iraq, or the Rohingyas from Burma, or the Burundians and Rwandans, are striking examples of the scale and violence of refugee movements over the past few years.

Only rapid action by the international community makes it possible to deal with such floods of refugees into regions which are sometimes difficult to reach and where conditions are already extremely precarious. Refugees are usually placed in camps in the host countries where protection and material assistance can be provided. The situation is often more difficult for people who are displaced within their own country, as they are not recognized as traditional refugees and often do not get the same attention and protection. Currently, the UNHCR estimates that there are about 23 million refugees and 26 million displaced persons in the world[1].

Women and children represent a high proportion of these uprooted populations. In many situations, there are more refugee women than men, and children make up about one-fifth to one-quarter of the population (Table 1). As the numbers of refugees have mounted, it has become very clear that such emergency situations pose particular threats to women, but issues relating to women in general and their reproductive health needs in particular have not received special attention until recently[2]. The gruesome experiences of the war in Bosnia and the Rwandan genocide and its consequences, however, confirmed again how much women and girls are vulnerable to gender-based discrimination, exploitation and violence, and are at risk in the communities from which they are fleeing, during flight, as well as in refugee camps or other places where they seek protection. Yet

Table 1 Demographic characteristics of selected refugee populations (1995). (From reference 1)

Country of asylum	Total refugee population	Ratio of women/men > 18 years	Percentage of children < 5 years
Kenya	232 400	1.46	19
Côte d'Ivoire	360 100	1.31	23
Pakistan	1 055 400	1.13	24
Iran	1 740 900	0.73	21

while women are at risk or under assault, they continue to remain responsible for the survival of their children and other members of their families.

This paper first highlights some examples of the special needs of women in these situations, before discussing possible interventions and lessons learned from past experiences. Among the most vulnerable groups are certainly women who are pregnant or in the process of childbirth or in postpartum recovery. Women and adolescents are also exposed to greater risks of sexual exploitation, abuse and violence. It has been shown in several studies that women in general experience particularly *high rates of mortality, morbidity and malnutrition* when compared with men[3,4]. This cannot be explained by physical vulnerability alone; discrimination is clearly a major factor. For example, it has been documented that female-headed households have a lower level of access to food and other distributed commodities and higher rates of malnutrition than those headed by a male. This was seen most recently in the Rwandan refugee camps near Goma in Zaire. A survey showed that 35% of the households in the camp of Kahindo were headed by a woman. The risk of inadequate access to food (less than 1000 kcal/persons/day as compared to an average ration of more than 2000 kcal/ person/day) was much greater for these families than for those headed by a man, and the risk was even greater if the family was large and included a child of less than 5 years[5].

Maternal mortality

Maternal mortality is a problem in most developing countries, even in stable situations. The World Health Organization (WHO) estimates that the mortality rates per 100 000 live births are approximately 640 for Africa, 420 for Asia and 270 for Latin America. Up to 80% of these maternal deaths are due to only a limited number of causes, many of which are preventable or treatable, such as obstructed labor, hemorrhage, infection, hypertensive disorders, anemia and complications of unsafe abortion[6].

Women in refugee camps may face increased risks in pregnancy because of a variety of additional factors such as the breakdown of health services, malnutrition, mental trauma and violence[7]. However, on a positive note, it has been shown recently that a significant proportion of maternal mortality can be avoided by a combination of adequately organized antenatal, delivery and postnatal care aimed at the detection and treatment of the problems previously mentioned. After stabilization of the health situation in the refugee camps around Goma and the initiation of adequate services, the maternal mortality rates in these camps were actually lower than in the surrounding population. Between January and September 1996, 22 453 infants were born alive in the Goma refugee camps, and 11 maternal deaths occurred during this period: a maternal mortality rate of 50 per 100 000 live births in Goma as compared to the 'usual' rate of about 600 in Africa[8].

Premature births and low-weight infants

Another indication of the health status of women, the support they get in the community and the adequacy of antenatal services is the proportion of *premature births* and of *low-weight infants*. The excellent surveillance system set up

19

in the camps around Goma was able to show that being pregnant as a refugee woman did not necessarily mean a lower health status with its negative consequences for the newborn. As shown in Figure 1, the proportion of newborns weighing less than 2500 g at birth was lower in the five camps around Goma, than in Malawi or even the West Bank.

Sexually transmitted diseases

Another issue that merits special attention is that of *sexually transmitted diseases* (STDs) including *human immunodeficiency virus* (HIV) and *acquired immunodeficiency syndrome* (AIDS). A major lesson of the AIDS epidemic so far has been that HIV spreads fastest in conditions of poverty, powerlessness and social instability – conditions that are often exacerbated during conflict and population movements, where the disintegration of community and family life means the break-up of stable relationships and the loss of

mutual support. Some of the factors that enhance the spread of HIV in situations of war and civil strife and are that:

(1) Women and children are at increased risk of violence and rape;

(2) Displaced women and girls may find themselves coerced into sex to gain access to basic needs such as food, water, shelter or security;

(3) Forced migration often entails people from rural areas with lower levels of HIV infection and also less awareness about the means of prevention, moving close to towns or mixing with people coming from urban areas; and

(4) Previously existing AIDS and STD control activities will have been severely disrupted or broken down, thus leaving little scope for women to protect themselves or have access to care.

It is well known that HIV and other STDs travel together and that the risk of HIV infection is increased if one of the partners has another STD at the time of sexual intercourse. However, little is known about rates of STD infection in refugee women and how little this affects their health. Some of the few data available[9,10] are shown in Table 2.

These figures indicate high rates of infection, more than half of the women having cervicitis and/or vaginitis. Because of the greatly increased risk of HIV transmission, the long term complications of STDs such as infertility, pelvic

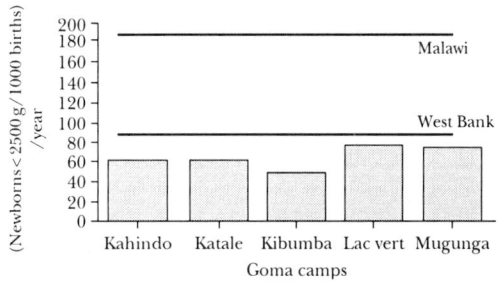

Figure 1 Rate of newborns < 2500 g in five Goma camps compared with Malawi and the West Bank

Table 2 Studies of STD infection in Turkish refugee women in Azerbaijan (1996)[9] and Rwandan refugee women in Tanzania (1994)[10]

	Study	
	Turkish refugees in Azerbaijan	*Rwandan refugees in Tanzania*
Women examined	all women aged 15–49 (n = 1465)	random sample of ANC attenders (*n* = 100)

Health findings	45.6% had cervicitis
	10% had candidiasis
	6.7% had vaginitis
	44% were anemic
	  (hemoglobin < 12 g/dl)
		over 50% had vaginitis
		4% had active syphilis
		3% were infected with Neisseria
		  gonorrhoeae

inflammatory disease, ectopic pregnancies and neonatal infections, and because 50–80% of women with gonorrhea and chlamydia are asymptomatic, early establishment of comprehensive STD services should be a priority.

Sexual violence

Sexual violence is an issue that has been ignored and sometimes denied for far too long. Rape and sexual abuse of women have been by-products of war and conflict throughout history. They are the most widely used types of violence against women and girls and yet remain the least condemned war crime. For example, 3% of Vietnamese boat women were reported to have been raped in 1985[11], and 192 cases of sexual abuse were documented among 210 000 Somali refugees[12]. However, it took the conflict in the territory of the former Yugoslavia and the treatment of women there to galvanize the international community into action. A team of experts appointed by the UN Commission on Human Rights concluded that 'rape had been used systematically as an instrument of ethnic cleansing and that women who had suffered from rape were severely traumatised by the experience and in need of health care and psychological and social rehabilitation'. It was estimated that anywhere between 20 and 50 thousand women had been raped during this conflict[13,14].

But what does the term sexual violence refer to? During armed conflict and displacement, existing forms of gender-based and sexual violence are often exacerbated because of the tensions of conflict, the frustration, powerlessness and loss of traditional male roles. Alcohol use may become more common, further increasing pre-existing domestic violence. In addition, the nature and scale of violence against women is different during conflict than before, ranging from random acts of assault by enemy troops, bandits, border guards, etc., to rape as a deliberate strategy of ethnic cleansing as in Bosnia. Some of the forms such violence takes include mass rape, rape camps, military sexual slavery, forced prostitution, forced 'marriages' and forced pregnancies. Multiple rape and gang rape are common. Sexual assaults are associated with violent physical assaults and many women die as a result. There may also be a resurgence of female genital mutilation, as a way to reinforce a sense of cultural identity or as a weapon of ethnic cleansing.

But, unlike with cholera or malnutrition where identifying the problem and counting the sick is a relatively easy task, gathering information on sexual violence is very difficult as victims may be reluctant to report abuse for fear of reprisals and social stigmatization, and figures can be manipulated to political ends. There are, however, some recent figures from refugee settings in Kenya and Zaire (Table 3) and Burundian refugees in Tanzania.

It is obvious that these figures tell very different stories. In the two stable refugee settings in Kenya and Zaire, the reported number of cases of rape varied between 1.5 and 2.5 per thousand women per year, apparently relatively low figures[15]. However, one must consider that these are only *reported* cases of rape, and that the figures do not include other forms of sexual violence.

A different situation was reported in a retrospective study concerning sexual violence during exodus, recently completed by the International Rescue Committee among Burundian refugees in Tanzania. A quarter of all women aged between 12 and 49 had experienced some form of sexual violence[16]. This happened at any stage in their quest for safety – in the conflict situation in Burundi, along the Tanzanian border, between the border and the refugee camps, and within and around the camps. Perpetrators included soldiers, policemen, fellow refugees, husbands and even security staff. In Rwanda, during the mass genocide, as a recent report commissioned by the Fondation de France suggests, 'virtually every adult woman or

Table 3 Reported cases of rape in two refugee settings (1995–96). (From reference 15)

	Number of women raped/year
Dadaab, Kenya	2.37/1000 women
Goma, Zaire	1.47/1000 women

girl past puberty who was spared from massacres by the militias had been raped'.

Some recent figures from Rwanda also tell the gruesome tale of the consequences of sexual violence. According to estimates of the National Population Office, two to five thousand children were born after the mass rape that occurred during the genocide. These children are called the children of bad memories or the children of hate. What future awaits these children? How will they be treated? How many of them will be abandoned by their mother? Interviews carried out by WHO showed that many women were not able to accept their child because the child was associated with the violence and torture perpetrated upon them and their families; some women abandoned their children in the hospitals or in the open fields after delivery, others committed infanticide and some decided to accept their child[17].

Health consequences of sexual violence

The *health consequences of sexual violence* are very diverse[18]. Unwanted pregnancies will lead to a rise in unsafe abortions, especially where abortion is illegal or unavailable. If the woman was pregnant at the time of sexual assault, a miscarriage may ensue. The damage to the genitals associated with sexual assault is terrible enough in itself, but the assault also increases the risk of transmission of HIV and other STDs, which may subsequently lead to pelvic inflammatory disease. Some women die from the direct consequences of rape: in one study in Somalia, of 16 documented rapes, half were reported to have resulted in the death of the victim[19].

Beyond the physical consequences, the psychological effects of sexual violence are profound. These may range from feelings of shock, a paralyzing fear of injury or death, and a profound sense of loss of control over one's life, to a decreased ability to respond to life generally, deep depression, an inability to live one's sexuality positively, and at the most extreme to thoughts or acts of suicide, homicide or infanti-

cide. The physical and psychological effects of sexual violence during armed conflict and displacement are worsened by the victims inability to access health services, by the breakdown of usual support systems and by the absence of a safe and supportive environment for healing.

Possible interventions

Following this brief review of some of the special problems that women face in times of conflict, *possible actions* to be taken and how these could be influenced by lessons learned from past experiences are discussed. Some health services should be provided right away, even during the first phase of an emergency. However, in these situations attention is often focused on immediate life-saving measures and insufficient priority is given to reproductive health care. In order to provide clear guidelines, UNHCR, the United Nations Family Planning Agency UNFPA and WHO recently agreed upon a Minimum Initial Service Package that includes advice on provision of antenatal, delivery and postnatal care, prevention of HIV transmission and prevention of the consequences of sexual abuse[20].

When considering antenatal and delivery care, it is essential to quickly identify previously trained personnel, including traditional birth attendants, and to provide them with a minimum of material. Now that HIV is present all over the world, universal precautions and safe blood transfusions must be guaranteed under any circumstance. In addition, the mass exodus from Rwanda demonstrated that even in the midst of grief and turmoil people request condoms, as life goes on. Finally, to prevent at least the most dreaded consequence of rape, emergency post-coital contraception should always be available, even before more sophisticated support services can be established[21]. Based on the data collected by the International Rescue Committee among Burundian refugees in Tanzania, referred to earlier, health staff at the way stations along the border as well as camp staff have been trained to make this method available to women who are raped.

Antenatal, delivery and postnatal care

Once the situation has stabilized, each of the elements of reproductive health care must be given more attention, and culturally appropriate and good-quality services should be established. One should remember that in stable refugee situations, complications of pregnancy and delivery are the leading causes of death and disease among women of child-bearing age. It is thus essential to establish comprehensive services for *antenatal, delivery and postnatal care*, including a referral system for the management of complications, as approximately 15% of women will develop complications and about 5% will require surgery. In establishing such services, priority should be given to female health workers including midwives, nurses and also traditional birth attendants (TBAs). TBAs are usually the key people at community level who will influence maternal and newborn care. In 1993 in the Somali refugee camps in Kenya, TBAs that carried out most deliveries and that were most accepted by the communities were chosen for training and supplied with delivery kits, and progressively improved the quality of care they were able to provide[22].

Breastfeeding is particularly important in conflict situations because of the increased risk of infectious disease for the newborn, because it may be the only sustainable food security for infants and young children, and because the bonding and care which it provides is crucial to mothers and children. The risks associated with bottle feeding are dramatically increased in precarious situations and usually outweigh the potential risk of HIV transmission via breastfeeding. Breastfeeding should thus be promoted and women should be assisted accordingly[23].

Dealing with sexual violence

Based on two decades of experience with providing antenatal, delivery and postnatal care in refugee settings, such services today can be established quickly and efficiently as demonstrated by the low rates of maternal mortality and low birth weights in the Goma camps in Zaire. However, there is much less experience when it comes to *dealing with sexual violence*. In 1992 a pilot project called the Women Victims of Violence Project was initiated in the Somali refugee camps (Dadaab) in north-eastern Kenya[12,24]. Early on in the refugee crisis, violence against refugees, and especially raping of women, was being reported at alarming rates. This project, the first of its kind, tried to assist women who had been raped and to prevent further attacks. Some of the key elements of this project are community-based security arrangements, anti-rape action committees, active co-operation with security personnel, focus on women's empowerment, and quality and compassionate health services for rape victims. The main lessons learned are that there needs to be community-based support for all security arrangements, that security personnel must collaborate actively and that quality and compassionate health services are essential. The project has not been able to prevent all cases of rape, as women still have to leave the camps in search of firewood and cannot always do this in groups. However, sexual violence within the camps has decreased and women now seek treatment and support rapidly.

Building on this experience and some more recent interventions in Rwandan refugee camps[25], some essential elements of a program targeted at preventing sexual violence have been identified[26]. They comprise the creation of an environment which is as secure as possible for women, including their participation in any decisions made and the direct distribution of food and other items to women, to preclude the use of coerced sex for access to these items. Overall awareness about the extent of sexual abuse and its terrifying consequences must be increased to counter denial and a possible feeling of impunity. This also involves the training of all parties concerned – military, police, refugee leaders, women's groups, etc., including the potential abusers.

While trying to put in place a system to prevent sexual violence, services must be made available to the victims. The biggest need identified in Rwanda was the need for counselling to overcome the psychological and social scars of the assault. At the same time, some women (especially those who have been raped) need access to emergency contraception, to STD services and, if necessary and possible, to safe abortion. Of course, abortion remains a subject of much debate. However, it seems that imposing the birth of a 'child of hate' on a woman who has already suffered the unspeakable, and who may not want or be able to care for this child in the future, is defensible neither from the ethical, nor the medical, nor the social point of view. Finally, to improve awareness about sexual violence and to be able to better assist the victims, it is very useful to document cases of abuse. But great attention must be paid to fully respect confidentiality, and it should only be done with the informed consent of the woman concerned.

Dealing with sexually transmitted diseases

What should be done about HIV/AIDS and STDs beyond the initial activities mentioned earlier? Condoms should be promoted more actively and the distribution system should be evaluated and improved to guarantee access to all youths and adults. This should be combined with information and education about HIV/AIDS and STD prevention, based on the level of awareness and knowledge in the population that prevailed before the exodus. In addition, much attention must be paid to ensuring access to comprehensive STD care using the syndromic approach and making essential drugs available[27,28]. Syphilis screening should be included systematically in antenatal care. As described earlier, 4% of Rwandan refugee women had active syphilis, thus indicating the need for detection and treatment. Finally, it should be mentioned that voluntary HIV testing and counselling is a low priority as long as all of the other services are not in place. HIV testing for diagnosis of HIV-related illness is only indicated if informed consent, counselling and confidentially can be assured and if confirmatory testing procedures can be carried out. People known to be infected with HIV or to have AIDS should remain within their communities, should have equal access to all available health care and should receive psychological support as needed.

Family planning services

This brief overview of reproductive health interventions concludes with a reference to *family planning services*. Beyond emergency contraception and condom distribution, the provision of a full range of family planning services is only warranted and feasible once the situation has stabilized. Before setting up such a program, it is important to assess whether the refugee population has already been exposed to family planning in the past and to which methods, to estimate the potential demand overall and the potential demand for specific contraceptives and to plan an information campaign that targets women as well as men.

Experience has shown that it is essential to provide a choice of birth control methods, preferably those that are already known[20]. Figure 2 shows the reaction to the initiation of a family planning program in the Goma camps. Both oral contraceptives as well as injectable preparations were in demand. The user rate increased over time with a clear preference for Depo-provera®. It is not known if this was mainly due to previous experience in Rwanda, as both methods were available in the camps and neither was favored by the health care staff.

Concluding remarks

Many of the issues discussed in this paper are remote from the everyday practice of most gynecologists and obstetricians. The situations of conflict and crisis referred to are clearly instances where society and its institutions have been severely disrupted and may be worst-case scenarios. However, in the same way that any physician would not dispute the necessity for an individual patient to have access to acute emergency care, the international medical community should by the same ethical and Hippocratic principles be committed to ensuring

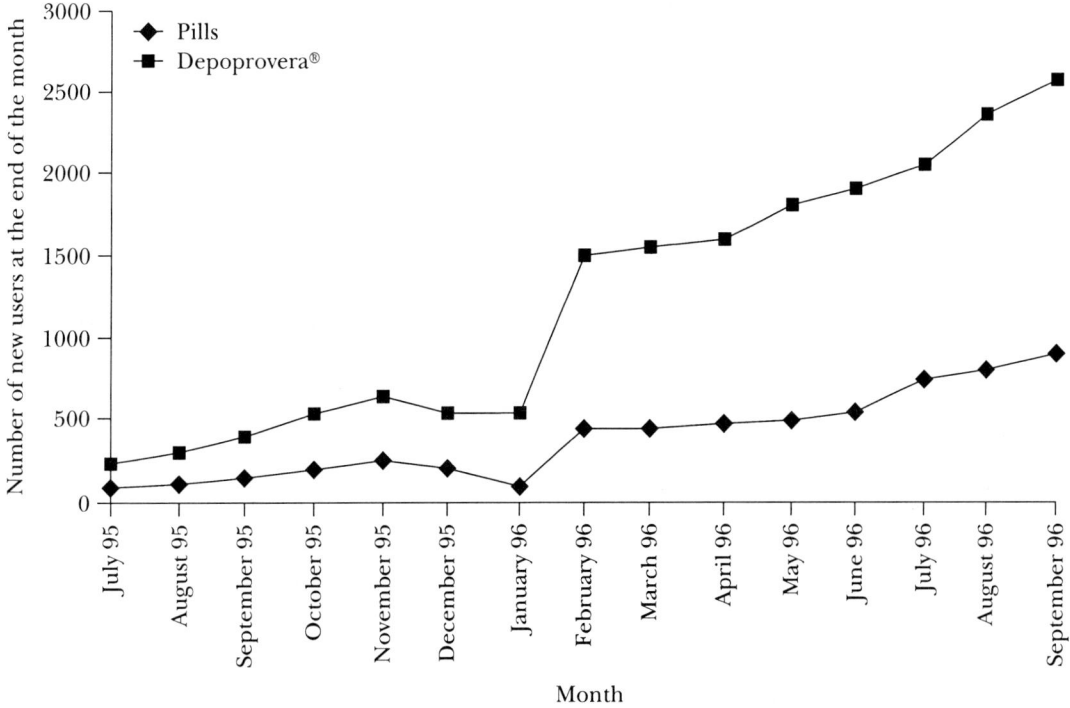

Figure 2 Comparison of birth control methods in Goma Mugunga camp from July 1995 to September 1996

that women whose lives are thrown into upheaval due to war and conflict well beyond their personal influence, get the support that they need.

Not providing assistance to girls and women in a crisis situation where they may have lost their social support network, have no economic means, have become solely responsible for their children and have even less protection than in their home environment, will have many lasting consequences for their health and well-being as well as for the health and well-being of their children. Over the past 15 years we have learned that even in desperate situations, well-organized and appropriate assistance can change the lives of women.

We should also acknowledge that many women living in resource-poor and socially unstable environments such as post-conflict areas, urban slums and marginalized minority groups, suffer the same problems as those discussed here. Some of the problems such as sexual violence or STDs and HIV are often denied or neglected. Hopefully the lessons learned in times of extreme vulnerability and suffering could also be applied to help women in other settings.

Acknowledgements

I am greatly indebted to Kate Burns (UNHCR/PTSS), Carole Djeddah (WHO/FRH), and Lorelei Goodyear (IRC), for providing me with much information which is difficult to otherwise access. I would also like to thank my collaborators at MSF for their continuous support in the preparation of this manuscript.

References

1. United High Commissioner for Refugees (1995). *The State of the World's Refugees. In search of solutions.* (Geneva: UNHCR)
2. Pierotti, D. and Malé, S, (1995). Refugee women: helping the helpless. *Entre Nous: Eur. Fam. Plann. Magazine,* No. 30–31. December
3. Rivers, J. P. W. (1994). Women and children last: an essay on sex discrimination in disasters. *Disasters,* **6**, 256–67
4. Forbes, M. S. *et al.* (1990). Issues in refugee and displaced women and children. *Expert Group Meeting on Refugee and Displaced Women and Children,* Vienna, 2–6 July
5. Suetens, C. and Dedeuwaerder, M. (1994). Food availability in the refugee camp of Kahindo, Goma, Zaire. *Med. News,* **3**, 16–22
6. World Health Organization (1994). *Mother–Baby Package: Implementing Safe Motherhood in Countries,* WHO/FHE/MSM/94.11. (Geneva: WHO)
7. Mears, C. and Chowdury, S. (1994). *Health Care for Refugees and Displaced People.* (Oxfam), Oxford
8. UNHCR (1995–96). Unpublished data collected during the Rwanda refugee crisis in Goma, Zaire
9. UNHCR/PTSS (1997). Azerbaijan, Armenia and Georgia: strengthening reproductive health services. *UNHCR/PTSS Mission Report,* February
10. Msuya, W., Mayaud, P., Mkanje, R. *et al.* (1996). HIV/STD intervention in Rwandan refugee camps in Tanzania, abstr. Tu.D.242. *XI International Conference on AIDS,* Vancouver, July
11. UNHCR (1986). *Services for Vietnamese Refugees who have Suffered from Violence at Sea: An Evaluation of the Project in Thailand and Malaysia,* February, 1986. (Geneva: UNHCR)
12. Musse, F. (1994). Women's Victims of Violence Project in Kenya. *Refugee Participation Network,* **16** (March), 17–20
13. Enloe, C. (1993). Have the Bosnian rapes opened a new era of feminist consciousness. In Stiglmayer, A. (ed.) *Mass Rape: The War Against Women in Bosnia-Herzegovina.* (University of Nebrovka Press)
14. Brautigam, C. A. (1996). Traumatised women: overcoming victimisation through equality and non-discrimination. In Danieli, Y., Rodley, N. S. and Weisaeth, L. (eds.) *International Responses to Traumatic Stress.* (New York: Baywood Publ.)
15. Unpublished UNHCT statistics, 1996
16. Nduna, S. and Goodyear, L. (1997). Pain too deep for tears: assessing the prevalence of sexual and gender violence against Burundian refugees in Tanzania. (New York: International Rescue Committee)
17. Djeddah, C. (1996). Wars and unaccompanied children in Africa: who they are and major health implications. *WHO/UNICEF/IPA Pre-Congress Workshop,* Kampala, Uganda, November
18. Heise, L. L., Pitanguy, J. and Germain, A. (1994). Violence against women. The hidden health burden. *World Bank Disc. Paper,* No. 255 (Washington D.C.: The World Bank)
19. Gersony, R. (1990). Why Somalis flee: A synthesis of conflict experience in northern Somalia by Somali refugees, displaced persons and others. *Int. J. Refugee Law,* **2**, 27
20. UNHCR (1995). *Reproductive Health in Refugee Situations. An Inter-Agency Field Manual.* (Geneva: UNHCR)
21. Consortium for emergency contraception (1996). *Emergency Contraceptive Pills: A Resource Packet for Health Care Providers and Program Managers.* (Welcome, USA)
22. Médecins Sans Frontières (1996). In Hanquet, G. (ed.) *Refugee Health: An Approach in Emergency Situations.* (Paris: Medecins Sans Frontières)
23. King, F. S. (1992). *Helping Mothers to Breastfeed.* (Nairobi, Kenya: AMREF)
24. IAWG (1997). Reproductive health in refugee situations. *IAWG Update Newslett.,* No. 2, January, p. 3
25. UNHCR/PTSS (1997). *Community-based Response to Sexual Violence. Crisis Intervention Teams, Ngara, Tanzania,* January. (Geneva: UNHCR/ PTSS)
26. United Nations High Commissioner for Refugees (1995). *Sexual Violence against Refugees: Guidelines on Prevention and Response.* (Geneva: UNHCR)
27. WHO, UNHCR and UNAIDS (1996). *Guidelines for HIV Interventions in Emergency Settings,* UNAIDS/96.1. (Geneva: UNAIDS)
28. Nersesian, P. and Brady, B. (1995). Controlling STDs/HIV within dynamic refugee settings. *Refugee Participation Network,* **20** (November), 26–9

Obstetrician-gynecologists: women's primary physicians

3

V. Seltzer

Thank you for giving me the opportunity to address the XV FIGO World Congress. It is quite a privilege for me. I have been greatly impressed by the excellent talks that I have heard this week, and it has been a pleasure to meet and speak with so many distinguished colleagues from around the world.

Since I am giving one of the last talks at the last FIGO meeting of the twentieth century, I am afforded the opportunity to reflect on the enormous challenges that need to be addressed in the next century.

As you all know, FIGO has been in existence for more than four decades. The organization is fortunate to be able to bring together some of the finest minds and most dedicated physicians from around the world. Because of the skill and commitment of the obstetrician-gynecologists who are involved in FIGO, there are considerable opportunities to advance the cause of improving the health care and well-being of women.

I am going to spend the next few minutes sharing with you my dreams and visions of what I hope FIGO can work toward in the twenty-first century. It may seem to be an overwhelming challenge. However, the stakes are high. Hundreds of millions of women are in need and can benefit.

I believe that obstetrician-gynecologists are really the most effective advocates for and providers of women's health care, and that to provide the best reproductive health care our role must extend far beyond the reproductive tract. To best address a woman's reproductive health, it is necessary to take into account the context of her general health. I believe that the obstetrician-gynecologist should emphasize preventive care, and make certain that our patients are being provided primary health care. I believe that it is necessary to address our patients' psychological as well as physical well-being.

I don't think we really can achieve enough for our patients if we focus only on a particular disease process, but do not view it in the context of our patients' general physical and mental health. In addition to our concern about our patients' physical and mental health, we must also be concerned about her status and rights in her home, family, and community, as so eloquently advocated by President Fathalla.

As each of us looks inward regarding what we can do for our individual patients to keep them healthy, we should also look outward to our local communities, our own nations, and to our colleagues around the world to determine how we can best work together to promote women's health.

Our local issues will vary, depending upon what the main problems are for a woman's health and well-being in our region. I am going to discuss what the American College of Obstetricians and Gynecologists has been doing in the past several years to enhance the general health and well-being of women in the United States, and then suggest what I hope we can all be involved with globally.

From a study of overall health statistics, it is estimated that, in the United States, one half of premature deaths, one-third of all cases of acute disability, and one half of all cases of chronic disability could be prevented by reducing behavioral risk factors. The American College of Obstetricians and Gynecologists has emphasized the importance of addressing the needs of the whole patient in addition to focusing on reproductive health. At present, more than half of the obstetrician-gynecologists in the United States who responded to our survey indicated that they spend more than half of their time providing primary-preventive care.

In addition, a few years ago, graduate medical education, what we call resident education, in Obstetrics and Gynecology in the United States was re-evaluated and redesigned to emphasize general women's health in addition to reproduction. In addition to the traditional focus on all aspects of women's reproductive health care, residents in Obstetrics and Gynecology are now educated in preventive and ambulatory primary health care for women. In order to have a residency program approved by our Obstetrics and Gynecology Residency Review Committee, the residency program director must demonstrate a breadth and depth of education in preventive and primary care and in behavioral medicine, in addition to education in all aspects of reproductive medicine.

During the past several years, the leadership of the American College of Obstetricians and Gynecologists has emphasized the importance of obstetrician-gynecologists giving serious attention to the main causes of morbidity and mortality in women, and doing what we can to prevent their occurrence, thereby reducing the burden of suffering for women.

Heart disease is the leading cause of death in women in the United States. It is responsible for 350 000 deaths each year in US women. As you all know, one of the most effective means of reducing coronary artery disease is the use of hormone replacement therapy (HRT) in post-menopausal women. Obstetrician-gynecologists have led the way in patient education regarding the use of hormone replacement therapy and in treating postmenopausal women with HRT. In addition, we are playing a major role in educating our patients regarding the importance of exercise, proper diet, and calcium intake. These efforts, of course, have had an impact not only on the prevention of heart disease, but also on reducing the risk of osteoporosis, which is another major contributor to disability and death in US women.

The second leading cause of death in women in the United States is cancer, resulting in the death of 250 000 women each year. Obstetrician-gynecologists have played a major role in reducing cancer mortality. Several decades ago, cervical cancer was a common cause of death for women in the United States. Due to the aggressive programs by the Ob-Gyn community of PAP smear screening, and colposcopy for women with abnormal PAPs, there are now fewer than 5000 cervical cancer deaths a year in US women.

One of our major cancer targets during the last two decades has been breast cancer. In the US, it has been the obstetrician-gynecologists who have played the most prominent role in patient education and screening for this disease. This has resulted in a decrease in the rate of occurrence of tumors larger than 3 cm in diameter, and an increase in the detection rate of small tumors and *in situ* lesions. Due in part to the organized, aggressive campaign by obstetrician-gynecologists to educate women about breast cancer and to screen them for the disease, mortality from breast cancer in the United States is finally declining.

Unfortunately, just as we have been seeing improvements in breast cancer mortality, we have been faced with an alarming increase in lung cancer mortality among women in the US. During the past decade, lung cancer replaced breast cancer as the leading cause of cancer deaths in women in the United States. As many as 90% of these cancer deaths may be associated with cigarette smoking. As more men have quit smoking, lung cancer deaths in US men have been declining. Women in the United States have not shown the same decline in cigarette smoking rates, and the number of teenage girls who are starting to smoke cigarettes is of great concern. Because of this very serious problem, obstetrician-gynecologists are undertaking a major effort to educate our patients about the risks of smoking and helping them to stop, or, even better, to not start smoking at all.

Of course, an increasingly alarming problem for women in the United States and around the world is infection with the human immunodeficiency virus. Obstetrician-gynecologists have been, and must continue to play a central role in reducing the risk of women and their children from becoming infected.

Clearly, mental health is a major component of a women's well-being. Depression is one of the most widespread and debilitating mental health problems for women in the United States and throughout the world. In the US, it is estimated that seven million women suffer from clinical depression at any given time. This illness occurs more than twice as often in women in our country as it does in men. The incidence peaks among women ages 25–44. Often obstetrician-gynecologists are the only physicians that women in this age group see on a regular basis. Obstetrician-gynecologists, both during their residencies and in practice, are increasingly being educated to diagnose and treat depression, in an effort to reduce the burden of suffering for these women.

Obstetrician-gynecologists in the United States have become involved in addressing previously unrecognized social problems such as domestic violence. This is a global problem that causes great suffering for millions of women. ACOG's 43rd President, Dr Richard Jones, who also appeared on this FIGO program, made this issue the focus of his term in office. He encouraged obstetrician-gynecologists to identify patients who are subjects of abuse and to develop programs that can identify and help them. We certainly have not solved this problem in our country, but our voice is being heard, and we have been able to help many women.

Please do not misunderstand what I am saying. There are many imperfections in the health-care system in the United States, and we are far from achieving ideal health for all women.

What I am saying is that, more and more, obstetrician-gynecologists in the United States have accepted the fact that we are not doing the best for our patients if we limit our focus to the narrowest scope of their reproductive health needs. We can most fully contribute to our patients' reproductive health when we focus, in addition, on their general wellness. This means

that we must be involved in understanding the main causes of morbidity and mortality for each individual patient and for women in the community in general, and do whatever we can to reduce or eliminate these problems by prevention and by early detection of disease, as well as by effective action.

This implies concern for the patient's psychological as well as physical well-being. And, it means that we must be concerned about how women are treated in their homes and within their communities. Unless our patients have knowledge and can have their needs met, they live in a state of suboptimal health, and this also has profoundly negative effects on their families and communities.

Since I have been accorded the privilege of giving one of the last talks at the last FIGO meeting of this century, I would like to take this opportunity to suggest what I hope we can do collectively to improve women's health in the twenty-first century. During this week in Copenhagen I have had the privilege of meeting many brilliant, and dedicated physicians from around the world. The women of the world are truly fortunate to have such an incredible nucleus of physicians concerned with their reproductive health.

We must work collectively to improve reproductive health for all women. To improve women's reproductive health and to insure safe motherhood we must, as individuals and as an international organization, focus on their general physical and mental well-being and on prevention of disease. I believe that we must work together to eliminate anything that constitutes a barrier to keeping women healthy, whether it is a woman's status in her home, her status within the community, or her lack of equal access to education or health care, including her lack of access to family planning education and resources.

I believe that each of us must feel a responsibility beyond the specific needs of the individual women whom we treat. We need to be concerned about and advocates for women's health and for improved status of women within society.

There are alarming statistics that are known to most of the people in this room, but they are not necessarily known by all obstetrician-gynecologists, and they should be. Each year approximately 585 000 women die of complications related to pregnancy and childbirth. That's almost one woman a minute. The five leading contributors to maternal mortality are hemorrhage, infection, hypertensive diseases of pregnancy, obstructed labor, and complications related to unsafe abortion. In addition to mortality related to pregnancy, many millions of women suffer serious morbidity from a wide range of problems such as fistulas and pain.

In some countries, women spend more than half of their lives between the ages of 15 and 45 either pregnant or breastfeeding. The World Health Organization has estimated that, if all women who wanted no more children were able to stop having children, the birth rate would fall by one-third in some parts of the world. What is even more significant is that maternal mortality could be reduced substantially. In one country it was estimated that, if women only had the pregnancies they planned, there would be almost a two-thirds reduction in maternal mortality.

Of course, a woman's likelihood of dying as a result of pregnancy relates both to her likelihood of dying during a particular pregnancy and to the number of pregnancies that she has. In some parts of the world, a woman's likelihood of having her cause of death be a maternal death may be more than 1 in 20. Especially high-risk pregnancies are often those in adolescents and in older women. These pregnancies are frequently unplanned or undesired.

The root of these problems is multifaceted, and there are no obvious or easy solutions. However, I do believe that FIGO, the world organization of obstetrician-gynecologists, can use its international authority to urge that each national society attempt to address these problems, both individually and collectively.

We must do all that we are able to do to reduce maternal mortality. A part of this is working to increase access to family planning education and resources. We can obviously do a lot to reduce maternal mortality just by reducing the incidence of unplanned and undesired pregnancy.

Another important issue is education. In most studies it has been shown that, as levels of education are increased, women are more likely to have their first child at a later age, have longer intervals between pregnancies, and have fewer children.

I believe that an essential component of the problem of maternal mortality and morbidity is the status of women in all countries, my own included. We probably cannot achieve the most for our patients unless we are willing to let our voices be heard on this issue as well.

Essentially all obstetrician-gynecologists entered the field because we are concerned with women's health. As I have indicated, I believe that, to have the best outcomes for women's reproductive health, we must be involved with women's general physical and mental health. Furthermore, we must be concerned with women's wellness in the context of their homes, communities, and society.

I believe that this is a challenge for each of us as we look towards the twenty-first century. Each of us has a lot to accomplish for our own patients, our own health-care facilities, and our own communities, as well as with our colleagues throughout the world.

I believe that the more than 150 000 obstetrician-gynecologists represented by the constituent societies of FIGO can accomplish a great deal if we work together, as well as cooperating with other international organizations such as the World Health Organization. The challenges are great, but I believe that we can meet them.

I wish to thank you again for the privilege of addressing the XV FIGO World Congress.

Recovering fetal cells in maternal blood for prenatal genetic diagnosis

4

J. L. Simpson and S. Elias

Introduction

Fetal cells circulate in the maternal blood during pregnancy. Isolation and analysis of these cells is rigorously being pursued for non-invasive prenatal genetic diagnosis. Increasingly, consensus has developed that fetal aneuploidy is detectable.

Several different fetal cell types exist in maternal blood: trophoblasts, lymphocytes, granulocytes and nucleated red blood cells. The most promising advances have been made with nucleated red blood cells; thus, the focus in this paper will be on that cell type. Key points for discussion include the consistency with which these fetal cells can be recovered and the reliability with which diagnosis can be made. Whether the sensitivity of detection is competitive with maternal serum analyte screening and ultrasonographic analysis will also be discussed.

Time of origin and disappearance of fetal cells

Using nested primer polymerase chain reaction (PCR) for Y-specific DNA, signals can be detected early in pregnancy in the peripheral blood of pregnant women carrying male fetuses. Such Y-specific signals were detected at 33 and 40 days' gestation by Thomas and colleagues[1]. Liou and co-workers[2,3] found Y sequences indicative of male fetal cells in 19 of 19 pregnancies by 10–11 weeks.

One concern is that fetal cells from a prior pregnancy could persist in the maternal circulation and, hence, interfere with diagnosis. This could be especially troublesome if aneuploid cells were to persist after a chromosomally abnormal live-born offspring or a chromosomally abnormal spontaneous abortion. To allay this concern, Hsieh and associates[4] followed 28 women delivered of a male fetus. One week after gestation, 26 of the 28 women delivered of males showed ZFY and SRY sequences in their blood. By 4 months, only 11 of the 28 showed Y-specific sequences; by 8 months, only two of 23. Our group has similarly not found prior male pregnancies to present diagnostic difficulties. Using Y-specific probes, no Y-specific cells were observed in eight women who were delivered of male babies (up to 22) years previously[5].

Bianchi and colleagues[6] have helped clarify the confusion by showing that the fetal cells persisting from prior pregnancies are recoverable, but not by the selection criteria commonly used to isolate erythroblasts for prenatal diagnosis. That is, positive selection for precursor stem cells is not achieved with CD71. Thus, status of prior pregnancies should not interfere with diagnosis.

Polymerase chain reaction-based diagnosis for Mendelian traits

Detection of fetal Mendelian disorders by PCR-based technology does not require enrichment. Because PCR sensitivity is so great, only a small amount of DNA is necessary to detect a given genotype. Moreover, the DNA may be derived from any type of fetal cell. Mendelian diagnosis thus does not necessitate targeting of any specific fetal cell type.

Fetal sex

Determining fetal sex is obviously useful in couples at risk for X-linked recessive traits. Nested primer analysis for Y-DNA sequences was used initially by Lo and co-workers[7,8] to establish that fetal cells exist in maternal blood. Detection rates for fetal cells increase as gestation progresses, approximating to 100% by the end of the first trimester[2,3].

Autosomal dominant and recessive disorders

Camaschella and associates[9] were the first to detect a Mendelian disorder by analysis of DNA of the fetal cells present in maternal blood; DNA obtained from maternal blood of three pregnancies at risk for β-thalassemia/hemoglobin Lepore~Boston~ were studied. Hemoglobin Lepore-Boston is a hybrid δ-β globin gene that results from unequal crossing-over between misaligned β- and δ-genes, leading to a 7-kb deletion. Camaschella and colleagues[9] used PCR to amplify for hemoglobin Lepore~Boston~-specific DNA in unsorted maternal blood of women whose male partners carried the Lepore~Boston~ mutation. The mutation was correctly identified in two fetuses, and excluded in a third. Camaschella and colleagues[9] made no attempt to enrich for any specific cell type, but Hawes and co-workers[10] later flow-sorted for trophoblasts before applying a similar molecular strategy to detect DNA indicating paternally transmitted β-thalassemia in the fetus.

An ideal circumstance for detecting a Mendelian disorder through analysis of fetal cells in maternal blood might exist when the father is heterozygous (Aa) and the mother homozygously abnormal (aa) for an autosomal recessive trait. The normal allele, which may or may not be transmitted by the heterozygous father, should be readily detectable. If blood from the homozygous mother reveals DNA of the normal paternal allele (A) the fetus can be deduced to be heterozygous (Aa).

Fetal rhesus (D) status

The genetic basis of Rh(D) negativity is usually a gene deletion, *d* representing lack of the gene encoding *D*. If the mother is Rh negative and the father homozygous for Rh(D) (Rh positive), all fetuses must be heterozygous (Dd); every pregnancy would then be at risk for RhD-isoimmunization. If the father is fortunately heterozygous, the likelihood is 50% that the fetus would inherit his RhD gene and, hence, be affected; the other 50% of pregnancies would not be at risk for Rh-isoimmunization. Lo and associates[11] determined fetal Rh(D) status in Rh-negative sensitized women whose spouses were heterozygous. Unsorted bloods from 21 RhD-negative women were subjected to PCR for Rh(D) sequences. Among 11 women showing a positive PCR signal, seven had a RhD-positive fetus; of the 10 not showing a signal, two had a RhD-positive fetus. Overall, eight of the 10 women carrying a RhD fetus showed a RhD signal. An improved set of primers was later recommended[12]. Geifman-Holtzman and colleagues[13] studied 18 RhD-negative pregnant women (one twin gestation). Thirteen infants were serotyped as RhD positive; in 10 of the cases, RhD-positive PCR signals were detected in maternal blood. Six infants were serotyped as RhD negative; none showed RhD-positive signals in maternal blood. A similar approach should allow determination of Rh(C) or Rh(E) status[13].

Enrichment of fetal nucleated red blood cells for cytogenetic diagnosis

Pursuing of the fetal nucleated red cell (erythroblast) is attractive because nucleated red blood cells (NRBCs) comprise about 10% of red cells in the 11-week fetus and 0.5% in the 19-week fetus. Yet NRBCs are rare in peripheral adult blood. Nucleated red blood cells do not persist longer than perhaps 5 days in the adult; thus, fetal NRBCs seem less likely to persist as clones from previous pregnancies than would be the case with lymphocytes.

Bianchi and co-workers[14] were the first to focus on NRBCs, flow-sorting for transferrin receptor (CD71) expression and examining by PCR for a Y sequence. In 1990, this group showed that after enrichment, Y sequences were found in six of eight pregnancies in which women were carrying male fetuses. Our initial experience failed to confirm this work, but we were soon successful when sorting not only for

CD71 but also for cell size, cell granularity and glycophorin-A positivity[15,16]. Using nested PCR primers for a Y-specific sequence, we correctly identified male fetuses in 12 of 12 flow-sorted samples[15]. We identified female fetuses in five of six samples.

Later, our group was the first to detect fetal aneuploidy by analysis of maternal blood, analyzing interphase cells by fluorescent *in situ* hybridization (FISH) with chromosome-specific probes. Analyzing blood obtained prior to chorionic villus sampling (CVS), we detected trisomy 18[16] and trisomy 21[17]. In 1993, we tabulated our experience with 69 maternal blood samples[18,19]. Of eight aneuploidies, only one was not detected. No false-positive results were observed. Since then work has proceeded on several fronts.

Methods of enrichment

Although fetal cells clearly exist in maternal blood, they are rare. The fetal:maternal cell ratio is approximately 1 per 100 000–10 000 000, although data of Wachtel and colleagues[20] would suggest that fetal cells are considerably more frequent. Assuming a consensus of no more than 1 fetal per 100 000 maternal cells, FISH analysis for fetal chromosomal abnormalities will require some type of enrichment. (As described above, PCR-based technologies can detect certain Mendelian disorders without enrichment.) The general strategy of enrichment is to obtain a sample that is relatively richer with respect to fetal cells than maternal cells. Even after enrichment, the final ratio is likely to be heavily maternal, perhaps 99:1. However, even the 1% of fetal cells can allow reasonably efficient search for aneuploidy using FISH with chromosome-specific probes.

Enrichment is accomplished sequentially. Techniques like Percoll-gradient separation are preliminary in most protocols. More thorough separation requires flow-sorting or magnetic activated cell-sorting (MACS). The principle is that one selects against (negatively) those cells of the undesired type and selects for (positively)

those cells of the desired type. Flow-sorting can process huge numbers of cells quite rapidly; however, the technology is expensive, and physical stress is exerted on separated cells. Nevertheless, flow-sorting technology is the method that appears to our group to be most useful.

Other groups have had success with utilizing the simpler technology of magnetic activating cell-sorting (MACS). In MACS antibodies directed against the cells sought for enrichment are conjugated to magnetic beads; these beads (and, hence, the desired cell type) are retained under magnetic field when cells in solution pass through a column surrounded by a magnet. Cells that do not have an antigen against the antibody in question do not attach to beads, are not retained in the magnetic field and pass through unimpeded to be discarded. After the magnet is deactivated, cells attached to beads can then be collected for subsequent analysis. The procedure of MACS is considerably cheaper than fluorescence activated cell-sorting (FACS) but has not proved as efficient to our group.

A variant of MACS, utilized by Jefferson Medical College, is to use ferro-fluids. Other techniques based on physical separation have been used; Wachtel and colleagues[20] use a counter current technology. The basis is the physical difference between fetal versus maternal cells.

Antigen selection criteria

No ideal selection criteria exist, although considerable progress has been made towards this end. Our own work initially dealt with positive selection for glycophorin-A and CD71 (transferrin). Flow-sorting has continued to involve selecting fetal cells on the basis of size (forward degree angle scatter) and various other characteristics. Since moving to Baylor in 1994, we have introduced selection for the nucleus (LDS751) and for γ-globin[21–23]. We abandoned glycophorin-A positive selection despite our initial success because available monoclonal antibodies against glycophorin-A caused cell clumping. We often utilize negative depletion, for example using anti-CD45 to remove lympho-cytes. The remaining cells should be relatively enriched in the desired fetal cell type (i.e. NRBC). However, negative selection methods probably inadvertently exclude many cells of interest. Although it has been estimated that a 20-cm^3 blood sample contains approximately 100 fetal cells, most investigators detect only one or two fetal cells in normal pregnancies (i.e. XY cells if the fetus is 46,XY) and 3–10 cells in aneuploid pregnancies (e.g. +21).

At present, we favor positive selection on the basis of CD71 and negative selection against CD45 cells. We are exploring use of sorting for various fetal hemoglobins (ε- and ζ-globin), but have not reached a final decision.

Multicolor FISH analysis

Detection of chromosomal abnormalities is likely to require recovery of fetal cells from maternal blood by FISH analysis of interphase cells. (However, see below for the prospect of culturing fetal cells.) The technique of FISH analysis has been used by our group since 1991, enabling us to achieve the first detection of fetal trisomy. However, in our earlier work, sequen-tial or selected use of probes for selected chro-mosome-specific probes were employed: X, Y and usually 21 or 18. On the other hand, a genuine screening program requires prospec-tive analysis of all chromosomes that would be detected in at least maternal serum screening programs (13, 18 and 21). Not only analysis of a single chromosome-specific probe in a given interphase nucleus is required, but rather simul-taneous analysis of at least numbers 13,18, 21, X and Y.

Until the past 12–18 months, application of five-color FISH technology to physically stressed flow-sorted fetal cells had proved technically difficult. However, Bischoff and co-workers of our unit have now demonstrated the abil-ity to analyze efficiently (98%) all these chromosomes simultaneously, using directly labeled probes that intercalate into DNA (Vysis Inc., Downers Grove, IL)[24].

Sensitivity of fetal aneuploidy detection

Having achieved the crucial step of simul-taneous five-color FISH analysis, the accuracy of detecting chromosomal abnormalities in fetal blood can be determined. Initially, the assump-tion was made that sensitivity could be deter-mined simply by calculating the number of preg-nancies in which male (XY cells) were correctly detected. Male cells, presumably fetal in origin, prove detectable in approximately 50–70% of cases during optimal runs; the number of false-positives found by our group is low (< 1%), providing overall correct identification at a level of approximately 75%. However, the number of fetal cells detected in normal male pregnancies is usually only one or two, among up to 3000 interphase cells screened.

Increasingly, it has become clear that more fetal cells are present in the maternal blood in aneuploid pregnancies than in euploid preg-nancies. No certain explanation for this differ-ential effect exists, but clearly it is salutary. Studies that simply report on the detection of male cells in maternal pregnant blood are thus no longer considered contributory because aneuploidy detection would be greatly under-estimated. In the United States, clinical evalua-tion is currently under way by the National Institute of Child Health and Human Develop-ment to determine the sensitivity and specificity of detection for aneuploidy. Participating cent-ers include our group at Baylor College of Med-icine/University of Tennessee, Memphis as well as groups at Tufts College of Medicine, Jefferson Medical College and Wayne State Univer-sity/University of Basel. The end-point will be numbers of pregnancies in which fetal trisomies are detected per numbers of pregnancies in which fetal trisomies exist.

Culturing fetal cells from maternal blood

Chromosomal analysis of fetal cells present in maternal blood has been based on FISH analy-sis. This approach was taken on the assumption that fetal metaphases could not be obtained from cells circulating in maternal blood because the latter could not be transformed. By contrast, Valerio and co-workers[25] have recently reported that fetal cells can be isolated and induced to proliferate. These investigators first separate maternal blood by density-gradient, and then identify fetal cells by biotin-labeled human erythropoietin. Enrichment is accomplished by magnetic separation using beads conjugated to streptavidin; streptavidin binds to biotin and, hence, recovers the erythropoietin-labeled cells. After magnetic deactivation, the labeled eluted cells in suspension are placed in a semi-solid medium containing various cytokines, stem cell factor and growth factors. Fetal-colony forming unit-erythroid and mature-burst forming unit-erythroid progenitor cells proliferate, and their origin verified by PCR or FISH. This exciting technology should detect aneuploidy. Progress in the area is awaited with great interest.

Post-sorting identification of fetal cells to facilitate FISH analysis

The technique of FISH analysis with chromosome-specific probes to detect fetal aneuploidy remains complicated by (1) the high proportion of maternal cells remaining after enrichment, and (2) the inability to distinguish maternal XX from fetal XX cells. We and others have sought to develop strategies for distinguishing maternal from fetal cells. At 12–32 weeks' gestation, fetal hemoglobin (HbF, $\alpha_2\gamma_2$) constitutes 90–100% of the total hemoglobin (Hb). By birth, the switch to production of predominantly adult Hb (HbA, $\alpha_2\beta_2$) has generally occurred. Because adult erythroid cells produce abundant amounts of HbA, β-globin expression serves as a marker for identifying adult erythroblasts; γ-globin serves as a marker for fetal erythroblasts.

A novel *in situ* method was developed in our laboratory for detection of cells transcribing γ-globin mRNA[23]. This method takes advantage of the formation of sense–antisense RNA duplexes that identify HbF-producing cells. An oligonucleotide antisense primer specific to γ-globin cDNA is added to a reaction mixture containing Taq polymerase, unlabeled deoxyribonucleoside triphosphate (dNTPs) and directly labeled deoxyuridine triphosphate (dUTP)-rhodamine (which emits red fluorescence). One-step annealing, extension and incubation is followed by standard FISH analysis. Visually detectable differences in γ-globin mRNA fluorescence intensities distinguish cells producing abundant HbF (fetal cells) from adult cells that produce HbA; FISH analysis can then be performed only on the former. In eight cases studied between 11 and 18 weeks' gestation, results were consistent with predictions. Only a small percentage of adult cells produce HbF (0–1.0%), but these also produce HbA and, hence, show FITC β-globin antibody. In three of five male pregnancies, 0.34% of cells (range of 1–3 cells/case) showed a signal for the Y-specific probe: these cells were negative for β-globin expression and positive for γ-globin mRNA, as predicted. In three female pregnancies, 0.42% of cells were also positive for γ-globin mRNA. In the two remaining male pregnancies, cells were neither positive for γ-globin mRNA nor found to have a signal for the Y-probe.

Incorporation of fetal cell analytes into clinical practice (non-invasive screening)

The various technologies for non-invasive screening (fetal cells in maternal blood, maternal serum analyte screening and ultrasound (nuchal translucency)) have generally been considered mutually exclusive. In fact, several could be combined using the principle of likelihood ratios that has made it facile to screen for multiple, as opposed to a single, maternal serum analyte. Indeed, analysis of fetal cells in maternal blood is likely to be especially useful in specific circumstances.

We believe that fetal cells are more likely recoverable earlier in gestation (say, 20 weeks or less, and probably < 15 weeks). We can thus envision concurrent application of nuchal translucency, first trimester maternal serum screening and analysis of fetal cells in maternal blood. If aneuploid fetal cells indeed prove more frequent in maternal blood than non-aneuploid fetal cells, an especially useful method would exist for diminishing false- positive screening results. The emotional savings of avoiding an invasive procedure would be great, as would the financial savings. For example, the current screening policy in many countries is predicated upon the total cost of prenatal diagnosis equaling no more than that incurred if 5% of the population were to undergo amniocentesis. If a greater aneuploidy detection rate could be obtained with a lower false-positive rate, consider-

able resources could be saved. Given that high-speed flow technology techniques now require only limited flow-sorting time (the major expense), and given that automation of FISH technology is certainly achievable, universal screening of fetal cells can indeed be envisioned. Fetal cells in maternal blood cells might be analyzed only after a positive serum or ultrasound findings. If fetal aneuploid cells are not recovered, an invasive procedure could be avoided. Universal fetal cell screening is the other, more direct, approach.

References

1. Thomas, M. R., Williamson, R., Craft, I., Yazhani, N. and Rodeck, C. H. (1994). Y chromosome sequence DNA amplified from peripheral blood in women in early pregnancy. *Lancet*, **343**, 413–14

2. Liou, J.-D., Pao, C. C., Hor, J. J. and Kao, S.-M. (1993). Fetal cells in the maternal circulation during first trimester in pregnancies. *Hum. Genet.*, **92**, 309–11

3. Liou, J.-D., Hsieh, T.-T. and Pao, C. C. (1994). Persistence of cells of fetal origin in maternal circulation of pregnant women. In Simpson, J. L. and Elias, S. (eds.) *Fetal Cells in Maternal Blood: Prospects for Noninvasive Prenatal Diagnosis*, pp. 237–41. (New York: New York Academy of Sciences)

4. Hsieh, T.-T., Pao, C. C., Hor, J. J. and Kao, S. M. (1993). Presence of fetal cells in maternal circulation after delivery. *Hum. Genet.*, **92**, 204–5

5. Elias, S., Lewis, D. E., Simpson, J. L., Nguyen, D. D., Murrell, S., Schober, W., Scott, J., Boinoff, J. and Bischoff, F. Z. (1996). Isolation of fetal nucleated red blood cells from maternal blood: persistence of cells from prior pregnancy is unlikely to lead to false positive results. *J. Soc. Gynecol. Invest.*, **3**, 359A

6. Bianchi, D. W., Zickwolf, G. K., Weil, G. J., Sylvester, S. and DeMaria, M. A. (1996). Male fetal progenitor cells persist in maternal blood for as long as 27 years postpartum. *Proc. Natl. Acad. Sci. USA*, **93**, 705–8

7. Lo, Y.-M., Patel, P., Wainscoat, J. S., Sampietro, M., Gillmer, M. D. G. and Fleming, K. A. (1989). Prenatal sex determination by DNA amplification from maternal peripheral blood. *Lancet*, **2**, 1363–5

8. Lo, Y.-M.-D., Pate, P., Sampietro, M., Gillmer, M. D. G., Fleming, K. A. and Wainscoat, J. D. (1990). Detection of single-copy fetal DNA sequence from maternal blood. *Lancet*, **335** 1463–4

9. Camaschella, C., Alfarno, A., Gottardi, E., Travi, M., Primignani, P., Calgaris-Cappio, F., and Sagglio, G. (1990). Prenatal diagnosis of fetal haemoglobin Lepore Boston disease on maternal peripheral blood. *Blood*, **75**, 2102–6

10. Hawes, C. S., Suskin, H. A., Kalionis, B., Mueller, U. W., Casey, G., Hall, J. and Rudzki, Z. (1994). Detection of paternally inherited mutations for β-thalassemia in trophoblast isolated from peripheral maternal blood. In Simpson, J. L. and Elias, S. (eds.) *Fetal Cells in Maternal Blood: Prospects for Noninvasive Prenatal Diagnosis*, pp. 181–5. (New York: New York Academy of Sciences)

11. Lo, Y.-M.-D., Bowell, P. J., Selinger, M., MacKenzie, I. Z., Chamberlain, P., Gillmer, M. D., Elliott, P., Littlewood, T. J., Fleming, K. A. and Wainscoat, J. S. (1993). Prenatal determination of fetal RhD status by analysis of peripheral blood of rhesus negative mothers. *Lancet*, **341**, 1147–8

12. Lo, Y.-M.-D., Bowell, P. J., Selinger, M., MacKenzie, I. Z., Chamberlain, P., Gillmer, M. D. G., Elliott, P., Pratt, G., Littlewood, T. J., Fleming, K. A. and Wainscoat, J. S. (1994). Prenatal determination of fetal rhesus D status by DNA amplification of peripheral blood of rhesus-negative mothers. In Simpson, J. L. and Elias, S. (eds.) *Fetal Cells in Maternal Blood: Prospects for Noninvasive Prenatal Diagnosis*, pp. 229–36. (New York: New York Academy of Sciences)

13. Geifman-Holtzman, O., Bernstein, I. M., Berry, S. M., Bianchi, D. W. and Holtzman, E. J. (1996). Rapid molecular determination of fetal rhesus E type. *Prenat. Diagn.*, **16** 489–93

14. Bianchi, D. W., Flint, A. F., Pizzimenti, M. F., Knoll, J. H. M. and Latt, S. A. (1990). Isolation of fetal DNA from nucleated erythrocytes in maternal blood. *Proc. Natl. Acad. Sci. USA*, **87**, 3279–83

15. Wachtel, S. S., Elias, S., Price, J., Wachtel, G., Phillips, O., Shulman, L., Meyers, C., Simpson, J. L. and Dockter, M. (1991). Fetal cells in maternal circulation: isolation by multiparameter flow cytometry and confirmation by PCR. *Hum. Reprod.*, **6**, 1466–9

16. Price, J., Elias, S., Wachtel, S. S., Klinger, S., Dockter, M., Tharapel, A., Shulman, L. P., Phillips, O. P., Meyers, C. M., Shook, S. and Simpson, J. L. (1991). Prenatal diagnosis using fetal cells isolated from maternal blood by multiparameter flow cytometry. *Am. J. Obstet. Gynecol.*, **165**, 1731–7

17. Elias, S., Price, J., Dockter, M., Wachtel, S., Tharapel, A. and Simpson, J. L. (1992). First trimester prenatal diagnosis of trisomy 21 in fetal cells from maternal blood. *Lancet*, **340**, 1033

18. Simpson, J. L. and Elias, S. (1993). Isolating fetal cells from maternal blood: advances in prenatal diagnosis through molecular technology. *J. Am. Med. Assoc.*, **270**, 2357–61

19. Simpson, J. L. and Elias, S. (1994). Fetal cells in maternal blood: overview and historical perspective. In Simpson, J. L. and Elias, S. (eds.) *Fetal Cells in Maternal Blood: Prospects for Noninvasive Prenatal Diagnosis*, pp. 1–8 (New York: New York Academy of Sciences)

20. Wachtel, S. S., Sammons, D., Manley, M., Wachtel, G., Twitty, G., Utermohlen, J., Phillips, O. P., Shulman, L. P., Taron, D. J., Muller, U. R., Koeppen, P., Ruffalo, T. M., Addis, K., Porreco, R., Murata-Collins, J., Parker, N. B. and McGavran, L. (1996). Fetal cells in maternal blood: recovery by change flow separation. *Hum. Genet.*, **98**, 162–6

21. Simpson, J. L. and Elias, S. (1995). Isolating fetal cells in the maternal circulation. *Hum. Reprod.*, **1**, 409–18

22. Lewis, D. E., Schober, W., Murrell, S., Nguyen, D., Scott, J., Boinoff, J., Simpson, J. L., Bischoff, F. Z. and Elias, S. (1996). Rare event selection of fetal nucleated erythrocytes in maternal blood by flow cytometry. *Cytometry*, **23**, 218–27

23. Bischoff, F. Z., Lewis, D. E., Nguyen, D., Murrell, S., Schober, W., Scott, J., Simpson, J. L. and Elias, S. (1995). Fetal cells in maternal blood: more efficacious FISH analysis by using gamma globin mRNA to identify fetal cells after flow-sorting. *Am. J. Hum. Genet.*, **57**, A33

24. Bischoff, F. Z., Lewis, D. D., Nguyen, S., Murrell, S., Schober, W., Scott, J., Leonard, K., Simpson, J. L. and Elias, S. (1997). Advances in prenatal diagnosis using fetal cells isolated from maternal blood: five-color FISH analysis of flow sorted cells for chromosomes X, Y, 13, 18 and 21. *Prenatal Diag.*, submitted

25. Valerio, D., Aiello, R., Altieri, V., Malato, A. P., Fortunato, A. and Canazio, A. (1996). Culture of fetal erythroid progenitor cells from maternal blood for non-invasive prenatal genetic diagnosis. *Prenat. Diagn.*, **16**, 1073–82

Genetics of gynecological cancer: molecular events implicated in trophoblastic neoplasia development

5

N. Wake, T. Matsuda, T. Arima and H. Kato

Background

Choriocarcinoma is a highly invasive tumor consisting of markedly anaplastic trophoblast totally lacking in residual villous structures. However, little is known about the molecular mechanism related to tumor development: these tumors may originate from the trophoblast of any type of conception. Although malignant complications only infrequently occur after abortion or after an apparently normal live birth, the risk of choriocarcinoma associated with complete mole is 2000–4000 times greater than that associated with an apparently normal live birth. However, there has been no direct proof in the majority of patients that choriocarcinoma indeed derives from complete mole. Genetically, complete mole that is androgenetic in origin can be placed into at least two classes[1–9]. The vast majority of complete moles result from fertilization of an egg devoid of nuclei (an empty egg) by a haploid spermatozoon. The paternally derived haploid set then duplicates and restores diploidy. Invariably, this class of moles has a 46,XX karyotype and is completely homozygous for paternally transmitted alleles, 46,YY conceptuses being non-viable. Fertilization of an empty egg by two spermatozoa is responsible for the rare class of complete moles. This mole is heterozygous at some gene loci but homozygous at others. The probability of this rare mole being homozygous at a particular gene locus is 50%. The genome of choriocarcinoma should reflect that of the pregnancy from which the tumor arose. After a live birth or spontaneous abortion, therefore, both maternal and paternal contributions of genome should be present in the tumor genome. Choriocarcinoma after complete mole conceptions, however, should carry only paternal genomes. The absence of a paternal contribution in the tumor genome is a feature of non-gestational choriocarcinoma.

Based on these genetic backgrounds, a small number of trophoblastic tumors have been examined using chromosomal heteromorphisms and enzyme or DNA polymorphisms[10–16]. However, the number of cases reported is too small to disclose the predominant association of complete mole with choriocarcinoma. First, we examined the genetic origin of a relatively large number of trophoblastic tumors in order to demonstrate the propensity to malignancy of complete moles. Demonstration of this association is required to explore the related molecular mechanism of choriocarcinoma development, as the putative forerunner carries unique genetic features as mentioned previously. The monoallelic contribution shown in the mole would render a certain gene susceptible to functional inactivation by 'one-hit' kinetics. Alternatively, uniparental transmission of genes that are subject to parental imprinting in humans would impair their regulation. Thus, the features exhibited by complete mole would be associated with inactivation of particular tumor suppressor genes, contributing to the propensity to malignancy.

Malignant trophoblastic neoplasms with different modes of origin

Genomic DNAs obtained from 24 fresh or paraffin-embedded tumors were successfully amplified by polymerase chain reaction (PCR). Based on pregnancy history, these tumors included nine postmolar trophoblastic tumors, 12 tumors preceded by live birth or abortion and three non-gestational tumors. Polymerase chain reaction-polymorphism data revealed the absence of a maternal genome in eight postmolar trophoblastic tumors. This was contrasted with the presence of a maternal genome in 12 tumors preceded by live birth or abortion and three non-gestational tumors. Thus, these eight postmolar trophoblastic neoplasms developed from malignant transformation of complete moles. Six tumors were homozygous at three or more gene loci in which the partners were heterozygous (Figure 1b). A female sex chromosome constitution was anticipated because PCR failed to amplify any fragment specific to the sex-determining region, Y (SRY) gene sequence in these tumors. These genetic features may be compatible with those of the complete mole that results from fertilization of an empty egg by an X-bearing sperm. The heterozygosity was recognized in two tumors at a few gene loci (Figure 1a). The 240-bp PCR product specific to the SRY gene sequence was present in one tumor but not in the other. It seemed likely that the two tumors originated from an XX or XY dispermic, androgenetic mole.

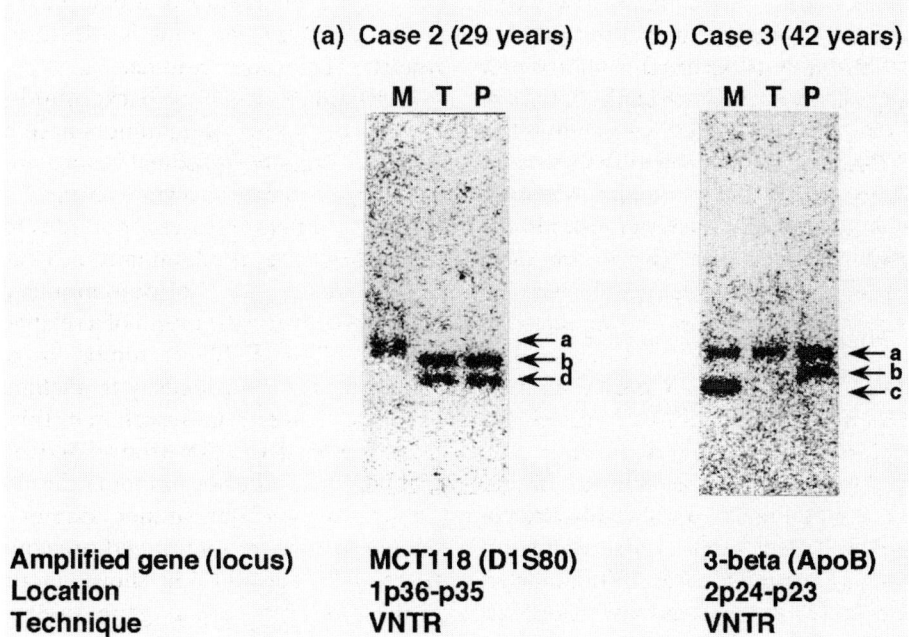

(a) Case 2 (29 years)   **(b) Case 3 (42 years)**

M T P   M T P

Amplified gene (locus)	MCT118 (D1S80)	3-beta (ApoB)
Location	1p36-p35	2p24-p23
Technique	VNTR	VNTR

Figure 1 Polymerase chain reaction (PCR) polymorphism of two choriocarcinomas: (a) Tumor showed two bands that were absent in maternal DNA, suggesting androgenetic origin. These bands with different mobilities that were also seen in partner's DNA indicated that tumor was heterozygous at this D1S80 gene locus. This tumor was also heterozygous at three other gene loci but homozygous at remaining loci. These observations suggested that tumor might originate from XX, heterozygous complete mole because of no amplification product with PCR using SRY gene-specific primer set; (b) PCR polymorphisms at ApoB gene locus shown by tumor indicated absence of paternal allele. This tumor was androgenetic in origin and homozygous at four gene loci in which partner was heterozygous. PCR targeted to SRY gene sequences failed to produce any amplified fragment. These features may be compatible with that of XX, heterozygous mole. P, PCR products from partner; T, PCR products from tumor; M, PCR products from patients; VNTR, variable number of tandem repeats

The remaining one choriocarcinoma contained an allele derived from the patient at a few gene loci. The finding is compatible with the assumption that the tumor did not arise from antecedent complete mole. A full-term delivery prior to a complete mole conception would explain this tumor development.

All 12 tumors in the second class had alleles of both paternal and maternal contribution. However, discordance of sex between the antecedent pregnancy product and the tumor was recognized in three choriocarcinomas. The absence of paternal contribution suggested a parthenogenetic origin of three non-gestational choriocarcinomas. The findings that PCR polymorphisms were either homozygous in certain loci or heterozygous in others may mean that the tumor was derived from a germ cell after meiosis I. As a result, at least three subtypes with different modes of origin were demonstrated in the 24 trophoblastic tumors. Although more than half the number of trophoblastic tumors collected here had a maternal contribution of genomes, the present data still give support to the suggestion that of all the forms of pregnancy that predispose patients to choriocarcinoma, the most likely is the complete mole.

Human chromosome 7 carries putative tumor suppressor gene involved in choriocarcinoma development

Many tumor suppressor genes are inactivated by intragenic mutations in one allele, accompanied by the loss of a chromosomal region containing the remaining allele, termed loss of heterozygosity. Mapping such deleted regions has been used to identify sequences involved in malignancies. However, the monoallelic contribution exhibited by the complete mole and its transformant would mask the chromosomal region where the allelic loss frequently occurs. To resolve the difficulty, we tried to identify a specific human chromosome on which putative tumor suppressor genes are located, by using microcell-mediated chromosome transfer. We introduced a single human chromosome

1,2,6,7,9 or 11 independently into CC1 choriocarcinoma cells by using a mouse A9–human chromosome library[17]. The mouse A9–human chromosome library consisted of cell clones with individual neomysin phosphotransferase gene (pSV2-neo) tagged human chromosomes. Thus, we carried out chromosomal *in situ* hybridization using a pSV2-neo as a probe to demonstrate the successful transfer of an intact donor chromosome into CC1 cells.

We evaluated tumorigenicity and *in vitro* transformed phenotypes in these microcell hybrids and compared the results with those for the parent CC1 cells (Table 1). The parent CC1 cells formed progressively growing tumors with 100% tumor-take incidence following subcutaneous inoculation of 1×10^7 cells into nude mice. All of the microcell hybrid clones containing a single chromosome 1,2,6,9 and 11 were

Table 1 Tumorigenicity of parental CC1 cells and microcell hybrids with introduced chromosome

Cell type	*Tumorigenicity (number of tumors/ number of inoculation sites)*	*Average time when long axis reached 10 mm* (days)
Parental cell		
CC1	10/10	26
Microcell hybrid clones (introduction of ch.1)		
1–1	6/7	16
1–2	6/6	13
Microcell hybrid clones (introduction of ch.2)		
2–1	6/6	16
2–2	8/8	31
Microcell hybrid clones (introduction of ch.6)		
6–1	6/6	19
Microcell hybrid clones (introduction of ch.7)		
7–1	0/9	> 80
7–2	2/11	70
7–3	3/10	47
7–4	7/12	49
Microcell hybrid clones (introduction of ch.9)		
9–1	5/6	64
9–2	5/5	24
Microcell hybrid clones (introduction of ch.11)		
11–1	2/2	32

tumorigenic; the tumor-take incidence ranged from 83 to 100% in these clones. The difference was not significant between the parent CC1 cells and the microcell hybrids. This was sharply contrasted with the suppression of tumorigenic potentials in the microcell hybrid clones that contained the transferred chromosome 7. Complete suppression of tumorigenicity was observed in one clone, from which no tumor was produced for up to 100 days following inoculation of 1×10^7 cells. Tumorigenic potentials were partially suppressed in the remaining three clones. Reduced tumor-take incidence (from 18 to 58%), as well as prolonged tumor growth, was demonstrated in these clones. We obtained tumorigenic revertant clones from tumors produced by the inoculation of these microcell hybrid clones. These revertants were highly tumorigenic, producing progressively growing tumors with 75–100% tumor-take incidence. Deletion of a transferred chromosome 7 was suggested in the tumorigenic revertant.

In vitro growth properties of the microcell hybrids that contained chromosome 1,2,6,9 or 11 were similar to those of the parent CC1 cells. However, significant prolongation of population doubling time and suppression of soft agar growth efficiency were demonstrated in the microcell hybrid clones that contained a transferred chromosome 7. These results indicated that a single human chromosome 7 derived from normal fibroblasts had a potential to suppress the tumorigenicity and the *in vitro* growth properties of human choriocarcinoma cells. This potential was clearly not shared by other kinds of human chromosome examined here. The observation is, thus, compatible with the idea that chromosome 7 carries putative tumor suppressor gene(s) that negatively regulate choriocarcinoma cell growth. Identification of the locus on chromosome 7 that is critical for choriocarcinoma is currently in progress.

Association of IGF2 and H19 imprinting with choriocarcinoma

Parental origin-specific functional differences between two alleles, known as genomic imprint-

ing, seem to be exploited for a regulatory mechanism crucial for the proper development of both embryonic and extraembryonic tissues[18–26]. The list of identified imprinted genes is lately growing rapidly in mouse and man. Among those genes, insulin-like growth factor (IGF)2 and H19 tightly linked on human chromosome 11 are of special interest because of their reciprocal imprinting and possible association with certain malignancy and congenital anomalies. The IGF2 gene is expressed from the paternally derived allele[27,28], whereas the H19 gene is expressed from the maternally derived allele[29–31]. The imprint-specific methylation in the 5′ region of H19 is considered to be important for this reciprocal regulation[32].

The complete mole characterized by grossly swollen villi in the absence of a fetus is proof of the vital importance of genomic imprinting in human embryogenesis. Since IGF2 acts as a dominant oncogene[33,34] and H19 as a tumor suppressor[35], imprinted regulation of these genes would affect the propensity to malignancy of complete moles. Thus, we studied IGF2 and H19 expression, and methylation status of H19 gene in complete mole and choriocarcinoma. All RNA samples were subjected to reverse transcriptase–polymerase chain reaction (RT–PCR) to study the expression of IGF2 and H19 in complete moles. The result of Apa I polymorphism of IGF2 genomic PCR products obtained from 10 complete moles and their parents revealed that all moles were androgenetic in origin. These moles expressed IGF2, in agreement with the imprinted expression of the paternally derived allele of this gene. Notwithstanding the paternal origin of H19 alleles, results of RT–PCR invariably showed that H19 was expressed in every case. Northern blot hybridization showed that the level of H19 expression in the mole was roughly comparable to that of normal placentae. It is evident that the paternal H19 allele, which was destined to become silent in normal zygotic development, remained active in the mole.

Differential methylation is reportedly established in the 5′ region of H19 in sperm, and a subset of CpG methylation is faithfully maintained after fertilization to suppress the paternal allele. Expression of the paternal H19 allele found in complete moles may be due to demethylation in this region. Hence, we examined CpG methylation at 10 sites encompassing the 5′ portion and the entire coding region. Southern blot hybridization showed that the amount of 1.8-kb H19 genomic DNA fragments in the 5′ portion and 1.7- or 1.3-kb fragments in the 3′ portion decreased almost by 50% after Hpa II digestion in androgenetic moles. Apparently one-half of the H19 gene was methylated and the remaining half was hypomethylated in these tissues *en masse* (Figure 2). The pattern was analogous to that in placenta that had most probably an allele-specific methylation profile with almost completely unmethy-

lated, active maternally derived allele and heavily methylated, inactive paternally derived allele. It is tempting to postulate, thus, that one H19 allele is maintained active in androgenetic moles irrespective of the primary imprint.

We examined the IGF2–H19 regulation in choriocarcinoma to address whether this unique pattern of expression in the mole would be responsible for choriocarcinoma development. In 10 of the choriocarcinoma samples examined, eight were derived from trophoblasts of normal placentae and two were sequelae to the complete mole. Northern blot hybridization revealed the considerably high expression of H19 and very low expression of IGF2 in these choriocarcinoma cell lines, irrespective of zygotic or androgenetic origin (Figure 3). The

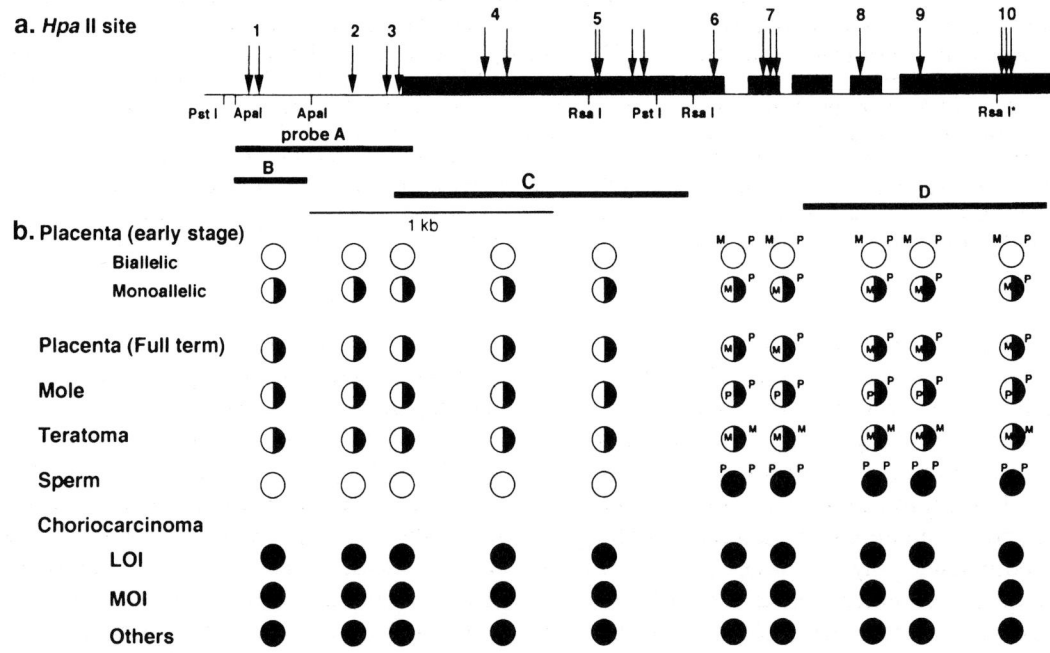

Figure 2 Methylation status at 10 Hpa II sites covering entire H19 gene regions. (a) Restriction map for Pst I, Apa I and Rsa I restriction enzymes, and exons are indicated by black-filled boxes. Rsa I* denotes polymorphic site at 3′ H19 terminal. Probes A–D are shown as horizontal lines; Hpa II sites are numbered 1–10. Each site was distinguishable by differences in fragment size on Southern blots. (b) Methylation status at 10 Hpa II sites of H19 gene in placenta early in development that expressed H19 biallelically or monoallelically, full-term placenta, androgenetic mole, parthenogenetic teratoma, sperm and choriocarcinoma. Filled and unfilled circles denote hypermethylation and hypomethylation of both alleles at each Hpa II site, respectively. Black/unfilled circles indicate allele-specific methylation in which one allele was hypermethylated and other was hypomethylated. Parental origin (P or M) of an allele was determined in 3′ portion of H19 using Rsa I site polymorphisms. LOI, loss of imprinting; MOI, maintenance of imprinting

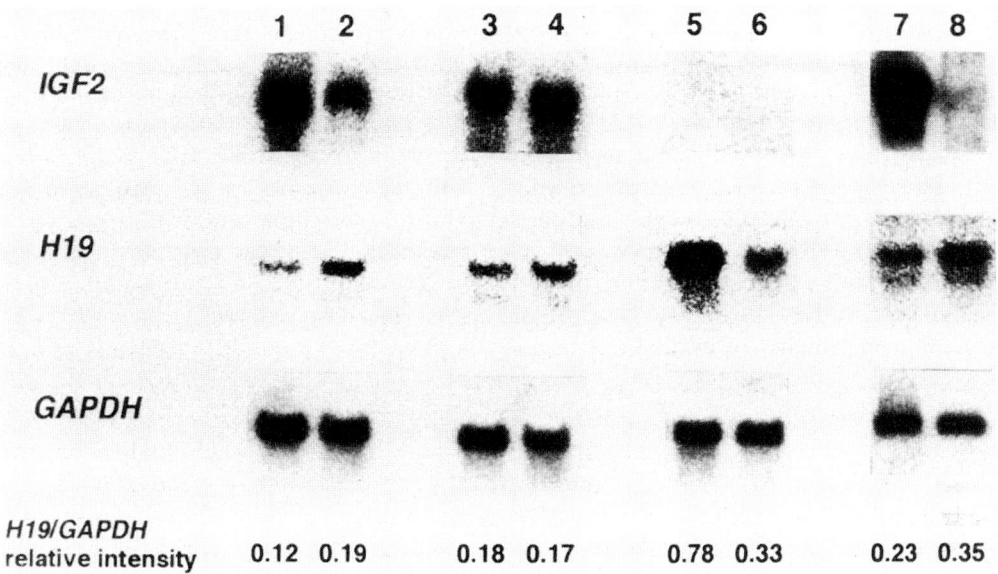

Figure 3 IGF2 and H19 expression levels on Northern blots in placenta, androgenetic mole and chorio-carcinoma. Significant differences in IGF2 and H19 expressions were not evident among placentae (1,2) and androgenetic moles (3,4). Abundance of H19 transcripts was accompanied by virtual abolition of IGF2 expression in choriocarcinoma with biallelic expression of IGF2 and/or H19 (5,6). Monoallelic expression of IGF2 and H19 resulted in abundance of IGF2 and H19 transcripts in CC3 cells (7). However, IGF2 expression was repressed in NUC1 cells that expressed IGF2 and H19 monoallelically (8). Relative intensity of H19 is shown at bottom of figure. RNAs obtained from placentae, androgenetic moles and choriocarci-nomas were resolved by electrophoresis, transferred to nylon membranes and hybridized with IGF2, H19 and glyceraldehyde-3-phosphate dehydrogenase (GAPDH) probes (control). Membranes were stripped after each hybridization and rehybridized. A BAS 1000 imaging analyzer (Fuji, Japan) was used for densitometric measurements

IGF2 and H19 transcripts were apparently intact in size. Thus, the activity state of two alleles was examined by means of Rsa I and Alu I polymor-phisms of H19, and Apa I and a CA repeat polymorphisms of IGF2. Although two cell lines were homozygous, the remaining eight chorio-carcinoma cell lines were heterozygous for one or both IGF2 polymorphisms. However, only five cells were heterozygous for H19 polymor-phisms. Analyses by RT–PCR revealed that two IGF2 alleles were expressed in six cell lines and only one allele was expressed in the remaining two. Expression of H19 was also biallelic in three lines and monoallelic in two. Thus, relaxation of IGF2 and H19 imprinting is a frequent, but not consistent phenomenon in choriocarci-nomas.

The methylation status of 10 CpG sites in the entire gene body of H19 was examined. There was no further digestion with Hpa II (Figure 2). Thus, we concluded that hypermethylation of CpG sites over the entire H19 gene is compatible with active expression, apparently at variance with the findings in normal placenta and mole. Methylation status is critical for H19 expression, methylation for repression and unmethylation for expression in placentae and moles. Ap-parently, the carcinoma cells are capable of overcoming the repressive effect of methylation. As to the mechanism responsible for the unique pattern of IGF2 and H19 expression in chorio-carcinomas, we now speculate that the mutated promoter overcomes transcriptional suppres-sion by CpG methylation in the H19.

The present findings in complete moles and choriocarcinomas suggest that H19 may, at least partly, be responsible for malignant as well as normal growth of trophoblasts. Jinno and colleagues[36] described intermediate trophoblasts and cytotrophoblasts to be the major cell types which express H19. In contrast to these proliferating trophoblasts, no H19 transcript was found in the non-dividing, terminally differentiated syncytiotrophoblasts. In growing trophoblasts, H19 is biallelically expressed early in development, but the paternally derived allele is inactivated later. These findings suggest that regulation of the H19 activity is critical for growth of trophoblasts. In addition to these findings, abundant H19 expression in choriocarcinomas lends support for the diversity of H19 function probably depending on the tissue type. Thus, it may not be surprising that escaping of the paternal allele from the imprinted silencing is required for trophoblastic cell growth in the mole, and this opposition to the imprinting facilitates enhanced H19 expression, resulting in the contribution to choriocarcinoma development.

References

1. Kajii, T. and Ohama, K. (1977). Androgenetic origin of hydatidiform mole. *Nature (London)*, **268**, 633–4
2. Wake, N., Takagi, N. and Sasaki, M. (1978). Androgenesis as a cause of hydatidiform mole. *J. Natl. Cancer Inst.*, **60**, 51–7
3. Wake, N., Shiina, Y. and Ichinoe, K. (1978). A further cytogenetic study of hydatidiform mole, with reference to its androgenetic origin. *Proc. Jpn Acad.*, **54**, 533–7
4. Lawler, S. D., Pickthall, V. I., Fisher, R. A., Frovey, S., Evans, M. W. and Szulman, A. E. (1979). Genetic studies of complete and partial hydatidiform moles. *Lancet*, **2**, 580
5. Yamashita, K., Wake, N., Araki, T., Ichinoe, K. and Kuroda, M. (1979). Human lymphocyte antigen expression in hydatidiform mole. Androgenesis following fertilization by a haploid sperm. *Am. J. Obstet. Gynecol.*, **135**, 597–600
6. Jacobs, P. A., Wilson, C. M., Sprenkle, J. A., Rosensheim, N. B. and Migeon, B. R. (1980). Mechanism of origin of complete hydatidiform moles. *Nature (London)*, **268**, 714–16
7. Ohama, K., Kajii, T., Ikamoto, E., Fukuda, Y., Imaizumi, K., Tsukahara, M., Kobayashi, K. and Hagiwara, K. (1981). Dispermic origin of XY hydatidiform moles. *Nature (London)*, **292**, 551–2
8. Wake, N., Seki, T., Fujita, H., Okubo, H., Sakai, K., Okuyama, K., Hayashi, H., Shiina, Y., Sato, H., Kuroda, M. and Ichinoe, K. (1984). Malignant potential of homozygous and heterozygous complete moles. *Cancer Res.*, **44**, 1226–30
9. Wake, N., Fujino, T., Hoshi, S., Shinkai, N., Sakai, K., Kato, H., Hashimoto, M., Yasuda, T., Yamada, H. and Ichinoe, K. (1987). The propensity to malignancy of dispermic heterozygous moles. *Placenta*, **8**, 319–26
10. Wake, N., Tanaka, K., Chapman, V., Matsui, S. and Sandberg, A. A. (1981). Chromosomes and cellular origin of choriocarcinoma. *Cancer Res.*, **41**, 3137–43
11. Fisher, R. A., Lawler, S. D., Povey, S. and Bagshawe, K. D. (1988). Genetically homozygous choriocarcinoma following pregnancy with hydatidiform mole. *Br. J. Cancer*, **58**, 788–92
12. Chaganti, R. S. K., Koduru, P. R. K., Chakraborty, R. and Jones, W. B. (1990). Genetic origin of a trophoblastic choriocarcinoma. *Cancer Res.*, **50**, 6330–3
13. Fisher, R. A., Paradinas, F. J., Newland, E. S. and Boxer, G. M. (1992). Genetic evidence that placental site trophoblastic tumors can originate from a hydatidiform mole or a normal conceptus. *Br. J. Cancer*, **65**, 355–8
14. Fisher, R. A., Nawlands, E. S., Jeffreys, A. J., Boxer, G. M., Begent, R. H. J., Rustin, G. J. S. and Bagshawe, K. D. (1992). Gestational and nongestational trophoblastic tumors distinguished by DNA analysis. *Cancer*, **69**, 839–45
15. Arima, T., Imamura, T., Amada, S., Tsuneyoshi, M. and Wake, N. (1994). Genetic origin of malignant trophoblastic neoplasms. *Cancer Genet. Cytogenet.*, **73**, 95–102
16. Sasaki, S., Katayama, P. K. and Roesler, M. (1982). Cytogenetic analysis of choriocarcinoma cell lines. *Acta Obstet. Gynaecol. Jpn*, **34**, 2253–6
17. Koi, M., Shimizu, M., Morita, H., Yamada, H. and Ohimura, M. (1989). Construction of mouse A9 clones containing a single human chromosome tagged with neomycin-resistance gene via microcell fusion. *Jpn J. Cancer Res.*, **80**, 413–18

18. DeChiara, T. M., Robertson, E. J. and Efstratiadis, A. (1991). Parental imprinting of the mouse insulin-like growth factor II gene. *Cell*, **64**, 849–59

19. Barlow, D. P., Stoger, R., Herrmann, B. G., Saito, K., and Schweifer, N. (1991). The mouse insulin-like growth factor type-2 receptor is imprinted and closely linked to the *Tme* locus. *Nature (London)*, **349**, 84–7

20. Bartolomei, M. S., Zemel, S. and Tilghman, S. M. (1991). Parental imprinting of the mouse H19 gene. *Nature (London)*, **351**, 153–5

21. Left, S. E., Brannan, C. L., Reed, M. L., Ozcelic, T., Francke, U., Copeland, N. G. and Jenkins, N. A. (1992). Maternal imprinting of the mouse *Snrpn* gene and consented linkage homology with the human Prader–Willi syndrome region. *Nature Genet.*, **2**, 265–9

22. Hatada, I., Sugama, T. and Mukai, T. (1993). A new imprinted gene cloned by a methylation-sensitive genome scanning method. *Nucl. Acids Res.*, **21**, 5577–82

23. Giddings, S. J., King, C. D., Harman, K. W., Flood, J. F. and Carnaghi, L. R. (1994). Allele specific inactivation of insulin 1 and 2 in the mouse yolk sac indicates imprinting. *Nature Genet.*, **6**, 310–13

24. Hayashizaki, Y., Shibata, H., Hirotune, S., Sugino, H., Okazaki, Y., Sasaki, N., Hirose, K., Imoto, H., Okuizumi, H., Muramatsu, M., Komatsubara, H., Shiroishi, T., Moriwaki, K., Katsuki, M., Hatano, N., Sasaki, H., Ueda, T., Mise, N., Takagi, N., Plass, C. and Chapman, V. M. (1994). Identification of an imprinted U2af binding protein related sequence on mouse chromosome 11 using the RLGS method. *Nature Genet.*, **6**, 33–40

25. Villar, A. J. and Pedersen, R. A. (1994). Parental imprinting of the *Mas* protooncogene in mouse. *Nature Genet.*, **8**, 373–9

26. Guillemot, F., Caspary, T., Tilgman, S. M., Copeland, N. G., Gilbert, D. J., Jenkins, N. A., Anderson, D. J., Joyner, A. L., Rossant, J. and Nagy, A. (1995). Genomic imprinting of *Mash-2*, a mouse gene required for trophoblast development. *Nature Genet.*, **9**, 235–42

27. Ohlsson, R., Nystrom, A., Pfeifer-Ohlsson, S., Tohonen, V., Hedborg, F., Schofield, P., Flam, F. and Ekstrom, T. J. (1993). IGF2 is parentally imprinted during human embryogenesis and in the Bechwith–Wiedemann syndrome. *Nature Genet.*, **4**, 94–7

28. Giannoukakis, N., Deal, C., Paquette, J., Goodyer, C. G. and Polyohronakos, C. (1993). Parental genomic imprinting of the human IGF2 gene. *Nature Genet.*, **4**, 98–101

29. Rachmilewitz, J., Goshen, R., Ariel, I., Scheneider, T., de Groot, N. and Hochberg, A. (1992). Parental imprinting of the human H19 gene. *FEBS Lett.*, **309**, 25–8

30. Zhang, Y., Shields, T., Grenshaw, T., Hao, Y., Moulton, T. and Tycko, B. (1993). Imprinting of human H19: allele-specific CpG methylation, loss of the active allele in Wilms' tumor, and potential for somatic allele switching. *Am. J. Hum. Genet.*, **58**, 118–24

31. Ferguson-Smith, A. C., Sasaki, H., Cattanach, B. M. and Surani, M. A. (1993). Parental-origin-specific epigenetic modification of the mouse H19 gene. *Nature (London)*, **362**, 751–5

32. Steenman, M. J. C., Rainier, S., Dobry, C. J., Grundy, P., Horon, I. L. and Feinberg, A. P. (1994). Loss of imprinting of IGF2 is linked to reduced expression and abnormal methylation of H19 in Wilms' tumor. *Nature Genet.*, **7**, 433–9

33. Rainier, S., Johnson, L. A., Dobry, C. J., Ping, A. J., Grundy, P. E. and Feinberg, A. P. (1993). Relaxation of imprinted genes in human cancer. *Nature (London)*, **362**, 747–9

34. Ogawa, O., Eccles, M. R., Szeto, J., Monoe, L. A., Yun, K., Maw, M. A., Smith, P. J. and Reeve, A. E. (1993). Relaxation of insulin-like growth factor II gene imprinting implicated in Wilms' tumour. *Nature (London)*, **362**, 749–51

35. Hao, Y., Crenshaw, T., Moulton, T., Newcomb, E. and Tycho, B. (1993). Tumor suppressor activity of H19 RNA. *Nature (London)*, **865**, 764–7

36. Jinno, Y., Ikeda, Y., Yun, K., Maw, M., Masuzaki, H., Fukuda, H., Inuzuka, K., Fujishira, A., Ohatani, Y., Okimoto, T., Ishimaru, T. and Niikawa, N. (1995). Establishment of functional imprinting of H19 gene in human developing placentae. *Nature Genet.*, **10**, 318–24

Reproductive impact of sexually transmitted infections

6

J. N. Wasserheit and H. T. MacKay

Introduction

Although human immunodeficiency virus (HIV) infection is the most recent and, in terms of deaths, the most devastating sexually transmitted disease (STD) epidemic of our era, it is not the only one. Other STDs lie at the crossroads of impaired fertility, adverse outcomes of pregnancy, reproductive tract cancer and sexual transmission of HIV itself (Figure 1). Therefore, effective prevention and management of STDs are strategic common elements in women's and infants' health, and in HIV prevention.

The frequency and reproductive impact of these infections defines a particularly critical role for obstetricians and gynecologists in STD detection, treatment and patient counseling. This role is made even more important because the majority of STDs are asymptomatic, and often escape detection unless providers of reproductive health-care, such as family planning,

antenatal, delivery and postpartum services, routinely address these issues. We will, therefore, begin by highlighting the high burden of sexually transmitted infections in developing and industrialized countries. We will summarize the reproductive consequences of these infections across the reproductive cycle, and discuss recent findings that affect clinical management. We will close by suggesting the types of STD clinical preventive services that should be offered to women as a minimum standard of care at each point in the reproductive health care continuum.

Incidence and prevalence of sexually transmitted infections

Estimates of the incidence and prevalence of sexually transmitted infections are just that – *estimates*. They vary depending upon the sources of data that are available and the methods used to detect cases. In much of the developing world, neither clinician- nor laboratory-based STD surveillance systems exist. Instead, estimates are usually extrapolated from special studies of selected, non-representative populations. These studies may also suffer from a range of problems in design, specimen collection and transport, laboratory methods and data analysis. In most industrialized countries, systems are in place for the routine reporting and analysis of data on several – usually bacterial – STDs. Data from nationally representative surveys, hospitals or specialized clinics and clinician visits may also be available. However, factors such as incompleteness or bias in reporting and lack of

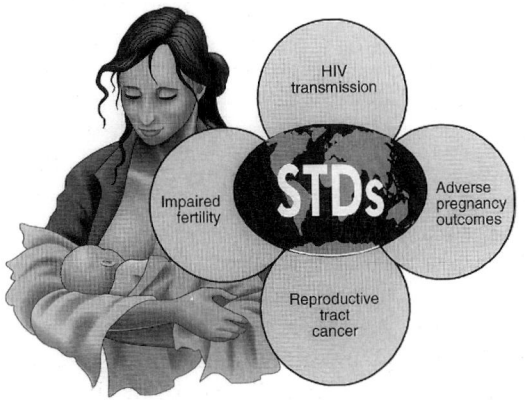

Figure 1 Reproductive impact of sexually transmitted diseases (STDs)

Table 1 Median sexually transmitted disease (STD) prevalences in Sub-Saharan Africa (per 100 women): low-risk population includes women visiting antenatal or family planning clinics or women sampled in community-based studies; high-risk population includes women attending STD clinics or women with symptoms suggestive of STDs; very-high-risk population includes women engaged in prostitution. Reproduced from reference 2 with permission

	Disease				
Population	Gonorrhea	Chlamydia	Trichomoniasis	Syphilis	HIV infection
Low risk	5	8	23	10	3
High risk	15	11	20	19	17
Very high risk	26	18	23	25	21

laboratory confirmation of diagnoses often compromise these data.

Despite these limitations, a very consistent picture emerges from the data that are available. Sexually transmitted infections are common in most countries around the world[1-4]. In Sub-Saharan Africa, for example, while median STD prevalences are predictably high among high-risk populations such as STD clinic patients or commercial sex workers (CSWs), they are also substantial among what has traditionally been considered 'low'-risk populations, such as women attending antenatal or family planning clinics (Table 1). To put these prevalences into perspective, where the prevalence of syphilis among pregnant women reaches 10% or more, it has been estimated that 5–8% of pregnancies extending beyond the first trimester will result in a syphilitic infant or in syphilis-related fetal or infant deaths[5]. In fact, STDs are among the top five reasons for clinic visits in many Sub-Saharan African countries[6]. In addition, median prevalences usually mask markedly higher levels of infection in some subpopulations. Studies in urban areas of countries such as Botswana, Burundi, Malawi, Rwanda, Swaziland, Zambia and Zimbabwe have documented that between one in five and one in three pregnant women is HIV infected[7].

Sub-Saharan Africa is not unique with respect to the frequency of sexually transmitted infections. Although data are more limited and, therefore, perhaps less reliable from other parts of the developing world than from Africa, the available data suggest that these infections, particularly chlamydia, trichomoniasis and

bacterial vaginosis, are also common among family-planning and antenatal-clinic clients in many parts of Asia and Latin America[1,3,4]. Using extrapolations from selected local prevalence studies, and sex- and region-specific estimates of the duration of gonorrhea, chlamydia, syphilis and trichomoniasis, the World Health Organization (WHO) estimated that in 1995 there were more than 330 million new cases of curable STDs among adults world-wide (Figure 2)[4]. While Sub-Saharan Africa had the highest estimated incidence rate, with 254 new cases per 1000 population (followed by 160 per 1000 in South and South-East Asia, and 145 per 1000 in Latin America and the Caribbean), South and South-East Asia led the world in terms of absolute numbers of new cases, with an estimated 150 million, compared with 65 million and 36 million in Sub-Saharan Africa and Latin America/the Caribbean, respectively.

Although in some parts of the industrialized world substantial progress has been made in reducing rates of some STDs, in other areas, these STDs persist and, in the majority of industrialized countries, other infections such as chlamydia, genital herpes, human papillomavirus (HPV) infection and bacterial vaginosis (BV) remain widespread. During the past 15 or 20 years, syphilis and gonorrhea rates have fallen dramatically in the industrialized countries in which sustained national prevention efforts have been implemented (Figure 3). In several of these countries, syphilis has been virtually eliminated and gonorrhea has become a rare disease. While reported rates have also declined in the United States, they remain as much as

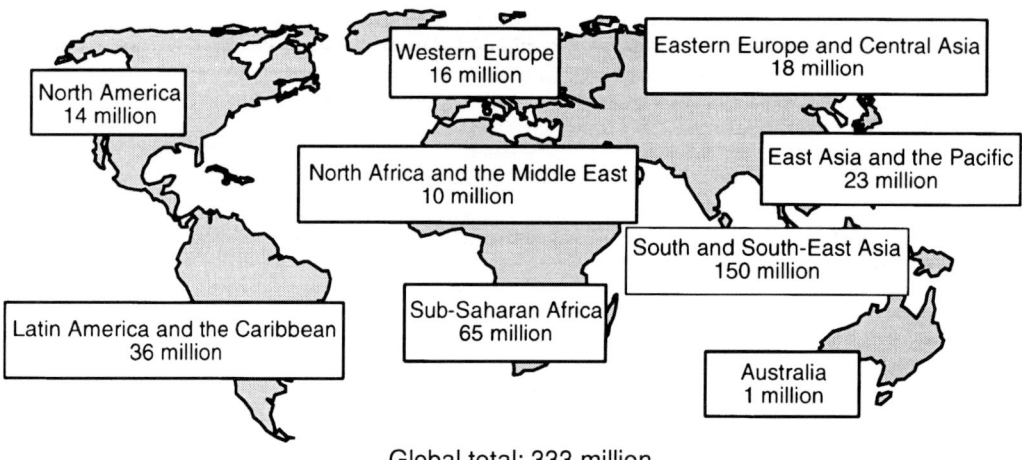

Global total: 333 million

Figure 2 Estimated new cases of curable sexually transmitted diseases (gonorrhea, chlamydial infection, syphilis and trichomoniasis) among adults, 1995. From reference 4

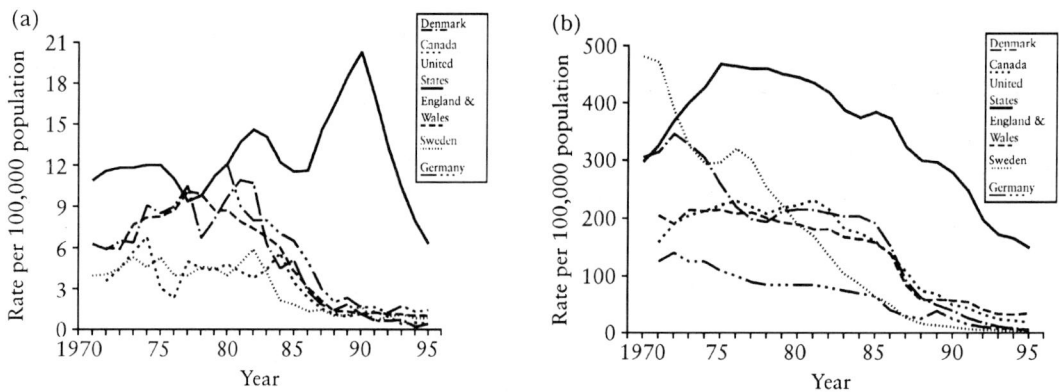

Figure 3 Syphilis (a) and gonorrhea (b) trends in industrialized countries

16 times higher for syphilis and 50 times higher for gonorrhea than in other industrialized countries[8]. Indeed, in the USA in 1995, STDs, including AIDS, accounted for 87% of cases of the 10 notifiable infectious diseases most frequently reported to the Center for Disease Control and Prevention (CDC), and chlamydia led the list[9]. Among 15–24-year-old women who were tested for chlamydia during family planning visits in 28 states across the USA, a median of 4.6% were positive[10]. Community or school-based surveys of adolescents have consistently demonstrated strikingly high chlamydia positivity rates of 5–12%[11].

While in industrialized countries routine surveillance is rarely conducted for viral STDs other than HIV infection or AIDS, it is these infections that probably represent the greatest morbidity burden in the USA and the rest of the industrialized world. For example, seroprevalence data indicate that about 22% of Americans over the age of 11 (or 45 million people) are infected with herpes simplex virus type 2 (HSV-2)[12]. We estimate that 24 million Americans are infected with HPV and up to a million additional infections may occur each year[8]. As of December 1996, almost 217 000 Americans were reported to be living with AIDS, roughly 37% of the

48

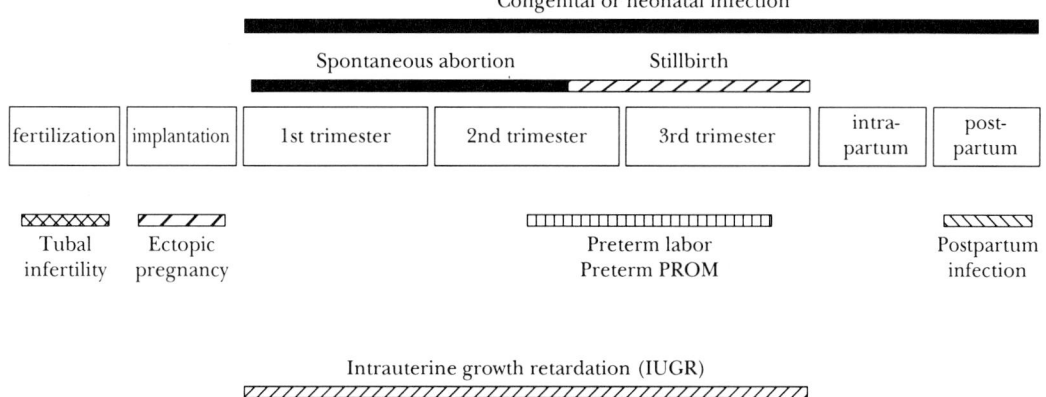

Figure 4 Overview of reproductive impact of sexually transmitted infections. PROM, premature rupture of membranes

581 000 AIDS cases reported since the beginning of the epidemic[13].

Reproductive impact of sexually transmitted infections

Sexually transmitted infections have the potential to compromise each phase of the reproductive cycle, from fertilization and implantation, through pregnancy to birth and the postpartum period (Figure 4).

Impact on fertilization and uterine implantation

The best documented and most widely recognized reproductive consequences of sexually transmitted infections are tubal infertility and ectopic pregnancy. The complete, bilateral tubal occlusion which prevents fertilization, and the partial tubal obstruction which prevents intrauterine implantation both occur primarily as a result of tubal dysfunction and scarring following pelvic inflammatory disease (PID) or, more specifically, salpingitis. Gonococcal or chlamydial cervical infections that ascend into the upper genital tract are the most common causes of PID and its sequelae among reproductive-aged women[14,15]. However, polymicrobial infection occurs frequently and often involves a combination of the anaerobes and facultative aerobes associated with bacterial vaginosis (Figure 5a).

Both infertility and ectopic pregnancy appear to be relatively frequent complications of PID. Data from a landmark Swedish cohort study of more than 1800 symptomatic women with laparoscopically verified PID indicate that, overall, 16% were unable to conceive following their infections[16]. Risk of tubal factor infertility increased with repeated episodes of PID and with delayed health-care. After a single episode, approximately 8% became infertile, and each additional episode roughly doubled that proportion (20% following two and 40% following three or more episodes). In addition, compared with women who sought more timely care, women who waited 3 days or more after the onset of symptoms to obtain care had twice the risk of infertility[17]. The Swedish study also suggests that almost one in 10 women with laparoscopically verified PID will experience an ectopic pregnancy as their first post-PID pregnancy[16]. However, the relative importance of infection in impaired fertility varies in different regions of the world. A number of studies, including a WHO multicenter investigation, have shown that, in Africa, as many as 80% of infertile couples had an infectious etiology, compared with up to 35–40% in Latin America and Asia, and 10–35% in industrialized countries[1,3]. In the USA, for example, at least 15% of infertile

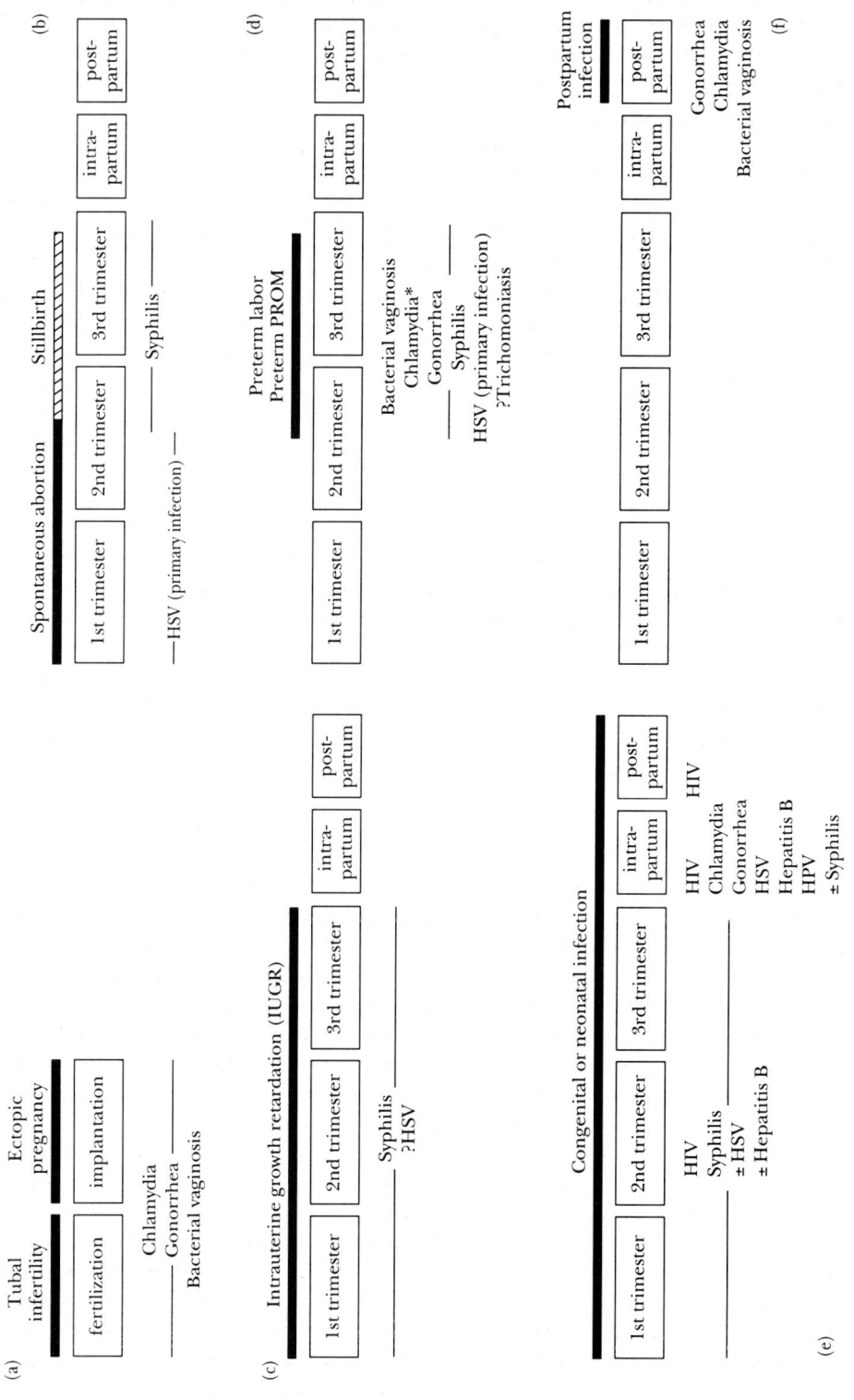

Figure 5 Reproductive impact of sexually transmitted infections; impaired fertility (a) and adverse outcomes of pregnancy (b–f). *IgM positive; HSV, herpes simplex virus; PROM, premature rupture of membranes; HIV, human immunodeficiency virus; HPV, human papilloma virus

women suffer from tubal damage secondary to PID[8]. It is equally sobering that ectopic pregnancy is the leading cause of first-trimester maternal deaths among American women.

A number of recent findings have advanced our understanding of the manifestations and effective management of PID and its consequences. First, the reproductive impact of 'silent' or 'atypical' PID is becoming better appreciated. Less than one-half of women with tubal occlusion report a history of PID, despite serological evidence of prior chlamydial or gonococcal infection[14]. Furthermore, among Seattle women diagnosed with chlamydial cervicitis, 40% had endometrial biopsies consistent with endometritis[18]. Second, while antibiotic treatment appears to prevent infertility and ectopic pregnancy if initiated within 2 days of the onset of lower abdominal pain, as many as 85% of women with PID may delay seeking care, particularly women with chlamydial infection because of the minimal or atypical nature of their symptoms[15,17]. Even among those who do obtain care, non-compliance with 10–14-day, multidose regimens may exceed 65%[15]. In aggregate, these data point to early detection of cervical infection as the key to prevention of PID and the resulting impaired fertility.

A third set of new findings address these issues by demonstrating the effectiveness of chlamydia detection and treatment, not only in reducing chlamydial cervicitis, but also in decreasing the incidence of PID. During the 7 years from 1988 to 1995, among women living in the Pacific Northwest region of the United States and attending family planning clinics that offered routine chlamydia screening and treatment, test positivity fell by 65% (from 9.3 to 3.3%)[19]. Implementation of similar programs in the Mid-Atlantic and Mountain states in 1994 resulted in equally dramatic declines (31 and 16%, respectively, among teens within just 2.5 years)[19]. In addition, a randomized controlled trial of chlamydia screening and treatment among 18–34-year-old women enrolled in a US health maintenance organization (HMO) showed almost a 60% reduction in PID incidence during the 12-month follow-up period[20].

The impressive declines in PID documented at a national level over the past decade in Sweden are consistent with these data[21].

Impact on fetal development

In contrast to the relatively extensive data supporting our understanding of the links between sexually transmitted infections and tubal infertility or ectopic pregnancy, data elucidating the impact of these infections on fetal development are quite limited both in quantity and quality. Both intrauterine infection during pregnancy and adverse outcomes, such as spontaneous abortion, stillbirth and intrauterine growth retardation (IUGR), are difficult to study, and establishing causal relationships in this area is an ongoing research challenge. However, while many controversies persist, several points should be recognized.

Intrauterine infection with sexually transmitted organisms occurs primarily by one of two routes: hematogenous spread or ascent from the lower genital tract. During pregnancy, organisms that are present in the maternal blood, such as herpes simplex virus (HSV) and *Treponema pallidum* (the etiological agent of syphilis), may infect the placenta, causing, at least in the latter case, focal proliferative villitis and vasculitis with plasma cell infiltration and Langerhans giant cell formation[22,23]. Fetal infection may follow placental infection either via fetal blood vessels or by direct extension to fetal membranes and amniotic fluid. While associations between STDs that ascend from the cervix (e.g. chlamydia or gonorrhea) and fetal wastage or fetal growth retardation continue to be debated, available data suggest that it is primarily hematogenously disseminated infections such as HSV infection and syphilis that are responsible for STD-related spontaneous abortion, stillbirth and IUGR (Figure 5b and c).

In the USA, second-trimester spontaneous abortions (pregnancy loss between 13 and 20 weeks of gestation) and stillbirths (fetal death after 20 weeks) each occur in about 1% of clinically recognized pregnancies[24,25]. They are probably more common in parts of the developing world where there is a higher incidence of bacterial STDs. It is these outcomes, more than first-trimester spontaneous abortions, in which STDs play a clinically important role. Although *T. pallidum* has been documented in tissue of spontaneously aborted fetuses as early as 9 weeks of gestation[26], evidence that syphilis plays a causal role in fetal wastage is strongest in relation to stillbirth. On the other hand, as many as 54% of pregnant women with symptomatic primary genital HSV infection before 20 weeks of gestation may experience a spontaneous abortion[27]. As is the case with IUGR and later manifestations of genital herpes in pregnancy, recurrent infection does not appear to increase risk of spontaneous abortion[28]. Data on the role of the other major STD that disseminates hematogenously, HIV infection, in fetal wastage and growth retardation remain inconclusive[22].

Impact on birth and neonatal health

The effect of sexually transmitted infections on low birth weight (less than 2500 g) due to preterm birth (birth occurring prior to 37 weeks' gestation) is beginning to be more widely appreciated. Roughly two-thirds of preterm births are related either to preterm labor or to preterm, premature rupture of membranes (PROM), and infection appears to play a critical role in these spontaneous, preterm births[22]. In the USA, 6–10% of births are preterm and approximately 1% occur at less than 30 weeks of gestational age (producing an infant weighing 1000 g or less), while in the developing world, up to 30% of births may be of low birth weight[5,22,24]. The premature infants that result from these births account for as much as 70–80% of neonatal deaths, excluding those in newborns with congenital malformations. Despite sophisticated and costly neonatal intensive care, in the United States, about 60% of neonatal deaths and substantial permanent disability are concentrated among the 1% of 'very-low-birthweight' babies. Because of these strong links

between prematurity and neonatal mortality, the growing evidence that, in some populations, sexually transmitted infections may represent a preventable cause of a substantial proportion of prematurity has sparked great interest.

Chorioamnionitis and amniotic fluid infection appear to be the principal correlates of spontaneous preterm birth. They are usually the result of ascending rather than hematogenous spread of pathogens, although a broad range of sexually transmitted pathogens has been associated with preterm labor and preterm PROM (Figure 5d). Histological evidence of chorioamnionitis increases from about 10% in placentas at term to more than 90% in placentas delivered before 24 weeks of gestation, and BV-associated organisms are most frequently isolated[22]. The distribution of frequency of amniotic fluid culture positivity by gestational age parallels that for histological chorioamnionitis, although at a lower level. Both bacterial or protozoal products (e.g. phospholipases and proteases) and infection-induced cytokines and prostaglandins may play a role in linking chorioamnionitis and amniotic-fluid infection with preterm birth[22].

While most sexually transmitted infections have been associated with spontaneous preterm birth, many studies in this area have been difficult to interpret because they did not adequately consider potentially confounding risk factors. However, recent data strongly support a causal role for BV in preterm delivery, and more equivocal evidence suggests that incident chlamydial infection, gonorrhea, syphilis and primary HSV infection may also contribute to preventable prematurity. The role of trichomoniasis remains controversial. Three recent antibiotic treatment trials, two of them randomized, support earlier epidemiological studies, and have demonstrated significant reductions in preterm birth among pregnant women at high risk for premature delivery who were treated systemically for BV[22,29–31]. Given the high frequency of BV, particularly among African–American women, it has been estimated that as much as 40% of early spontaneous preterm birth might be prevented with treatment of this infection[24]. Although the results of studies of the relationship between chlamydial infection and prematurity have been conflicting, a consistent association has emerged between the subset of pregnant women with serological evidence of acute, primary infection by IgM positivity[22,32–34]. Finally, the role of trichomoniasis in preterm birth is an area of ongoing investigation. The multicenter Vaginal Infections and Prematurity Study of 13 816 pregnant women in the USA demonstrated a 1.3-fold increased risk of preterm birth among women infected with *Trichomonas vaginalis*[35]. However, it is still unclear whether associated vaginal anaerobes or trichomonads, themselves, are responsible for this effect.

Congenital or neonatal infections are the most widely appreciated impacts of sexually transmitted infections on birth and neonatal health. Infection may occur throughout pregnancy, in the course of delivery and, in the case of HIV infection, during the postpartum period via breast feeding. Almost every STD can result in congenital or neonatal infection, and the timing of infection depends on the STD involved (Figure 5e). Detailed discussion of the manifestations of these infections is beyond the scope of this short review, but can be found in reference 22. However, the effects of sexually transmitted infections are substantial both in terms of severity and frequency (Table 2).

The most important recent advances in this area relate to HIV infection. The Pediatric AIDS Clinical Trials Group 076 trial of zidovudine prophylaxis for HIV-infected pregnant women demonstrated a two-thirds reduction in vertical transmission of HIV[36]. Equally important but less widely appreciated are the findings of a landmark community-level randomized trial conducted in Tanzania that demonstrated that even basic STD detection and treatment can achieve a 40% reduction in new HIV infections[37]. The results of this trial emphasize the critical importance of STD diagnosis and treatment in the primary prevention of HIV infection in women.

Impact on postpartum health

Postpartum endometritis is a common cause of maternal morbidity, and sepsis associated with endometritis is an important cause of maternal mortality in both industrialized and developing countries. In industrialized countries, the majority of cases of postpartum endometritis are associated with Cesarean section, and infection after vaginal delivery is uncommon (1–3%)[38,39]. In developing countries, Cesarean delivery is less frequent, but postpartum endometritis following vaginal delivery is 10 times as frequent as in industrialized countries[40].

The causal association of sexually transmitted organisms as primary pathogens in postpartum infections is still to be completely defined. However, the same cervicovaginal infections that result in pelvic inflammatory disease in nonpregnant women, *C. trachomatis*, *N. gonorrhoeae* and bacterial vaginosis, appear to be primarily responsible for postpartum infections (Figure 5f). A study from Kenya demonstrated either *Neisseria gonorrhoeae*, *Chlamydia trachomatis* or both in 14% of women with clinical postpartum endometritis[41]. Another study from Kenya showed a 4.4-fold increased risk of postpartum upper genital-tract infection in women with *N. gonorrhoeae* and a 1.7-fold increase in those with *C. trachomatis*[40]. Chlamydia has been specifically associated with late postpartum endometritis, occurring from 7 to 42 days after delivery[42]. Anaerobic organisms associated with bacterial vaginosis are frequently isolated in postpartum endometritis, and bacterial vaginosis has been demonstrated to be a risk factor for post-Cesarean endometritis[43]. In industrialized countries, these organisms rather than *C. trachomatis* or *N. gonorrhoeae* are usually isolated in post-Cesarean endometritis and do not appear to be related to subsequent tubal infertility. In contrast, the very high rates of tubal infertility in some developing nations may be related to postpartum infections with *C. trachomatis* or *N. gonorrhoeae* occurring after vaginal delivery. Detection and treatment of gonorrhea and chlamydia during pregnancy may prevent secondary

Table 2 Effects of sexually transmitted infections on birth and neonatal health: implications for clinical preventive services. Adapted from reference 3, with permission

Organism or syndrome	Maternal infection rate (%)	Infant effects	Transmission risk from infected mother	Detection in pregnancy	Management of maternal infection	Management of neonatal infection
Neisseria gonorrhoeae	1–30	conjunctivitis, sepsis, meningitis	~30%	screening: culture, or antigen detection test; first visit and 3rd trimester	cefixime, ceftriaxone, spectinomycin partner management	ocular prophylaxis; treatment with ceftriaxone
Chlamydia trachomatis	2–25	conjunctivitis, pneumonia, bronchiolitis, otitis media	25–50% conjunctivitis, 5–15% pneumonia	screening: culture, or antigen detection test; 3rd trimester	amoxicillin, erythromycin, part-ner management	ocular prophylaxis; treatment with erythromycin
Treponema pallidum	0.01–15	congenital syphilis, neonatal death	50%	serological screening, first visit (universal), 3rd trimester (high risk)	penicillin, partner management	penicillin
Herpes simplex virus	1–30	disseminated central nervous system, localized lesions	3% recurrent at delivery, 30% primary at delivery	diagnosis: culture of lesions	acyclovir for first episode Cesarean section if lesions present at time of delivery	acyclovir
Human immuno-deficiency virus	0.01–20	pediatric AIDS	22–39%	screening: HIV ELISA, first visit	zidovudine prophy-laxis, counseling, partner management	zidovudine
Bacterial vaginosis	16–29	prematurity	NA	screening: wet mount, gram stain early 2nd trimester	metronidazole	NA
Trichomonas vaginalis	3–48	prematurity	rare	evidence is inadequate for recommendations	metronidazole, partner management	NA

NA, not applicable

infertility, as well as morbidity associated with postpartum and neonatal infection.

Clinical preventive services for sexually transmitted infections in reproductive health care continuum

Prevention of the adverse outcomes of sexually transmitted infections can and should occur wherever reproductive health services are provided. Discussion of the STD clinical preventive services that should be offered in each of the settings in the reproductive health-care continuum may provide a useful framework. For example, in family planning and other primary care settings, screening for *Chlamydia trachomatis* and *Neisseria gonorrhoeae* and treatment of clients and their partners can significantly reduce pelvic inflammatory disease and its long-term consequences[20]. Prevention counseling, including 'safe sex' strategies and dual contraceptive use with male or female condoms, will provide clients with methods to reduce the risk of acquisition of most sexually transmitted infections. Women positive for HIV should be counseled about the risk of vertical transmission and the potential benefit of zidovudine therapy during pregnancy.

Antenatal care provides an opportunity to prevent many of the infection-related adverse pregnancy outcomes discussed above. Early in prenatal care, all women should be screened for syphilis and hepatitis B, and all women should be offered screening for HIV. Women found to be HIV-positive should be offered zidovudine prophylaxis, if available. All women should be questioned about a prior history of herpes simplex and should be advised to report any suspicious symptoms that arise during pregnancy. An area of ongoing applied research is the identification of serodiscordant couples in an effort to provide targeted interventions for women at risk of primary infection in pregnancy. Women at risk on the basis of age, risk behaviors or local disease prevalence should be screened for *C. trachomatis* in the third trimester and for *N. gonorrhoeae* at the first prenatal visit. Repeat screening for *N. gonorrhoeae* and syphilis should

be performed in the early third trimester for women at continuing risk of acquiring these infections. Partners of infected women should be identified and treated, and both the woman and her partner should be counseled to reduce the risk of subsequent sexually transmitted infections.

Screening and treatment for bacterial vaginosis in women with previous spontaneous preterm delivery may reduce the risk of a preterm delivery in the current pregnancy[31]. At the present time, there is inadequate evidence to recommend routine screening for *T. vaginalis* in pregnancy. There is an ongoing randomized clinical trial looking at the value of routine screening and treatment in pregnancy of both trichomoniasis and bacterial vaginosis.

Additional opportunities for prevention exist at the time of delivery. Women without prenatal care should be screened for all of the STDs described under prenatal care. The results of a syphilis serology should be available prior to the patient returning home. Women with a history of genital herpes infection should be questioned about symptoms and examined for lesions. Women with active lesions of primary or recurrent genital herpes at the time of labor should undergo Cesarean section. Women without lesions but with a history of genital herpes or with an infected partner should be cultured at the time of vaginal delivery. A positive culture would indicate an exposed infant who requires close observation[22].

During the postpartum period, all infants should receive ocular prophylaxis for gonorrhea and chlamydia. Women who are HIV-positive should be counseled on the risk of HIV transmission through breast-feeding. Women with documented STDs and women at risk of acquiring STDs should be counseled on the use of dual contraceptive methods including the male or female condom.

In summary, the frequency and severity of sexually transmitted infections in terms of their impact on reproductive health demands increased attention on the part of providers of quality reproductive health services. The availability of the numerous effective interventions described above creates both an opportunity and a responsibility for each provider to carefully assess individual patient risk and provide appropriate screening and treatment at each stage of the reproductive health continuum.

References

1. Germain, A., Holmes, K. K., Piot, P. and Wasserheit, J. N. (eds.) (1992). *Reproductive Tract Infections.* (New York: Plenum Press)
2. Howson, C. P., Harrison, P. F., Hotra, D. and Law, M. (eds.) (1996). *In Her Lifetime: Female Morbidity and Mortality in Sub-Saharan Africa,* pp. 242–72. (Washington, DC: National Academy Press)
3. Tsui, A. O., Wasserheit, J. N. and Haaga, J. G. (eds.) (1997). *Reproductive Health in Developing Countries: Expanding Dimensions, Building Solutions,* pp. 41–86. (Washington, DC: National Academy Press)
4. Global Programme on AIDS (1995). *An Overview of Selected Curable Sexually Transmitted Diseases.* STD/GPA/WHO/Estimates/95.1. (Geneva: World Health Organization)
5. Schulz, K. F., Schulte, J. M. and Berman, S. M. (1992). Maternal health and child survival: opportunities to protect both women and children from the adverse consequences of reproductive tract infections. In Germain, A., Holmes, K. K., Piot, P. and Wasserheit, J. N. (eds.) *Reproductive Tract Infections,* pp. 145–82. (New York: Plenum Press)
6. Meheus, A. (1992). Women's health: importance of reproductive tract infections, pelvic inflammatory disease and cervical cancer. In Germain, A., Holmes, K. K., Piot, P. and Wasserheit, J. N. (eds.) *Reproductive Tract Infections,* pp. 61–91. (New York: Plenum Press)
7. US Bureau of the Census (1997). *Recent HIV Seroprevalence Levels by Country: January 1997.* Research Note No. 23. (Washington, DC: Health Studies Branch, Center for International Research)
8. Eng, T. R. and Butler, W. T. (eds.) (1997). *The Hidden Epidemic: Confronting Sexually Transmitted Diseases.* (Washington, DC: National Academy Press)
9. Center for Disease Control and Prevention (1996). Ten leading nationally notifiable infectious diseases – United States, 1995. *MMWR,* **45**, 883–4
10. Center for Disease Control and Prevention (1996). *Sexually Transmitted Disease Surveillance 1995.* (Atlanta: Department of Health and Human Services)
11. Wasserheit, J. N. (1996). Setting the stage for STD prevention in the next millennium. Presented at *1996 National STD Prevention Conference,* Tampa FA, December
12. Fleming, D. T. (1997). Herpes simplex virus type 2 sero-epidemiology in the United States, 1978 to 1991. Presented at *EIS Conference,* Atlanta, GA, April
13. Center for Disease Control and Prevention (1996). *HIV/AIDS Surveillance Report,* **8**, 1–39
14. Cates, W. and Wasserheit, J. N. (1991). Genital chlamydial infections: epidemiology and reproductive sequelae. *Am. J. Obstet. Gynecol.,* **164**, 1771–81
15. Hillis, S. D. and Wasserheit, J. N. (1996). Screening for chlamydia – a key to the prevention of pelvic inflammatory disease. *N. Engl. J. Med.,* **334** 1399–1400
16. Westrom, L., Joesoef, R., Reynolds, G., Hadgu, A. and Thompson, S. E. (1992). Pelvic inflammatory disease and fertility: a cohort study of 1,844 women with laparoscopically verified disease and 657 control women with normal laparoscopic results. *Sex. Transm. Dis.,* **19**, 185–92
17. Hillis, S. D., Joesoef, R., Marchbanks, P. A., Wasserheit, J. N., Cates, W. and Westrom, L. (1993). Delayed care of pelvic inflammatory disease as a risk factor for impaired fertility. *Am. J. Obstet. Gynecol.,* **168**, 1503–9
18. Paavonen, J., Kiviat, N. B., Brunham, R. C., *et al.* (1985). Prevalence and manifestations of endometritis among women with cervicitis. *Am. J. Obstet. Gynecol.,* **152**, 280–4
19. Center for Disease Control and Prevention (1997). *Chlamydia trachomatis* genital infections – United States, 1995. *MMWR,* **46**, 193–8
20. Scholes, D., Stergachis, A., Heidrich, F. E., Andrilla, H., Holmes, K. K. and Stamm, W. E. (1996). Prevention of pelvic inflammatory disease by screening for cervical chlamydial infection. *N. Engl. J. Med.,* **334**, 1362–6
21. Kamwendo, F., Forslin, L., Bodin, L. and Danielsson, D. (1996). Decreasing incidences of gonorrhea- and chlamydia-associated acute pelvic inflammatory disease: a 25 year study from an

urban area of Central Sweden. *Sex. Transm. Dis.,* **23**, 384–91

22. Watts, D. H. and Brunham, R. C. (1997). Sexually transmitted diseases including HIV infection in pregnancy. In Holmes, K. K., Sparling, P. F., Mardh, P. A., Lemon, S. M., Stamm, W. E., Piot, P. and Wasserheit, J. N. (eds.) *Sexually Transmitted Diseases,* 3rd edn. (New York: McGraw-Hill), in press

23. Sanchez, P. J. and Wendel, G. D. (1997). Syphilis in pregnancy. *Clin. Perinatol.,* **24**, 71–90

24. Goldenberg, R. L., Andrews, W. W., Yuan, A. C., MacKay, H. T. and St. Louis, M. E. (1997). Sexually transmitted diseases and adverse outcomes of pregnancy. *Clin. Perinatol.,* **24**, 23–41

25. Hsieh, H.-L., Lee, K.-S., Khoshnood, B. and Herschel, M. (1997). Fetal death rate in the United States, 1979–1990: trend and racial disparity. *Obstet. Gynecol.,* **89**, 33–9

26. Harter, C. A. and Benirschke, K. (1976). Fetal syphilis in the first trimester. *Am. J. Obstet. Gynecol.,* **124**, 705–11

27. Nahmias, A. J., Josey, W. E., Naib, Z. M., Freeman, M. G., Fernandez, R. J. and Wheeler, J. H. (1971). Perinatal risk associated with maternal genital herpes simplex virus infection. *Am. J. Obstet. Gynecol.,* **110**, 825–37

28. Brown, Z. A., Benedetti, J., Selke, S., Ashley, R., Watts, D. H. and Corey, L. (1996). Asymptomatic maternal shedding of herpes simplex virus at the onset of labor: relationship to preterm labor. *Obstet. Gynecol.,* **87**, 483–8

29. McGregor, J. A., French, J. I., Parker, R., Draper, D., Patterson, E., Jones, W., Thorsgard, K. and McFee, J. (1995). Prevention of premature birth by screening and treatment for common genital tract infections: results of a prospective controlled evaluation. *Am. J. Obstet. Gynecol.,* **173**, 157–67

30. Morales, W. J., Schorr, S. and Albritton, J. (1994). Effect of metronidazole in patients with preterm birth in preceding pregnancy and bacterial vaginosis. *Am. J. Obstet. Gynecol.,* **171**, 345–9

31. Hauth, J. C., Goldenberg, R. L., Andrews, W. W., Dubard, M. B. and Cooper, R. L. (1995). Reduced incidence of preterm delivery with metronidazole and erythromycin in women with bacterial vaginosis. *N. Engl. J. Med.,* **333**, 1732–6

32. Harrison, H. R., Alexander, E. R., Weinstein, L., Lewis, M., Nash, M. and Sim, D. A. (1983). Cervical *Chlamydia trachomatis* and mycoplasma infections. Epidemiology and outcomes. *J. Am. Med. Assoc.,* **250**, 1721–7

33. Sweet, R. L., Landers, D. V., Walker, C. and Schachter, J. (1987). *Chlamydia trachomatis* infection and pregnancy outcome. *Am. J. Obstet. Gynecol.,* **156**, 824–33

34. Berman, S. M., Harrison, H. R., Boyce, W. T., Haffner, W. J., Lewis, M. and Arthur, J. B. (1987). Low birth weight, prematurity, and postpartum endometritis. Association with prenatal cervical *Mycoplasma hominis* and *Chlamydia trachomatis* infections. *J. Am. Med. Assoc.,* **257**, 1189–94

35. Cotch, M. F., Pastorek, J. G., Nugent, R. P., Yerg, D. E., Martin, D. H. and Eschenbach, D. A. (1991). Demographic and behavioral predictors of *Trichomonas vaginalis. Obstet. Gynecol.,* **78**, 1087–92

36. Connor, E. M., Sperling, R. S., Gelber, R., Kiselev, P., Scott, G., O'Sullivan, M. J., VanDyke, R., Bey, M., Shearer, W., Jacobson, R. L., *et al.* (1994). Reduction of maternal–infant transmission of human immunodeficiency virus Type 1 with zidovudine treatment. Pediatric AIDS Clinical Trials Protocol 076 Study Group. *N. Engl. J. Med.,* **331**, 1173–80

37. Grosskurth, H., Mosha, F., Todd, J., Mwijarubi, E., Klokke, A., Senkoro, K., Mayaud, P., Changalucha, J., Nicoll, A., ka-Gina, G., *et al.* (1995). Impact of improved treatment of sexually transmitted diseases on HIV infection in rural Tanzania: randomized controlled trial. *Lancet,* **346**, 530–6

38. Gibbs, R. F., Rodgers, P. J., Castaneda, Y. S. and Ramzy, I. (1980). Endometritis following vaginal delivery. *Obstet. Gynecol.,* **56**, 555–8

39. Duff, P. (1986). Pathophysiology and management of postcesarean endomyometritis. *Am. J. Obstet. Gynecol.,* **67**, 269–76

40. Plummer, F. A., Laga, M., Brunham, R. C., Piot, P., Ronald, A. R., Bhullar, V., Mati, J. Y., Ndinya-Achola, J. O., Cheang, M. and Nsanze, H. (1987). Postpartum upper genital tract infections in Nairobi, Kenya: epidemiology, etiology, and risk factors. *J. Infect. Dis.,* **156**, 92–8

41. Temmerman, M., Laga, M., Ndinya-Achola, J. O., Paraskevas, M., Brunham, R. C., Plummer, F. A. and Piot, P. (1988). Microbial aetiology and diagnostic criteria of postpartum endometritis in Nairobi, Kenya. *Genitourinary Med.,* **64**, 172–5

42. Hoyme, U. B., Kiviat, N. and Eschenbach, D. A. (1986). Microbiology and treatment of late postpartum endometritis. *Obstet. Gynecol.,* **68**, 226–32

43. Watts, D. H., Krohn, M. A., Hillier, S. L. and Eschenbach, D. A. (1990). Bacterial vaginosis as a risk factor for post-cesarean endometritis. *Obstet. Gynecol.,* **75**, 52–8

Minimal access surgery: cost effectiveness implications

7

O. M. Petrucco

Introduction

The majority of advanced laparoscopic surgical procedures are as invasive as open operation, and it is far more appropriate to refer to this surgery as 'minimal access surgery'[1].

Use and application of minimal access surgery has grown rapidly over the past 10 years in many branches of surgery, especially gynecology. Gynecologists are attracted to minimal access surgery because of improvement in cosmetic result and, more significantly, the more rapid recovery, shorter hospitalization and therefore potential cost savings associated with this surgery.

Advanced endoscopic surgery has found application in the management of diverse gynecological conditions including those listed in Table 1.

Added to the recuperative advantages, other benefits of minimal access surgery include improved visibility, assessment of pathology and potential for therapy at diagnosis.

In most countries, however, minimal access surgery has been introduced and practiced widely without adequate assessment of efficacy and safety, thus creating dissension between enthusiasts of the technique and gynecologists who continue to use laparotomy for their surgery. Added to this argument is the fact that, while some minimal access surgery procedures are fulfilling early expectations, others have been associated with new complications other than those expected for traditional surgery. The question of whether the majority of minimal access surgical techniques have proven advantages and cost effectiveness over traditional

Table 1 Gynecological conditions: endoscopic surgery

Disease process	Endoscopic technique
Menorrhagia	Laparoscopic assisted hysterectomy
	Hysteroscopic endometrial ablation/resection
Ectopic pregnancy	Laparoscopic salpingotomy/salpingectomy
	Laparoscopic injection methotrexate/other destructive agents
Urinary stress incontinence	Laparoscopic Burch colposuspension
Benign ovarian tumors	Laparoscopic cystectomy/oophorectomy
Pelvic and rectovaginal, gastrointestinal and bladder endometriosis	Laparoscopic laser/electrosurgical ablation, laparoscopic excision
Vaginal prolapse	Laparoscopic pelvic floor reconstruction
Pelvic malignancy	Laparoscopic lymphadenectomy
Uterine fibroids	Laparoscopic myomectomy/hysteroscopic myoma resection
Congenital uterine abnormalities (recurrent miscarriages)	Hysteroscopic resection uterine septum
Uterine synechiae	Hysteroscopic division adhesions
Infertility related to adhesions, hydrosalpinx, sterilization	Laparoscopic adhesiolysis, salpingostomy, salpingectomy, laparoscopic tubal anastomosis
Polycystic ovarian disease	Laparoscopic laser/electrocautery drilling

techniques is still to be resolved. These arguments have stimulated consideration of evidence-based decision-making in gynecology. Assessment of minimal access surgery based on review of clinical literature often reveals data accumulated from retrospective studies or anecdotal personal experience and very few randomized controlled clinical trials. Unlike the systemic reviews seen in other branches of medicine, and in particular the Cochrane Pregnancy and Childbirth database, the application of epidemiological principles to assess the effectiveness of gynecological treatments is only just beginning. Unless proven safe and clinically effective new minimal access surgical procedures must be considered experimental.

Added to issues of efficacy and patient safety, escalating health-care expenditure requires close scrutiny of new surgical procedures so that cost effectiveness is assured. Quality assessment in women's health-care, therefore, must examine efficacy, effectiveness and efficiency in relation to clinical outcome. To examine the role of minimal access surgery in gynecological practice we should therefore assess the following:

(1) Performance outcome;

(2) Clinical effectiveness and appropriateness;

(3) Risks, benefits and complication rates;

(4) Cost effectiveness.

Because many minimal access surgical procedures are performed in day surgery centers, costs incurred in the postoperative care of patients at home must be included. The time to full recovery and ability to return to work can then be fully assessed in comparison with conventional surgery.

Using these guidelines it is useful to review some of the gynecological conditions currently treated by minimal access surgery.

Role and impact of laparoscopic-assisted hysterectomy

Disorders of menstruation resulting from dysfunctional uterine bleeding and fibroids remain the most common indications and affect up to 20% of women. The costs associated with consultations, investigations and management of menorrhagia account for a sizeable proportion of health-care budgets in developed countries. A total of 821 700 prescriptions costing UK£7 176 596 as well as 128 000 diagnostic procedures and 73 000 hysterectomies were associated with the treatment of menorrhagia in England and Wales in 1993[2].

Reich and colleagues[3] introduced laparoscopic-assisted hysterectomy with the objective of transforming abdominal hysterectomy via laparotomy to an endoscopic technique. The majority of laparoscopic-assisted hysterectomy procedures are currently performed as laparoscopic assisted vaginal hysterectomies. Several reports in the literature confirm that a trend towards a decrease in abdominal with a concomitant increase in vaginal and laparoscopic-assisted hysterectomy procedures is occurring[4-6]. Proponents of vaginal hysterectomy, however, point to the fact that vaginal hysterectomy is usually possible in the presence of previous pelvic surgery and sepsis, endometriosis and uterine fibroids, which are usually considered indications for abdominal hysterectomy[7-9].

To date in Australia, laparoscopic-assisted hysterectomy has not gained widespread acceptance. The Medicare database for 1994–95 indicates that laparoscopic-assisted hysterectomy accounted for 8% of hysterectomies. Less than 10% of gynecologists had performed fewer than three laparoscopic-assisted hysterectomy operations[10].

Types of laparoscopic-assisted hysterectomy

Classifications of surgical approaches for laparoscopic-assisted hysterectomy are dependent on the extent of surgery performed vaginally and particularly whether the uterine artery is divided laparoscopically or vaginally. An extensive body of literature has now accumulated detailing number of procedures, technique, operative time, hospital stay, complications and recovery interval.

Table 2 Randomized controlled trials of abdominal versus laparoscopic hysterectomy

	Raju and Auld (1994)[11]		Phipps and Nayak (1993)[12]	
	LAVH/BSO	TAH/BSO	LAVH/BSO	TAH/BSO
Sample size (n)	40	40	24	29
Operating time (min)	100	57	65	30
Analgesia	6.6 (days)	13.3	1.5 (doses)	4.5
Hospital stay (days)	3.5	6.0	2	6
Return to work (days)	21	42	14	42
Complications	minimal, no difference		nil	nil
Cost				
Disposables (UK£)	225	30	500	50
Total (UK£)	1260	1750	substantially less for LAVH	

LAVH, laparoscopic-assisted vaginal hysterectomy; BSO, bilateral salpingo-oophorectomy; TAH, total abdominal hysterectomy

Only a small number of prospectively randomized trials, however, comparing laparoscopic-assisted hysterectomy with abdominal and vaginal hysterectomy are available for review. Two studies comparing total abdominal hysterectomy and bilateral salpingo-oophorectomy, and two more comparing vaginal hysterectomy, with laparoscopic-assisted vaginal hysterectomy are summarized in Tables 2 and 3.

Patient selection, laparoscopic techniques and degree of vaginal surgery differed in these studies. All four studies, however, demonstrated a doubling of the operating time for laparoscopic-assisted hysterectomy compared with abdominal and vaginal approaches. Abdominal hysterectomies were associated with a significant increase in analgesia requirements compared with laparoscopic-assisted hysterectomy and vaginal procedures. Patients with abdominal operations required a significantly longer stay in hospital; however, vaginal and laparoscopic-assisted hysterectomy procedures had similar postoperative bed days. Laparoscopic-assisted hysterectomy and vaginal procedures were associated with a statistically shorter interval for returning to work or normal activity in comparison with abdominal hysterectomy.

An increased cost for laparoscopic-assisted hysterectomy was demonstrated in all four studies largely due to the use of disposable equipment. The potential does exist, however, for indirect savings associated with decrease in hospitalization and quicker return to work.

Results of non-randomized prospective or retrospective studies have tended to be similar in terms of patient outcome and cost. Selection bias and small numbers make overall interpretation more difficult.

Table 3 Randomized controlled trials of vaginal (VH) versus laparoscopic hysterectomy (LH)

	Richardson et al. (1995)[7]		Summitt et al. (1992)[13]	
	LH	VH	LAVH	VH
Sample size (n)	22	23	29	27
Operating time (min)	131	77	120.1	64.7
Analgesia (days)	2.9	2.6	not recorded	
Hospital stay (days)	3.2	3.3	0.5	0.5
Return to activity (days)	23.1	22.2	not recorded	
Return to work (weeks)	6.4	5.7	not recorded	
Complications	36%	30%	1	2
Cost (US$)	not recorded		7905	4891

LAVH, laparoscopic-assisted vaginal hysterectomy

Complications of laparoscopic-assisted hysterectomy

A meta-analysis review of 29 studies involving laparoscopic-assisted hysterectomy procedures was carried out by Garry and Phillips[14]. Skilled laparoscopic surgeons contributed 3184 cases.

The most common complications were febrile morbidity (4.3%) and conversion to laparotomy (3.45%). Trochar injuries (2.57%), bowel injury (0.47%) and urinary tract damage occurred in 1.38% of cases. Comparison with the benchmark study of Dicker and co-workers[15] of complications for abdominal and vaginal hysterectomy indicates a lower febrile morbidity and need for transfusion, and comparable rates for unintended major surgery, bowel and urinary tract trauma and incidence of pulmonary embolus. Laparoscopic-assisted hysterectomy was associated with a complication rate of 15.6/1000 compared to 24.5 for vaginal and 42.8 for abdominal hysterectomy.

Small uncontrolled retrospective studies have similarly found little difference in complication rate between groups[16–19]. Of some concern, however, have been reports of ureteric and bladder injuries of greater incidence (up to 4.8%[20]) than expected for abdominal (0.5%) and vaginal hysterectomy (1.66%)[15]. These injuries have been associated with the use of the linear stapler or attempts to divide or control hemorrhage from the uterine artery pedicle.

To assess the effect of the 'learning curve' for the incidence of major and minor complications associated with performance of laparoscopic-assisted hysterectomy in South Australia, an audit of medical records of all hospitals where this technique was performed was undertaken between 1991 and 1994. The overall complication rate for 760 cases was 110/1000 comprising febrile morbidity (41.5/1000) hemorrhage (30/1000) and bowel injury (6.2/1000). Urinary tract injury occurred in 2.4% of cases (ureteric injury 0.5%, bladder injury 0.9%, late diagnosis 1.1%). The results of this audit confirmed that, particularly in the learning phase, attempts to occlude the uterine artery were associated with greater morbidity to ureter and bladder than abdominal hysterectomy.

Apart from procedure-specific complications, those associated with laparoscopy itself have to be considered (vascular and bowel injury, gas embolism, etc.).

Subtotal versus laparoscopic-assisted hysterectomy

Laparoscopic subtotal hysterectomy was first described by Semm[21] and subsequently promoted by several endoscopic surgeons[22–24]. Operating times similar to those for laparoscopic-assisted vaginal hysterectomy were reported by these authors (60–188 min). Removal of the uterus from the abdominal cavity has been facilitated by use of electronic morcellators. Lyons[25] found a statistically significant reduction in blood loss, operating time, hospital bed days and return to normal activities when compared with patients having laparoscopic-assisted vaginal hysterectomy. The same author found costs to be lowest for the subtotal procedure when compared with laparoscopic-assisted vaginal and abdominal hysterectomy.

Ablation of the endocervical canal with laser or roller-ball diathermy has been performed in the majority of cases. Reported studies were too small to make meaningful comparison of complication rate; however, serious complications were not reported in any of the above series.

Conclusions

Laparoscopic-assisted hysterectomy procedures have become popular with patients and endoscopists because of less pain and shorter hospitalization and return to full activity. Because of the paucity of randomized prospective controlled trials comparing different types of hysterectomy, available reports need to be complemented by nationally co-ordinated clinical trials. Complications of laparoscopic-assisted hysterectomy will require continued monitoring, particularly when clinicians are past the 'learning curve' stage of experience, but, however, currently do not seem to be significantly higher than for abdominal and vaginal hysterectomy. As well as providing tuition for advanced laparoscopic techniques, gynecologists in training should be taught to become expert vaginal surgeons so that the vaginal approach can be fully exploited as a means of performing hysterectomy.

Laparoscopic management of ectopic pregnancy

The performance of laparoscopic salpingectomy by Shapiro and Adler in 1973[26] and salpingotomy by Bruhat in 1977[27] transformed laparoscopy from a diagnostic to a therapeutic procedure for ectopic pregnancy. World-wide controversy, however, still exists concerning the most cost-effective approach to management with a substantial number of patients managed by laparotomy. Australian Medicare figures indicate that only 50% of patients with ectopic pregnancies are managed laparoscopically[10].

Laparoscopic-administered methotrexate

The results of two randomized trials[28,29] comparing laparoscopic surgery with laparoscopic administration of methotrexate confirmed that instillation of methotrexate was equally effective to surgery in terms of (1) persistent trophoblastic activity, (2) time interval to disappearance of β human chorionic gonadotropin (hCG) and (3) subsequent intrauterine pregnancy rate.

A third randomized trial was discontinued because of poor results in the methotrexate group[30].

Laparoscopic surgery for ectopic pregnancy

Assessment by Garry[31] of six major series of laparoscopic treated patients ($n = 952$) reported in the interval 1986–94 was summarized thus: success rate, 95–100%; complications, 0–3.6%; operating time, 36–62 min; and hospital stay, 0.8–2 days.

The same editorial described six studies ($n = 660$) treated by laparoscopy or laparotomy, respectively, with the following conclusions reached: operating time, 55–75 min for laparoscopy, 51–103 min for laparotomy; analgesic requirement (three studies), less, greater; hospital stay, 1.0–1.7 days, 3.3–5.2 days; return to full activity, 10–12 days, 23–42 days; and complications were not significant for either laparoscopy or laparotomy.

Faulk and Steiger[32] in a retrospective study assessed cost of laparoscopic and laparotomy management of 177 patients. They confirmed a 25% saving in favor of laparoscopy. Cost savings were not reduced, however, because of a 21% rate of conversion to laparotomy for 'ineffective laparoscopic excisions'.

Laparoscopic salpingotomy versus salpingectomy

Retrospective non-randomized studies comparing laparoscopic salpingotomy (five series, 520 cases) and salpingectomy (two series, 157 cases) indicated an intrauterine pregnancy rate in 58% for salpingotomy and 31% for salpingectomy cases. A review of fertility in patients with ectopic pregnancy in a solitary tube treated by salpingotomy (20 studies) confirmed a subsequent intrauterine pregnancy rate of 55% (range 13–100%)[33].

For patients not wanting to remain fertile, or those with severe tubal disease or rupture, a clear indication to perform salpingectomy exists. On the other hand, for patients desiring to remain fertile there is a need for objective evidence to decide whether removal or conservation of the Fallopian tube is the treatment of choice.

Risks of conservative management include:

(1) Incomplete evacuation of trophoblast;

(2) Trophoblast seeding in the peritoneal cavity;

(3) Persistence of tubal disease;

(4) Inactive ectopic with expected spontaneous resolution.

Persistence of trophoblast has been reported to occur in 0–20% of cases with an average of 5%[34].

Conclusions

Evidence from review of the literature indicates that laparoscopic management of ectopic pregnancy should be the preferred method of treatment in the majority of cases. Clinical outcome is similar to that for laparotomy-treated patients with similar or better opportunity for future fertility. Laparoscopy-treated patients have less pain and requirement for analgesia, and have shorter hospital stay and interval to resumption of full activity.

The need for prospective randomized clinical studies to determine the role of expectant, methotrexate and laparoscopic conservation or removal of the affected Fallopian tube continues to exist.

Role of minimal access surgery for management of adnexal tumors

Clinicians using ultrasound-directed, laparoscopic and minilaparotomy surgery for aspiration or removal of ovarian tumors face the difficulty of being able to differentiate between functional cysts and ovarian neoplasms. The use of diagnostic ultrasound, radiological modalities and the measurement of tumor markers have only limited diagnostic potential.

Simple unilocular cysts, however, occur in 60% of premenopausal women and up to 6% of asymptomatic postmenopausal women. Approximately 1% of simple cysts in pre- and postmenopausal women are malignant (0.3% invasive and 0.5% tumors of low malignant potential)[35].

Lack of vegetation within cystic tumors usually indicates benign nature; however, in postmenopausal women two of three cystic tumors with solid components are likely to be malignant. The most useful predictor of malignancy in cystic tumors greater than 30 mm in size is the ultrasound-determined morphological appearance of the cyst. Endovaginal ultrasound is also more reliable than aspiration cytology to investigate suspicious cystic tumors.

The incidence of ovarian malignancy in 5307 laparoscopy-managed patients with ovarian tumors was found to be 1.5% by Blanc and colleagues[36]. Over a 12-year period of laparoscopic management of adnexal cystic masses, Canis and associates[37] encountered an overall incidence of malignancy of 2.5%. Immediate laparotomy was performed in all cases of suspected or confirmed malignancy.

The use of endo-bags and extra-abdominal cyst drainage reduces the risk of tumor spread. The finding by Volz and co-workers[38] that CO_2 pneumoperitoneum encourages tumor-cell implantation is of some concern.

Conclusions

Transvaginal or abdominal ultrasound is mandatory for the investigation of ovarian tumors. The aim of laparoscopic surgery, as in open laparotomy, is to achieve complete removal of the tumor tissues without rupture. Should malignancy be confirmed at frozen section, formal oncological surgery should be performed. Aspiration of ovarian cysts with equivocal cytological results and possibility of tumor spread should be discouraged whenever malignancy is a possibility.

Future directions for minimal access surgery

Technological advances

Despite the introduction of high-resolution three-chip endocameras and on-line digital enhancement, improvement in image quality, image resolution, stereopsis and camera manipulation will be required to improve endoscopic surgery. High-definition television including high-resolution monitors is already enhancing the improved performance of endocameras.

Laboratory techniques and clinical studies comparing two- and three-dimensional viewing technology have demonstrated that three-dimensional video-endoscopy improves surgical manipulations and intraoperative procedures[39]. Spatial visual perception of stereoscopic images may, however, cause depth-perception problems to some users.

A system ('Vistral') which abolishes the flatness of vision imposed by a video monitor automatically enhancing depth perception has already had experimental and clinical evaluation and has been shown to diminish eye strain and fatigue[40]. The University of Dundee research group achieve projection of the endoscopic image in space over the patient.

Computer-programmed voice-activated robotic arms, recently introduced to endoscopic surgery, efficiently alter camera position, obviating the need for an assistant at the operating table.

An endoscopic guidance system controlled by the surgeon via a joy-stick adapted to the handle of the surgical instrument allows the tip of the endoscope to follow movements of the surgeon's finger. This 'Cam Track' input device achieves efficient and intuitive endoscope operation by the surgeon[41]. Efforts to reproduce the essential components of human visual sense by the same group have led to research into creating a multifunctional visual tool incorporating panoramic view, maintenance of clear vision and endoscope guidance.

Systems providing 'remote tracking' responding to head and eyeball movements with secondary activation of the camera will further facilitate surgical manipulations. Virtual reality technology has enhanced teaching of endoscopic techniques in a very realistic fashion. We also await with interest further advances in tele-robotic, telepresence and immediate remote surgery[42].

Accreditation and credentialling for minimal access surgery

A controversial aspect of minimal access surgery relates to accreditation and credentialling of gynecologists wanting to perform this surgery. Historically, enthusiasts having learnt new techniques by observation of colleagues eventually formed endoscopy societies in different countries. Having established forums for meetings and education, the need to establish guidelines for credentialling and accreditation of individuals to perform advanced endoscopic surgery became apparent.

In 1992 the Australian Gynaecological Endoscopy Society (AGES) proposed 'Guidelines for training in Advanced Operative Laparoscopy in the speciality of Obstetrics and Gynaecology', which were accepted by the Royal Australian College of Obstetricians and Gynaecologists (RACOG). The guidelines suggested levels of training for safe conduct of new operations. In 1993 and 1994 the RACOG further outlined the responsibility of Fellows and Health Authorities in relation to advanced endoscopic surgery by issuing a 'Policy Statement for Implementation of Advanced Endoscopic Surgery'. Inherent in these guidelines is the need to appoint preceptors to teach new techniques, and the establishment of Accreditation Committees to approve new gynecologists to perform advanced endoscopic surgery.

Similar approaches have been introduced by sister endoscopy societies in the UK, Canada, USA and Europe. This positive attitude to training accreditation and credentialling will hopefully ensure that the next generation of gynecologists will be competent in all aspects of gynecological surgery, i.e. abdominal, vaginal and endoscopic.

References

1. Cuschieri, A. (1992). 'A rose by any other name . . .' Minimal access or minimally invasive surgery? *Surg. Endosc.*, **6**, 214
2. Nuffield Institute for Health, NHS Centre for Reviews and Disseminations, Royal College of Physicians (1995). *Effective Health Care*, (London: Churchill Livingstone)
3. Reich, H., McGlynn, F. and Sekel, L. (1993). Total laparoscopic hysterectomy. *Gynaecol. Endosc*, **2**, 59–63
4. Querleu, D., Cosson, M., Parmentier, D. and Debodinance, P. (1993). The impact of laparoscopic surgery on vaginal hysterectomy. *Gynaecol. Endosc.*, **2**, 89–91

5. Casey, M. J., Garcia-Padial, J., Johnson, C., Osborne, N. G., Sotolongo, J. and Watson, P. (1994). A critical analysis of laparoscopic assisted vaginal hysterectomies compared with vaginal hysterectomies unassisted by laparoscopy and transabdominal hysterectomies. *J. Gynecol. Surg.*, **10**, 7–14

6. Johns, D. A., Carrera, B., Jones, J., DeLeon, F., Vincent, R. and Safely, C. (1995). The medical and economic impact of laparoscopically assisted vaginal hysterectomy in a large, metropolitan, not-for-profit hospital. *Am. J. Obstet. Gynecol.* **172**, 1709–19

7. Richardson, R. E., Bournas, N. and Magos, A. L. (1995). Is laparoscopic hysterectomy a waste of time? *Lancet*, **345**, 36–41

8. Browne, D. S. and Fraser, M. I. (1991). Hysterectomy revisited. *Aust. NZ J. Obstet. Gynaecol.*, **31**, 148

9. Kovac, S. R. (1995). Guidelines to determine the route of hysterectomy. *Obstet. Gynecol.*, **85**, 18–23

10. Molloy, D. and Crosdale, S. (1996). National trends in gynaecological endoscopic surgery. *Aust. NZ J. Obstet. Gynaecol.*, **36**, 27–31

11. Raju, K. S. and Auld, B. J. (1994). A randomised prospective study of laparoscopic vaginal hysterectomy versus abdominal hysterectomy each with bilateral salpingo-oophorectomy. *Br. J. Obstet. Gynaecol.*, **101**, 1068–71.

12. Phipps, J. H., John, M. and Nayak, S. (1993). Comparison of laparoscopically-assisted vaginal hysterectomy and bilateral salpingo-oophorectomy with conventional abdominal hysterectomy and bilateral salpingo-oophorectomy. *Br. J. Obstet. Gynaecol.*, **100**(7), 698–700

13. Summitt, R. L., Stovall, T. G., Lipscombe, G. H. and Ling, F. W. (1992). Randomized comparison of laparoscopically-assisted vaginal hysterectomy with standard vaginal hysterectomy in an outpatient setting. *Obstet. Gynecol.*, **80**, 895–901

14. Garry, R. and Phillips, G. (1995). How safe is the laparoscopic approach to hysterectomy? *Gynecol. Endosc.*, **4**, 77–9

15. Dicker, R. C., Greenspan, J. R., Strauss, L. T., Cowatt, M. R., Scally, M. J., Peterson, H. B., DeStefano, F., Rubin, G. L. and Ory, H. W. (1982). Complications of abdominal and vaginal hysterectomy among women of reproductive age in the United States. *Am. J. Obstet. Gynecol.*, **144**, 841–8

16. Calandra, C. (1995). Laparoscopically-assisted vaginal hysterectomy. *Aust. NZ J. Obstet. Gynaecol.*, **35**, 78–82

17. Jones, R. A. (1995). Complications of laparoscopic hysterectomy: 250 cases. *Gynaecol. Endosc.*, **4**, 95–9

18. Angle, H. S., Cohen, S. M. and Hidlebaugh, D. (1995). The initial Worcester experience with laparoscopic hysterectomy. *J. Am. Gynecol. Laparosc.*, **2**, 155–61

19. Redwine, D. B. (1995). Laparoscopic hysterectomy compared with abdominal and vaginal hysterectomy in a community hospital. *J. Am. Assoc. Gynecol. Laparosc.*, **2**, 305–10

20. Baggish, M. S. (1992). The most expensive hysterectomy. *J. Gynecol. Surg.*, **8**, 57–8

21. Semm, K. (1993). Hysterectomy by pelviscopy: an alternative approach without colpotomy (CASH). In Garry, R. and Reich, H. (eds.) *Laparoscopic Hysterectomy*, pp. 118–32. (Oxford, UK: Blackwell Scientific Publications)

22. Donnez, J. and Nisolle, M. (1993). Laparoscopic subtotal hysterectomy (LASH). *Gynaecol. Endosc.*, **2**, 77–8

23. Hasson, H. (1993). Experience with laparoscopic hysterectomy. *J. Am. Assoc. Gynecol. Laparosc.*, **1**, 1–11

24. Ewen, S. P. and Sutton, C. J. G. (1994). Initial experience with supracervical laparoscopic hysterectomy and removal of the cervical transformation zone. *Br. J. Obstet. Gynaecol.*, **101**, 225–8

25. Lyons, T. L. (1993). Laparoscopic supracervical hysterectomy using the contact Nd:YAG laser. *Gynaecol. Endosc.*, **2**, 79–81

26. Shapiro, H. I. and Adler, D. H. (1973). Excision of an ectopic pregnancy through the laparoscope. *Am. J. Obstet. Gynecol.*, **117**, 290–1

27. Bruhat, M. A., Manhes, H., Choukroun, J. and Suzanne, F. (1977). Essai de traitement per coeleoscopique de la grossesse extra-uterine. A propos de 26 observations. *Rev. Fr. Gynecol. Obstet.*, **72**, 667–9

28. O'Shea, R. T., Thompson, G. R. and Harding, A. (1994). Intra-amniotic methotrexate versus CO_2 laser laparoscopic salpingotomy in the management of tubal ectopic pregnancy – a prospective randomised trial. *Fertil. Steril.* **62**, 876–8

29. Zilber, O., Pansky, M., Bukovski, I. and Golan, A. (1996). Laparoscopic salpingostomy versus laparoscopic local methotrexate injection in the management of unruptured ectopic gestation. *Am. J. Obstet. Gynecol.*, **175**, 600–2

30. Mottla, G. L., Rulin, M. C. and Guzick, D. S. (1992). Lack of resolution of ectopic pregnancy by intratubal injection of methotrexate. *Fertil. Steril.* **57**, 685–7

31. Garry, R. (1996). The laparoscopic treatment of ectopic pregnancy: the long road to acceptance. *Gynaecol. Endosc.*, **5**, 65–8

32. Faulk, R. A. and Steiger, R. M. (1996). Operative management of ectopic pregnancy: a cost analysis. *Am. J. Obstet. Gynecol.*, **175**, 90–6

33. Thornton, K. L., Diamond, M. P. and De Cherney, A. H. (1991). Linear salpingostomy for ectopic pregnancy. *Obstet. Gynecol. Clin. North Am.*, **18**, 95–109

34. Parker, J. L. and Thompson, D. J. (1994). Persistent ectopic pregnancy after conservative management: successful treatment with single-dose intramuscular methotrexate. *Aust. NZ J. Obstet. Gynaecol.*, **34**, 99–102

35. Osmers, R. G. W., Osmers, M., Von Maydell, B., Wagner, B. and Kuhn, W. (1996). Preoperative evaluation of ovarian tumours in the premenopause by transvaginosonography. *Am. J. Obstet. Gynecol.*, **175**, 428–34

36. Blanc, B., D'Ercole, C., Nicoloso, E. and Boubli, L. (1995). Laparoscopic management of malignant ovarian cysts: a 78 case national survey. 2. Follow up and final treatment. *Eur. J. Obstet. Gynaecol. Reprod. Biol.*, **61**, 147–50

37. Canis, M., Mage, G., Pouly, J. L., Wattiez, A., Manhes, H. and Bruhat, M. A. (1994). Laparoscopic diagnosis of adnexal cystic masses: a 12 year experience with long term follow up. *Obstet. Gynecol.*, **83**, 707–12

38. Volz, J., Koster, S., Weiss, M., Schmidt, R., Urbaschek, R., Melchert, F. and Albrecht, M. (1996). Pathophysiologic features of a pneumoperitoneum at laparoscopy: a swine model. *Am. J. Obstet. Gynecol.*, **174**, 132–40

39. Von Pichler, C., Radermacher, K. and Rau, G. (1996). The state of 3-D technology and evaluation. *Min. Invas. Ther. Allied Technol.*, **4**, 419–26

40. Cuschieri, A. (1996). Visual display technology for endoscopic surgery. *Min. Invas. Ther. Allied Technol.*, **5**, 427–34

41. Schurr, M. O., Buess, G., Kunert, W., Flemming, E., Hermeking, H. and Gumb, L. (1996). Human sense of vision: a guide to future endoscopic imaging systems. *Min. Invas. Ther. Allied Technol.*, **5**, 410–18

42. Cushieri, A. (1994). Shape of things to come. *Surg. Endosc.*, **8**, 83–5

Screening for gynecological cancer 8

W. T. Creasman

Cervical cancer

Gynecology is the classic example of a screening test that has had a major impact on the cancer so evaluated. In fact, in the case of cervical cancer, the Pap smear has been the only screening test for any cancer that has resulted in decreases in the incidence and mortality rate. It is appreciated that the incidence of cervical cancer varies tremendously around the world. As a generalization, the industrialized world has the lowest incidence while it is highest in the third-world countries. There are, however, variations within a given population. For instance, in New Orleans in the black population, there is a three-fold increased incidence of cervical cancer compared with that in the white population. A similar situation is seen in Singapore where the Indian population has about a three-fold increased incidence compared with that in the Malaysian population. Why such a disparity in the incidence of cancer within a well-defined locality in which medical care is readily available is unanswered. It is appreciated that breast cancer is the number one cancer in women worldwide, with cervical cancer being number two. Worldwide cervical cancer incidence approaches 500 000 new cases each year with approximately one-half of those individuals dying from their disease.

It is appreciated that, not only can there be a variation in incidence between races, but incidence can vary within different age groups. The Surveillance, Epidemiology, End Result (SEER) databank from the United States notes that white women under the age of 50 have a very low incidence and mortality from cervical cancer. In white women more than 50 years of age, the incidence of mortality increases several fold. This is also true for the black population with the incidence and mortality higher for both the young and older population compared with those for the white population.

When one looks at the *Annual Report* data of FIGO, it is appreciated that, over the last half century or so, improvement in the diagnosis and management of cervical cancer has been achieved. For instance, back in the early 1950s, data reported to the *Annual Report* noted that < 25% of all cervical cancer was stage I and this has increased to almost 40% by the 1990s. As a result, there has been a concomitant decrease in the numbers of stage II and III cancers reported. Not only has the incidence of early stage cervical cancer increased but, within a given stage, survival has improved. In the early 1950s, a 75% 5-year survival was reported for stage I carcinoma of the cervix and this has improved to about 85% in the early 1990s. Improvements in both stage II and stage III have also been appreciated.

It is well recognized that there are multiple risk factors for cervical cancer. It has been known for almost a century and a half that cervical cancer is a sexually transmitted disease. Ragoni-Stern, in the mid-19th century was the first to describe the sexual aspects of this disease, although it was not until the late 20th century that the sexual connotation was so stated. Coitus in the mid-adolescent years and multiple sexual partners are well recognized as epidemiological risk factors. Over the last decade or so, the role of human papilloma virus (HPV), particularly 16 and 18, has been implicated in the disease process. The laboratory data are very strong in this regard, although the epidemiological data have lagged behind the laboratory information. One of the risk factors which is very seldom stated is whether or not an individual has had a Pap smear. Probably the greatest risk factor for cervical cancer is an individual who has never had a Pap smear. If one evaluates data, even in the industrialized world, considerable benefits have been identified because of screening activities. If one evaluates the data from the United States over the past 25 years, there has been a decrease in the incidence of cervical cancer of about 25% but, more importantly, the death rates have decreased by about 50%. In the late 1960s and early 1970s, it was estimated that only about one-half of adult women in the United States had ever had a Pap smear and, today, that number is over 90%. If the incidence in death rates had remained at the level of 1970, during the subsequent 25 years in the United States, there would have been approximately 88 000 more cervical cancers and some 47 000 more cervical cancer deaths than were actually seen. The benefits of Pap smear screening are evident.

An example of the benefits of screening become more apparent when one looks at data from the Nordic countries. In many countries, medical decisions are made for political reasons. A decision, for instance, was made in Iceland in which 100% of the population would be targeted for screening. During the subsequent years, an 80% reduction in mortality was achieved. On the other hand, in Norway, only 5% of the population was targeted and they were only able to achieve a 10% reduction in mortality. Screening frequency also becomes important. Data from Sweden would suggest that in the one-time screened population, cervical cancer was seen one-third as frequently as in the non-screened population. If patients were screened every 3 years, the incidence was about one-tenth of that in the non-screened population. Recent data from Iceland noted that, in cancers identified at the time of screening, about one-half of all cervical cancers were stage I and, of that number, one-half were microinvasion. In the interval cancers or non-screened population, only 11% of the cervical cancers were stage I. So, cervical screening has resulted in a decrease in the incidence and mortality of

cervical cancer. Concomitantly, there has been a significant increase in the diagnosis of cervical intraepithelial neoplasia (CIN) and, of course, that is the whole purpose of the Pap smear, to identify preinvasive disease, treat with conservative methods and essentially eliminate the risk for that patient developing invasive cancer. If, in fact, invasive cancer is identified at the time of the screen, the diagnosis is made of earlier-stage disease. It should be remembered that nowhere in the world has there been a decrease in the mortality of cervical cancer without a large ongoing screening program.

As previously indicated, age seems to be an important criterion regarding the diagnosis of cervical cancer. When one again evaluates the data from the *Annual Report* of FIGO, it is noted that the number of patients reported are greatest in the four decades from age 40 to age 80. Although many would suggest that, once a woman reaches a certain age, screening can be stopped, it should be noted that by far the greatest number of patients reported with cervical cancer were 60 years of age or older. Stage of disease also correlates with age. The average age for patients with stage I is the late 40s, whereas in stage IV it is the late 50s. In the United States, 25% of all cervical cancers are in patients 65 years of age or older, yet 41% of all cervical cancer deaths are in this age range. Most of these individuals have never had a Pap smear. The prevalence of abnormal Pap smears is greater in the older population and this is irrespective of the Pap smear screening history in that individual. There appear to be two main age-peak incidences for cervical cancer, one being in the mid-to-late 40s and the other being in the mid-to-late 60s. When one evaluates the age for patients with carcinoma *in situ*, there appears to be a peak about 15 years of age earlier than the first age peak in relation to invasive cancer. The relationship between the two is well known. The second age peak, however, does not have a concomitant peak for carcinoma *in situ*. This may be because older individuals with invasive cancer have the disease arise *de novo* or the older population does not obtain Pap smears as frequently as the younger population and, therefore, preinvasive disease is not identified. It does appear, however, that there is a greater decrease in identifiable disease in the young patient who is screened, compared with the older patient.

The interval of screening has also been evaluated. A study from the University of Washington looked at their patients with squamous carcinoma of the cervix in relation to the last Pap smear. In evaluating their data, they noted that, if there had been a Pap smear taken at 3 years or a longer interval before the diagnosis of squamous carcinoma, there was approximately a threefold greater chance of having cancer than if optimal screening (1–2 years) was obtained. They then looked at a high-risk group of patients using four to nine sexual partners as an aggregate. With suboptimal screening in this high-risk category, there was a fivefold greater chance of having cervical cancer than if optimal screening was utilized. In a study from Duke University, interval screening was evaluated in relation to stage at the time of diagnosis. If a Pap smear had been done less than 3 years prior to the diagnosis of cervical cancer, 85% of the cancers were stage I. If the Pap smear that been done 3 years or longer prior to the diagnosis of cervical cancer, stage I was identified only in about 50% of patients.

It is appreciated that the Pap smear screening interval is determined not only by age but also by income of the household. This is true in the United States in which there is not universal medical coverage. In all age categories, the more affluent patient had a Pap smear more frequently than did the less affluent patient. Even in households with an income of $50 000 or more a year, the prevalence of screening in the older patient was only about one-third. The younger, more affluent patient appreciates the importance of the Pap smear and very few of these individuals have never had a Pap smear. In contrast, in the older, less affluent patient, approximately one-fifth have never had a Pap smear. It would appear that a golden opportunity is lost because, irrespective of age or affluence, patients come in contact with

health-care providers each year on an equal basis.

In the United States, it is reported that 9% of the adult women have never had a Pap smear. However, of the 90% who have had a Pap smear, about two-thirds have not had a Pap smear in the recent past. Unfortunately, this translates into rather large numbers in that 2.5 million adult women have never had a Pap smear in the United States and there are another 12 million women who are unaware of the importance of the Pap smear. In a recent survey of young co-eds at an Ivy League institution, interviews were held to determine knowledge concerning benefits of Pap smear screening. Only 61% of those interviewed knew that the Pap smear was to detect cancer, but only one-half of those knew that cervical cancer was the cancer being screened. There were some individuals who even thought that the Pap smear could identify breast cancer. Very few of these individuals knew the risk factors for cervical cancer.

A recent consensus conference held at the National Institutes of Health in Washington, DC, on cervical cancer noted that all cervical cancer could be eliminated or prevented with optimal Pap smear screening. They also noted that about one-half of all cervical cancer deaths were in women who had never had a Pap smear. it was also stated that about one-third of women in the United States had not had a Pap smear in the past 4 years.

It is appreciated that the optimal screening interval for the Pap smear is varied from country to country depending, to a certain degree, on governmental policy and economical considerations. The recommendation of the American College of Obstetricians and Gynecologists, the American Cancer Society and the National Cancer Institute of the United States is that all women who are or who have become sexually active or who have reached age 18 should have an annual Pap smear and pelvic examination. After a woman has had three or more consecutive, satisfactory, normal, annual examinations, a Pap smear may be performed less frequently at the discretion of the physician.

Ovarian cancer

In the industrialized world, ovarian cancer is more frequently seen than cervical cancer. In the female pelvis, corpus cancer is the most frequent cancer seen; however, in the United States, ovarian cancer kills more women than cervical and corpus cancer combined. It is appreciated that there are risk factors in ovarian cancer. Older age increases the chance of developing ovarian cancer yet the overall incidence is quite low. In the United States, it is said that one out of 70 women will develop ovarian cancer over their lifetime, yet at age 65, the chances of a women having ovarian cancer is < 1%. Infertility, late age at first pregnancy and late age at menopause have all been suggested as risk factors. Recently, a considerable amount of attention has been paid to the genetic aspect of ovarian cancer, particularly since the identification of the *BRCA-1* and *BRCA-2* genes.

For a screening test to be effective, several criteria need to be met:

(1) The disease should have a serious consequence and, certainly, ovarian cancer qualifies here;

(2) Treatment is more effective in screen-detected disease than in symptom-detected. It would appear that ovarian cancer satisfies this prerequisite if, in fact, stage I cancers can be identified with screening, compared with symptom-detected stage III. On the other hand, data is lacking on whether or not stage I detected by screening has a different prognosis than symptom-detected stage I, or stage III for that matter;

(3) Finally, there needs to be a high prevalence of detectable preclinical phase of the disease. Ovarian cancer has some problems in qualifying as a disease that can be easily screened. For instance, data is not available to suggest that ovarian cancer proceeds very orderly from a stage I to a stage II to a stage III or even a stage IV disease. Stage III disease could arise *de novo*. Certainly, extra-ovarian peritoneal carcinomatosis is a well-known entity in which, histologically and clinically, the disease looks like ovarian cancer, but in which the ovaries are minimally or not involved with cancer. Current data suggest that low-malignant potential tumors and invasive epithelial carcinomas are different, and low-malignant potential tumors do not necessarily transform into invasive cancer. A preinvasive lesion date has not been identified in ovarian cancer.

Although it would appear that there are major problems in trying to develop screening tests for ovarian cancer, nevertheless, attempts have been made using the CA125 test and ultrasound. Jacobs in London screened 22 000 women with the CA125 test. Through a process of elimination, 45 of these came to surgery for suspected ovarian cancers, yet only 11 ovarian cancers were found, for an incidence of 0.05%. Unfortunately, seven of the 11 patients had stage III disease, which is what would be expected in the normal population. In this case, three out of four surgeries performed because of a high suggestion of ovarian cancer resulted in no cancer being identified.

Campbell has evaluated a large group of women with ultrasound. A self-referred population of almost 5500 women were screened on three occasions approximately 1 year apart. During this time interval, almost 30 000 ovaries were identified. About 4% of these patients had a positive scan, of which, on rescan, about one-half were normal. Over 300 of these patients came to surgery, yet only five cancers were noted. Therefore, 66 out of 67 surgeries that were carried out identified no ovarian cancer. Several investigators have evaluated the use of ultrasound. Four different investigators have evaluated approximately 15 000 women for whom 560 came to surgery but only eight epithelial invasive cancers were identified. This, again, indicates that the incidence is only 0.05%.

Another study by Jacobs evaluated multiple potential screening tests. Four thousand women were screened with pelvic examination and CA125 test. Over 98% of these women had normal examinations. Of 22 patients who came to surgery because of an abnormality of multiple screening, only one patient had cancer. She had an abnormal pelvic examination, CA125 test and ultrasound scan and had a stage IA cancer. The incidence of cancer in this study was 0.02%.

It is now recognized that hereditary ovarian cancer syndrome has three subsets: breast–ovarian, site-specific ovarian and Lynch syndrome II. These three groups characteristically show clusters of cancers in families extending over the last two to four generations. Cancers also appear a decade or so at an earlier age than in the general population. This is thought to be caused by an autosomal dominant inheritance. In one population-based study of approximately 500 ovarian cancers, it was noted that < 7% of these patients gave a family history of ovarian cancer and only one (0.2%) possibly had hereditary ovarian cancer. In a high-risk group of patients in which there was one or more ovarian cancers in a first-degree relative of 391 patients so identified, about three-quarters were found to have no clear inheritance pattern (sporadic). The other one-quarter did appear to have either a multiple-site cancer or site-specific ovarian cancer, but the latter group represented only about 5% of the entire group of high-risk women. Therefore, it would appear that the chance of having genetic-linked ovarian cancer is probably no more than 1–2% of all ovarian cancers.

The question arises that if one is going to screen, who should be screened? According to the *Annual Report*, approximately one-half of all ovarian cancer is identified in women over 60 years of age. In the Campbell group which was self-referred, only 11% of all their patients were in the older age range. Van Nagel restricted his screening to postmenopausal women and, therefore, would have missed about 25% of the cancers. Borne, who evaluated high-risk women with limited screening to this group, missed > 95% of all ovarian cancer. It should be remembered that the chance of developing ovarian cancer, having one relative with ovarian cancer,

is 5%, while the chance of developing breast cancer without any risk factors is 10%.

It is well recognized that the birth control pill can prevent ovarian cancer. As the length of time of pill-taking increases, the risk decreases so that, at 10 years or longer of use, the risk for ovarian cancer is only about 20% of that for individuals not taking the pill. It would appear that the use of the birth control pill may have a greater impact upon the incidence and mortality of ovarian cancer than any screening test yet evaluated or any treatment developed to date.

It is estimated that a test with 100% sensitivity would require a 99.6% specificity to achieve a positive-predictive value of 10%. This would mean, therefore, that nine out of ten surgeries would not identify ovarian cancer. If the specificity drops to 97%, then there would be 75 false-positive results for each ovarian cancer identified. The problem with screening for ovarian cancer, therefore, is numbers. The incidence is low and, to date, there are no screening tests which would come close to giving a 10% positive-predictive value. This in itself is unacceptable. Therefore, unfortunately, it would appear at the present time that there are no available techniques suitable for routine screening of ovarian cancer.

Conclusion

In summary, the benefits of Pap smear screening are unrefutable. The issue that needs to be addressed is better education of patients as to the need of screening and its benefits so that this disease can be prevented and essentially eliminated. Unfortunately, adequate screening techniques have not been developed for ovarian cancer. To suggest to patients that current tests be applied for routine screening is neither prudent nor evidence-based, with a resultant large cost to patients and society as a whole. Hopefully, this will be rectified as our knowledge concerning ovarian cancer is enhanced.

Electronic publishing

9

J. J. Sciarra, L. G. Keith and C. L. Beecher

Historical introduction

Throughout history, the object of medical publishing has been both to record clinical and research observations and to disseminate information. Many of the first medical papers, written in Latin, were proceedings of learned societies. As the need for disseminating medical information became more widespread, medical articles became more common and societies emerged that were specifically devoted to medical specialties. These societies were initially responsible for publishing the majority of medical journals. This remains true today. Medical publishing falls into two categories: medical textbooks and reference books; and scientific journals. This chapter will focus on the latter, since it is in this area that electronic publishing has had the greatest impact.

The first scientific journals, as we know them today, emerged almost simultaneously in Britain and France. The *Journal des Scavans* appeared in 1665 in Paris and, at the same time, the Royal Society of London began to publish *Philosophical Transactions*. Following these examples, Germany also published its first medical journal in the same year. The first medical journal in Russia appeared in 1778 and in Sweden in 1799. In these formative years of medical publishing, editorial quality was not controlled as it is today. During the mid-18th century, a general dissatisfaction with the quality of scientific publication was discussed at the Royal Society of London. Because of this, the Earl of Macclesfield, then President-elect of the Royal Society of London, persuaded his colleagues to form a committee to review all scientific papers prior to their publication in the *Philosophical Transactions*, a procedure that the *Journal des Scavans* in Paris initiated in 1702. Thus, peer review became a standard in

medical publishing that has continued to the present time.

Until the 18th century, the United States, separated physically from England by an ocean, lagged behind Europe in the development of scientific journals. In 1743, however, the American Philosophical Society in Philadelphia was founded by Benjamin Franklin, who, in 1771, played an important role in publishing *Transactions*, a scientific journal in the United States. This publication provided the stimulus to develop additional scientific and medical journals in the United States. *The Medical Repository*, published in 1779, was the first American medical journal, followed in 1809 by the *New York Medical and Philosophical Journal*. The *New England Journal of Medicine*, begun in 1812, continues today as the oldest medical journal continuously published since its inception[1].

During the next two centuries, medical publishing was influenced by a myriad of historical events, medical and surgical innovations and technological advances. One of the most memorable technological advances occurred in the United States in 1893 when, during the Chicago World's Fair, people were able to witness first-hand the latest developments in the field of communication.

If, for example, a writer, while visiting the Chicago World's Fair, wanted to write an article on one of the new inventions, such as the incandescent light bulbs that lit the Fair, the writer could have purchased a ball-point pen with which to take notes. Then, the author could have used a new communication device, the telephone, to call a publisher in New York. If the publisher expressed disbelief about the invention, the writer then could purchase one of the new Kodak cameras available at the Fair, could snap a few pictures of the great hall lit by the new incandescent bulbs and have the photographs developed. The author could type the story using a manual typewriter, and use Gray's new teleautograph to send the story and photos from Chicago to the publisher in New York as proof that the information was indeed true. All of these technologies: the typewriter, teleautograph, Kodak camera, ball-point pen and long-distance telephone connections were available at the 1893 Chicago World's Fair[2]. A communication revolution of this magnitude had not occurred since Gutenberg invented the printing press with movable type in the 15th century. However, few people at that time could have foreseen how these technological innovations would change their lives, or could have imagined the impact that these technological advances would have on medical communication in the 20th century.

Today, just over 100 years later, we are faced with another technological revolution. Once again, it is difficult to anticipate exactly what impact the advent of the Internet, CD-ROM and e-mail will have on the future. However, like the innovations in communication in the late 19th century, it is likely that these innovations will significantly change our lives and our way of communication and publication.

Electronic publishing

Electronic publishing is defined here as any publication that can be read from a computer screen. This includes the Internet, CD-ROM and e-mail publications. Suprisingly, electronic publishing is not a new invention; in 1958, Hans Peter Luhn of Germany first used a computer to create abstracts and indexes of textual works written in the late 1950s. During the next 40 years, numerous advances necessary for producing electronic publications were made, and computer tools were developed to make the successful transition from print-on-paper to electronic publishing.

Computer hardware or software will not be considered here because these items are constantly changing[3,4]. The focus of this chapter will be the advantages and disadvantages of electronic publishing, as well as how this technology will affect the lives and clinical practices of obstetricians and gynecologists, and enhance research in the specialty of obstetrics and gynecology. A variety of presently available electronic products will be discussed.

Historically, medical publishing has involved a tangible object: a textbook or reference book, a journal or a newsletter. Since the advent of computer technology, however, the end results of publishing are not tangible, except in the case of the CD-ROM. Electronic publishing represents a truly new process for transferring information around the world, without paper.

Internet, CD-ROM and e-mail

There are three forms of electronic publishing: the Internet, CD-ROM and e-mail. Each modality has advantages and disadvantages which will be discussed below.

Internet

The Internet is a global communications network that began in 1957 following the launch of the Russian satellite, Sputnik. The Russian achievement prompted the United States to form the Advanced Research Projects Agency (ARPA) within the Department of Defense. The ARPA was charged with developing an interconnected computer network, called the Internet, assuring that the network would not cease if part of it were damaged. The Internet was designed as a network without a central governing body. Because the Internet was an open network, it began to grow. Today, tens of thousands of nodes on the Internet are scattered in virtually all countries; an estimated 25–30 million people world-wide have access to the Internet, and these numbers grow daily[5].

CD-ROM

The CD-ROM (compact disk read–only memory) has many of the same capabilities as the Internet, but has two main differences: (1) a CD-ROM disk has a finite amount of space: although this space is quite large, once it is filled, no more information can be stored on the disk; and (2) a CD-ROM is a tangible object that is manufactured and distributed. The production process does not provide either immediate publishing or global access, as is the case with either the Internet or e-mail. The CD-ROM is likely to be an intermediate step in electronic publishing; much of the information currently available on CD-ROM will probably become available on the Internet or e-mail within the next decade.

E-mail

E-mail, shorthand for electronic mail, dates back to approximately 1969. Like traditional mail services, e-mail is intended to be a private communication between sender and recipient. It is estimated that trillions of e-mail messages are exchanged annually be individuals worldwide. Unlike traditional mail services, e-mail is quick, usually reaching the recipient's computer, anywhere in the world, within minutes. E-mail requires no stamps or envelopes and multiple copies of the same message can be distributed with little effort or expense. In fact, the recipient of the message need not be at home to receive e-mail; the person can retrieve e-mail from anywhere in the world with a computer and telephone line.

Recently, the security of e-mail messages has been a concern. Eavesdropping on an e-mail message as it is in transit is possible, although somewhat difficult. Also, a sender can easily impersonate another sender and, thus, confuse the recipient. Despite these pitfalls, e-mail provides a unique way to quickly and efficiently communicate with a vast number of people around the world.

Change to electronic publishing

The transition from traditional paper publication to electronic publishing will take time. Although the technology is rapidly being developed and refined, those involved in the publishing industry, as well as editors, authors and the subscribers to scientific journals, must undergo changes in their thinking, expectations and behaviors.

In traditional publishing, a book, like a fetus in the uterus, usually undergoes a 9-month gestation period. The publishing process moves in a predictable linear sequence from manuscript to copyediting, design, typesetting, proofreading, indexing, printing and binding, and then distribution through traditional channels. Along the way, each person has a clearly defined job to perform.

During the past decade, electronic publishing has brought about decentralization in the publishing process and faster production schedules. This has meant that book publishing has developed a parallel processing mode, whereby copyediting, design, typesetting, proofreading and indexing may be performed simultaneously by the same person. As a result, the publisher's role has moved from typesetting and page layout, now easily accomplished by the author on the computer, to the organization and management of the publication process.

Concepts of electronic publishing

The differentiation of electronic publishing from paper publishing in most instances rests on four fundamental concepts. Electronic publishing is:

(1) Immediate;

(2) Global;

(3) Interactive;

(4) Multimedia.

Immediacy

In theory, an author can immediately publish his manuscript by posting it on the Internet. However, this new capability raises the question of whether this process is indeed publishing at all. A recent comment from the *New England Journal of Medicine* provides insight on this issue[5]. The *New England Journal of Medicine* recently announced that a manuscript posted on the Internet is equivalent to prior publication and, therefore, is ineligible for submission to the *New England Journal of Medicine*. Such a policy clearly acknowledges that the Internet is a legitimate venue for publication, but it leads directly to two important questions. First, how is editorial content regulated in an electronic medium? Second, how is peer review accomplished in this new publishing environment?

Regulation   As the Internet is not owned or regulated by any agency, no one is responsible for the quality of the information that is published on the Internet. As a result, many people view the editorial content of articles on the Internet with skepticism. One must travel with caution on the Internet. Anyone who has computer 'savvy' can appear to be a medical authority by designing an impressive looking Internet site. Thus, a publisher offering information that is false or biased may appear as prominent as, or even more prominent than, the most reputable information source. Concern over medical misinformation has prompted the US Food and Drug Administration (FDA) to consider regulating medical information that is disseminated over the Internet. Although publishing medical information in a textbook or journal is time-consuming and expensive, this traditional method of publishing has served as a gatekeeper for the flow of medical information to healthcare professionals and the public. The publisher has supported this gatekeeper function by recruiting reputable authors and editors. Publishers also can control the subject matter of books and journals by choosing whether or not to publish a particular book or journal. Although some Internet readers may be cautious about the source and validity of electronically available information, an audience unfamiliar with the rigors of the scientific method and the peer review process may not be as critical. Regulation of scientific information on the Internet is a significant problem.

Peer review   Many of the on-line scholarly journals are merely electronic versions of the paper journals. For these journals, the peer-review process has not changed; but how is the peer-review process handled by the growing number of journals that operate solely in an electronic environment?

Peer review is the process aimed at making a publication reflective of the peer community, not the editor's individual preferences and scope of knowledge. The traditional implementation of peer review is as follows:

(1) The editor receives a manuscript;

(2) The editor selects reviewers for the manuscript from a preselected review board;

(3) The reviewers make recommendations about whether the editor should accept the manuscript, reject it or ask for revisions from the author.

The peer-review process is usually anonymous and the reviewers are not known to the author. This method of peer review is somewhat cumbersome and involves the opinions and thoughts of a few individuals.

Electronic publishing raises a number of problems and questions with regard to traditional peer review. Since electronic publishing is global, theoretically, a working paper can be posted and an open forum created for peer commentary on the manuscript. In such a manner, the manuscript can receive immediate comment by all individuals interested in the subject. Even with an open forum, it is still possible to maintain anonymity for both the author and the reviewers, through computer programming. This method of peer review, theoretically, would make the manuscript truly reflective of the global peer community, and establish a rapid, collective, interactive process that is unattainable in any other medium[6].

There are, however, practical drawbacks to electronic peer review. For example, theft of scientific material is easily possible. One way to avoid this problem would be to have a secure area for review that would require a person interested in reviewing submitted manuscripts to apply to be a reviewer. This reviewer could be issued a code name or number by which all their comments would be listed. This way, anonymity would be preserved.

Global aspect

The global access of electronic publishing is a remarkable feature. With electronic publishing, publishers can achieve world-wide distribution of their products with little cost. Also, the global aspect of e-mail allows individuals to communicate with others around the world quickly and easily at a fraction of what it would cost to communicate the same information by telephone or fax.

Interactivity

Electronic publishing allows interactivity among individuals, but it offers much more. For example, users no longer sit passively in front of a book and read in a linear fashion from the beginning to the middle to the end. Electronic publishing allows users to actively direct their thoughts and reading paths in whatever direction they choose. The linear thought process of beginning, middle and end is no longer required. Instead, while viewing an electronic document, the reader may experience the beginning of several ideas or subjects, choose to conclude with one subject before returning to the middle of another or not choose to reach the end of a subject. The choice depends on the interests of the reader.

Multimedia capabilities

The reader's thought process can be affected by the multimedia capabilities of electronic publishing. Anything than can be captured electronically, such as words, diagrams, photographs or sounds, can be incorporated into an electronic document. Also, color can be added to an electronic document with no additional cost. With electronic publishing, the reader, no longer just reading words and forming pictures in his or her imagination, can actually hear the sound and view the image. For example, with only a printed description of laparoscopic sterilization, the reader would have only the words of the author to create a mental image which may or may not be accurate. With electronic publishing, however, it is possible to read the author's description while viewing a video of the surgery through the laparoscope and simultaneously listening to the surgeon, thus having a clear picture of what is being conveyed. The multimedia capabilities of electronic publishing are also useful in describing diagnostic tests such as ultrasound, magnetic resonance imaging (MRI) and computer assisted tomography (CAT) scans.

The interactivity and multimedia capability of electronic publishing have pitfalls. Without proper organization and planning, a reader, taking a link to another site, may not return to finish the original document. Therefore, planning is the key to the successful use of electronic publishing.

As electronic publishing gains ascendancy, traditional publishers may lose some of their control as the gatekeepers of medical information, but they will gain greater distribution of their products. Without question, in the next century, publishers will need to incorporate electronic publishing into their publication process. Many publishing companies are already doing this.

Electronic resources for obstetricians/gynecologists

There are many electronic resources for obstetricians and gynecologists, among them MEDLINE access, electronic journals, electronic textbooks and e-mail discussion groups. More information about some of the electronic resources listed below can be found in the 'Appendices' to this chapter.

Many universities provide MEDLINE access at no charge to faculty and staff members. Also, MEDLINE can be accessed electronically through the US National Library of Medicine (NLM) at no cost.

Many textbooks and reference books for the specialty of obstetrics and gynecology are being distributed electronically in the form of CD-ROM. These new electronic forms are not mere reproductions of the paper textbook, but have added features. For example, the CD-ROM version of the Sciarra loose-leaf series, *Gynecology and Obstetrics*, incorporates multimedia and also has MEDLINE abstracts and citations from 21 of the world's leading journals over the past 5 years.

Many electronic publications allow obstetricians and gynecologists to earn continuing medical education (CME) credits at home at their own pace. One such learning tool produced by the Royal College of Obstetricians and Gynaecologists (RCOG) is a CD-ROM program entitled DIALOG. DIALOG is a distance learning program worth 30 RCOG CME credits per year. DIALOG contains 50 fully interactive case studies based on real-life clinical scenarios per CD-ROM. These scenarios are supported by fully interactive color images, video and audio clips, and cover general obstetrics, general gynecology, fetal and maternal medicine, reproductive medicine, urogynecology and gynecological oncology.

Many journals, such as *Fertility and Sterility*, the *American Journal of Obstetrics and Gynecology*, *Obstetrics and Gynecology*, the *European Journal of Obstetrics and Gynecology* and the *International Journal of Gynecology and Obstetrics*, have web sites containing general information about the journal, such as the table of contents for past issues, subscription information and instructions to authors. The *American Journal of Obstetrics and Gynecology* has produced a searchable CD-ROM containing full journal articles from 1994 to 1995 that can be ordered from their web site. Also of note is the web site for *Obstetrics and Gynecology*. *Obstetrics and Gynecology* has developed a new section of their web site whereby manuscript reviewers can review manuscripts and submit their comments over the Internet. This new section is password-restricted and, therefore, can be accessed only by a reviewer after obtaining a password.

In addition to electronic journals and textbooks, there are e-mail discussion groups for obstetricians and gynecologists. These discussion groups usually have a specific topic that is discussed. Some of the topics include general obstetrics, gynecological oncology and reproductive endocrinology. These discussion groups are a good way to stay abreast of current medical information as well as to see how other colleagues world-wide are managing patients.

Electronic resources for health professionals

In 1994, the United States National Information Infrastructure Interagency Task Force stated that the health sector lagged 'far behind the other sectors of our economy in applying information and communication technologies'. In contrast, the importance of the Internet as a way to disseminate the exchange of information is now clearly recognized by both governmental and non-governmental organizations. The National Institutes of Health, the National Cancer Institute, the National Library of Medicine, the Center for Disease Control and the Food and Drug Administration in the United States, and the World Health Organization in Geneva, Switzerland are just a few of the organizations that use the Internet to publish vast amounts of up-to-date health-related information.

Various electronic publications of interest to practicing obstetricians and gynecologists are contained in the 'Appendices'. These 'Appendices', although by no means a complete listing of all electronic resources available to obstetricians and gynecologists, list the major publications, resources and societies in our specialty at the time of this publication, and can be used as a staring point for persons wishing to search for electronic resources.

Role of health-care providers

Obstetricians and gynecologists of the future will need to learn how to utilize these new forms of electronic communication and implement them in clinical practice and research. In this regard, it is important that physicians take an integral role in the development and creation of medically accurate electronic publications, since most electronic material is available to everyone throughout the world. Accordingly, we as clinicians also need to educate the public on the peer-review process and to instruct them on how to distinguish reliable medical information from bogus information.

The future: XVI FIGO World Congress

At the FIGO World Congress in the year 2000 in Washington, DC in the United States, announcements regarding the Congress could be sent to individuals by e-mail, registration could be submitted through the Internet, session chairs and co-chairs could co-ordinate their efforts by utilizing e-mail, outlines and manuscripts could be submitted to the Secretariat by e-mail, the final program could be sent to individuals by an e-mail newsletter and the proceedings of the Congress and abstract book could be electronically published over the Internet or be produced on CD-ROM. By utilizing electronic media, it would be possible for the XVI FIGO World Congress to be virtually paperless. Although this concept may be too advanced for many individuals and is unlikely to come to fruition in the next 3 years, an electronically enhanced FIGO World Congress is in the future – if not in the year 2000, in the next century.

Conclusion

It is possible today for obstetricians and gynecologists to begin implementing and utilizing electronic publishing and electronic communications in their own practice. Electronic publishing is immediate, global, interactive and multimedia-capable, making it possible to disseminate complex information quickly and efficiently to obstetricians, gynecologists and other women's health-care professionals throughout the world. This efficient and relatively inexpensive communication modality is an important step in advancing the specialty of obstetrics and gynecology and improving women's health world-wide.

Appendix A

Internet resources as of 20 May 1997

American College of Obstetricians and Gynecologists
http://www.acog.com

American Journal of Obstetrics and Gynecology
http://www.mosby.com/Mosby/Periodicals/medical/AJOG/ob.html

Centers for Disease Control
http://www.cdc.gov

CME on the Net: Specialty Categorized
http://www.execpc.com/~msmc/special.html

European Journal of Obstetrics and Gynecology and Reproductive Biology
http://www.elsevier.nl/inca/publications/store/5/0/5/9/6/1/505961.pub.shtml

Fertility and Sterility
http://www.asrm.com/profession/fertility/fspage.html

Food and Drug Administration
http://www.fda.gov

ICD-9-CM International Classification of Diseases
http://econ-www.newcastle.edu.au/hsrg/hypertexts/icd9cm.html

International Journal of Gynecology and Obstetrics
http://www.elsevier.nl/inca/publications/store/5/0/6/0/3/7/506037.pub.shtml

Medical Matrix
http://www.slackinc.com/matrix/

Medweb Clinical Practice
http://www.cc.emory.edu/WHSCL/medweb.clinical.html

Medweb Oncology
http://www.cc.emory.edu/WHSCL/medweb.oncology.html

National Institute of Environmental Health Sciences
http://www.niehs.nih.gov

National Institutes of Health
http://www.nih.gov

National Library of Medicine
http://www.nlm.nih.gov

New England Journal of Medicine
http://www.nejm.org

Obstetrics and Gynecology
http://www-east.elsevier.com/ong/Menu.html

OncoLink (University of Pennsylvania Cancer Center)
http://www.oncolink.upenn.edu/

Royal College of Obstetrics and Gynecology
http://www.rcog.org.uk

Society of Obstetricians and Gynecologists of Canada
http://www.medical.org

World Health Organization
http://www.who.ch/

Appendix B

CD-ROM resources (1997)

Subscriptions to the Royal College of Obstetricians and Gynaecologists' DIALOG (Distance InterActive Learning in Obstetrics and Gynaecology) are available at Noor Informatics Ltd, Wadbrough Road, Sheffield S11 8RG, UK; Fax: +44 (0) 114 243 0613.

The following CD-ROM materials are available through the Parthenon Publishing Group in the United States at One Blue Hill Plaza, PO Box 1564, Pearl River, New York, NY 10965, USA; Telephone: 914-735-9363; Fax: 914-735-1385; or in the UK at Casterton Hall, Carnforth, Lancashire LA6 2LA, UK; Telephone: 015242 72084; Fax: 015242 71587.

(1)   The Anatomy Project on CD-ROM;

(2)   The Reproductive System and Pelvis;

(3)   Basic Human Anatomy: Nomenclature, Systems and Tissues.

Or you may visit their Internet site at http://www.parthpub.com

The following CD-ROM materials are available through Lippincott-Raven Publishers, PO Box 1600, Hagerstown, MD 21741-1600, USA; Telephone: 301-714-2300; Fax: 301-824-7390; e-mail: lroders@phl.lrpub.com.

(1) Gynecology and Obstetrics;

(2) Comprehensive Review of Endometriosis;

(3) Laparoscopic Hysterectomy;

(4) The Complete Interactive Guide to Your Pregnancy;

(5) 1996 Interactive Review of Obstetrics and Gynecology;

(6) Anatomy of the Female Pelvis;

(7) Urogynecology: Evaluation and Treatment of Urinary Incontinence.

Appendix C

E-mail lists as of 20 May 1997

OB-GYN-L: Obstetrician–Gynecologist Mail List
    subscription address: listserv@bcm.tmc.edu
    subscription message: subscribe ob-gyn-l <your name>
    discussion topics include practices, research, interesting patients and lifestyle

GYN-DOCS: Gynecology Discussion Group
    subscription address: majordomo@oac1.oac.tju.edu
    subscription message: subscribe gyn-docs [address]
    discussion of general and subspecialty topics in gynecology

REPRENDO: Reproductive Endocrinology
    subscription address: listserv@umab.umd.edu
    subscription message: subscribe reprendo <your name>
    this mailing list is for medical professions interested in reproductive endocrinology

Continuing Medical Education (CME) Mail List
    subscription address: listserv@listerv.net
    subscription message:subscribe CME-L
    notifies physician users of CME sites

References

1. Booth, C. C. (1990). The origin and growth of medical journals. *Ann. Intern. Med.,* **113**(5), 398–402

2. Heyn, E. V. (1992). *A Century of Wonders.* (New York, NY: Doubleday)

3. Smith, R. P. and Edwards, M. J. A. (eds.) (1990). *The Internet for Physicians.* (New York, NY: Springer-Verlag)

4. Pareras, L. G. (1996). *Medicine and the Internet.* (New York, NY: Little, Brown and Co.)

5. Benjamin, I. (1997). The Internet: an introduction to cyberspace for the obstetrician–gynecologist. *Contemp. Obstet. Gynecol.,* **42**, 30–50

6. Peek, R. P. and Newby, G. B. (eds.) (1996). *Scholarly Publishing: the Electronic Frontier.* (Cambridge, MA: The MIT Press)

Telemedicine in gynecology and obstetrics in France

10

H. J. Philippe and C. Brunel

Progress in medicine should be sought only together with improved care. Politicians talk about controlling the costs of medical care, and lawyers make much fuss about medical complications, implying that medical care should be perfect. The two new goals of doctors have become saving money and avoiding lawsuits. Contrary to all expectations, medicine has improved under these two constraints (economic and legal). Telemedicine is one of the methods that can reduce health-care costs. It probably also improves the quality of care by expanding access to specialists and dissemination of information, and in developing networked medical practices.

What is telemedicine?

There are two types of telemedicine:

(1) Between patient and doctor, who are physically distant from one another and communicate by various means including telephone or fax. This is a form of medical practice from which clinical examination is, of course, missing. Genetic consultations, on the other hand, can sometimes take place this way.

(2) Between health-care professionals, involving collaboration between practitioners in the same or different specialties. In fact, improvements in means of communication and in the kinds of data that can be transmitted have led to another concept, that of 'telemedical' services. These can be divided into three categories: teleconsultation (diagnosis, treatment or surveillance), telemedical continuing education (video-phones, videoconferences, image banks or clinical cases) and collaborative remote evaluations. Teleconsultation can be a real remote consultation, or telesurveillance (that is, remote monitoring) or treatment at a distance (remote surgery, which is currently still fiction). It can also be a remote specialist referral (for diagnosis or treatment advice). Teletraining includes all the methods and services useful for developing continuing education at a distance by various means of telecommunication. The principal objective is the interactive diffusion of knowledge to many sites. 'Tele-evaluation' is intended to allow medical information to be shared towards the end of assessing the efficacy of medical practices. It requires a common language embodied by a shared medical chart.

Why telemedicine?

Telemedicine's role will depend on various aspects within the health-care system (including medical demography, hospital equipment, geographical distribution and means of communication) and the type of disorder. In France, the geographical distribution of gynecologist–obstetricians is unbalanced, but there are currently enough practitioners overall; none the less, there will be a shortage in several years. Seventy new specialists complete training annually, while between 400 and 800 will retire in the next 5–10 years. Maternity hospitals will probably be consolidated or merged in order to assure treatment of obstetric emergencies. None the less, there are institutions with varying equipment levels, requiring a network of collaboration. Moreover, the number of maternity hospitals with a neonatal intensive-care unit is decreasing; fewer pediatricians are willing to work schedules that include weekend and night on-call coverage, perhaps related to the increasing percentage of women specializing in pediatrics.

In France, midwives play an important role in monitoring pregnancies in both normal and difficult deliveries. In some situations they need to consult physicians. Telemedicine could be important in these situations. Anesthesiologists and obstetricians are co-operating ever more closely concerning anesthesia and the management of problem pregnancies; in many departments anesthesiologists also take on the role of the internist. The percentage of births with peridural analgesia averages 33% in France and reaches 85% in some departments. Again, all of this justifies the need to establish facilities of different levels that function as a network. Hospital equipment is not uniform; until now, it has depended upon the choices made by departmental heads in each hospital. Certainly the reorganization of the health-care system and the creation of regional health agencies will affect this distribution. Each kind of major new equipment (ultrasonic scanners, high-frequency respirators or cytogenetic laboratory) will be debated at a regional level from now on. It will therefore be necessary to define the facilities intended for treatment of pregnant women with different risk levels.

The distance between maternity hospitals is not a priority problem except sometimes in winter, when roads can be blocked and transportation is difficult. Some of these hospitals are, incidentally, small, minimally equipped and have small numbers of staff. In such circumstances, their survival can only be planned within a system of close liaison with larger institutions. Economic constraints stimulate both health-policy makers and doctors to make investment decisions that are within their means.

The value of telemedicine varies substantially according to the type of disorder. Its general objective is to improve overall access to useful information for health-care teams, regardless of their geographical situation or of the time of day. It allows medical specialists to work within networks and, therefore, concerns most particularly those specialties that deal with emergencies, such as obstetrics, and those dealing with a broad range of procedures, such as gynecology–obstetrics (with its four subspecialties: gynecological oncology, fetal medicine, reproductive medicine and urogynecology). To illustrate these points, the role of telemedicine in perinatal medicine will be analyzed.

The principal areas of application are maternal and perinatal emergencies and antenatal diagnosis. Some maternal emergencies can justify transfer to units that are better equipped or have more highly specialized staff (radiologists for embolizations, emergency specialists, nephrologists or cardiologists). In these situations, detailed discussion allows the manner and moment of transfer to be decided. Similarly, it is certain that in some situations, the fetus benefits by an *in utero* transfer. Most often, the transfer is not carried out on an emergency basis, but telecommunications allow the file to be transmitted as well as direct contact between the two treatment teams and, in some cases, with the mother-to-be.

Sometimes, as when fetal cardiac monitoring reveals anomalies, emergency transfer may be considered, by means which include helicopters. In other situations, telemedicine can help prevent transfers that are either dangerous or useless. In antenatal diagnosis, the tools of telemedicine allow experts in fetal medicine to be consulted about the ultrasonographic image or the appropriate management. Moreover, this can be done both rapidly and without transferring the patient, thereby reducing the anxiety related to repeated consultations and to delay before a definitive recommendation.

Moreover, the use of telemedicine in perinatology should help improve perinatal outcome. The levels of success have been only moderate, which may be explained by several factors, including most notably the absence of any network in most regions and competition between public and private sectors that should be complementary. For example, only 15–20% of infants weighing less than 1500 g are born in maternity hospitals with neonatal intensive-care units. In other European countries, this figure reaches 80%.

In summary, telemedicine is the tool that allows medical expertise to be put into networks and thereby multiplied. Knowledge can no longer be the exclusive property of a single person. The primary benefit is related to the continuity of care by the treating physician.

How is a telemedicine network established?

Setting up a telemedicine network will depend on which services are given the highest priority: consultation, education or evaluation. The investment is sufficiently high that these three functions optimally should be exploited simultaneously but also that these tools be available to other departments. If only a single area were considered, this method would require a cost–benefit analysis, since neither the costs nor the benefits have been assessed in France.

Establishing a telemedicine network requires determination of the issues, participants, general organization, equipment, type of data and documents to be transmitted, software for managing the documents and the images, and the transmission system and route.

Participants

The participants in a telemedicine network depend on its objectives. In perinatal medicine, general practitioners and gynecologists monitor pregnant women until the sixth month, and thereafter care providers include centers for the protection of mothers and infants (PMI) centers (which include midwives, obstetricians and pediatricians), private obstetrician–gynecologists, mobile units or emergency medical services (SAMU), clinics, general hospitals, referring departments and university hospital departments. Each of these should be able to contact a reference person for advice or transfer, or to set up

particular monitoring for or gather data about all the pregnant women in the network. Such data charts include the mother–child pair.

General organization

Facilities In theory, each participant should be able to be linked to the others. A multipoint unit allows videoconferencing when desired. There should also be a central unit that administers the common information from shared files, a data bank and clinical cases containing reference images for training.

Functioning Functioning requires a project director who brings together within the network all the institutions favorable to the project, and then organizes the stand-by duty schedules for remote examinations and consultants, the videoconferences and regular assessments of the network's functioning (number of transfers, number of recommendations, progression of the pregnancies, concordance of pre- and postnatal diagnoses, development of medical interventions and change in perinatal indicators). Facilities participating in the project must fulfill certain 'demands':

(1) Real participation (that is, there must be at least a tacit moral and legal contract and an understanding about the management of communications among different participants);

(2) A minimum shared file must exist and, if possible, be accessible by all (while respecting the confidentiality of the information).

Equipment (with cost of use and maintenance)

Personal computer It is possible to use a personal computer with a video capture card, 'meet-me' type communication software and a camera. The images can thus be digitized and then transmitted to or received from another system. The screen size determines the number of participants, two or three at most. This equipment costs approximately 15 000 fr.

Videoconference unit The system is the same but the screen quality and computer capacity allow participation by more people and more direct interaction with the remote expert. This equipment costs 200 000 fr.

Videoconference room This is a conference room where an image transmission system has been installed together with all of the image capture systems: camera, videocassette recorder, slides, scanner and microscope.

Type of data and documents transmitted

Any kind of document can be transmitted. Files are transmitted as computer files. The sound or video documents must first be digitized and then compressed, with help from an encoding–decoding device (CODEC).

Transmission system

Numéris (ISDN) Transmission by Numéris (the French equivalent of Integrated Services Digital Network (ISDN) lines in the US and 64 kbit transmission lines in the UK) resembles telephone communication and begins by dialing the other party's ISDN number. The constraint is technical: the quality of the transmission is directly related to the number of lines. With a line at 128 kbit/s (equivalent to two channels), the transmission of still images is excellent, but moving images (ultrasound, video or conference) require three lines for a rate of 384/kbit/s. Both the number of installed lines and the cost of communications thus increase. This transmission system allows communication between two facilities and is most often used for requesting opinions and recommendations. For videoconferences, it is often more useful to have more than two facilities involved. In this case, each participant interested in the video-conference must be connected to a multipoint bridge that allows a connection between all of the participants. This equipment includes installation of a Numéris line and a monthly charge of 300 fr.

Communication costs depend on distance (72 fr./h if < 5 km to 265 fr./h at distances between 50 and 100 km). Multipoint communication, that is between several sites, includes a surcharge of 180 fr./h

Internet Since there are currently at least 30 million Internauts (as Internet users are evocatively known in French), this network is of obvious interest. Connection costs can easily be reduced by connecting through an Internet service provider (ISP), if possible, geographically close to the medical facility. A standard telephone line is sufficient. None the less, the quality of transmission depends directly on the network's load, especially for moving images. Problems of Internet access and load disappear if the same computer network is used without connecting to the Internet – a system called Intranet.

What are the risks of telemedicine?

These risks are the same as those incurred by remote telephone consultations. The expert may err. Responsibility – and liability – remain with the professional in direct contact with the patient; it is this professional who may be blamed for not consulting an expert about a medical problem with which the attending physician or caregiver had insufficient experience. In France, to avoid complicating the distribution of liability, it has been decided that the experts consulted are not remunerated.

How can telemedicine be evaluated?

These new tools require assessment of their effect. The quality of the relationship between doctor and patient, and between doctors and expert specialists, the quality of the images transmitted, the medical results and, finally, the balance sheet can be evaluated.

What are the limits of telemedicine?

Clearly, a direct relationship between the doctor and the patient must be preserved. Confidence between these two partners has a major role in recovery. Teletransmission-assisted medical practice entails a risk of losing this contact and of losing information because of poor quality or patchy transmission. These three reasons could negatively affect the quality of care.

On the other hand, a doctor or surgeon treating, alone, a disorder he or she has not often encountered, can also entail a risk for the patient. Transfer is a solution with three disadvantages: the delay attached; loss of contact with the attending physician; and the cost linked to transfer, to travel and to the new consultation.

The solution offered by telemedicine is possible only if the attending physician remains the only person responsible to and for the patient. In such a case, contact between doctor and patient is preserved, and the attending physician has every motivation to provide the expert with the maximum amount of information, so that the recommendation is most appropriate to the patient's situation.

Considering the possibility of remote surgery, a large proportion of current surgery is performed by endoscopy; the surgeon operates by monitoring his gestures on the screen and by the feeling of contact with the organs involved. It can easily be imaged that an inexperienced surgeon might, then, appropriately position the surgical and optical instruments that will allow imaging of the abdominal cavity; from a distance, the expert may manipulate the instruments, viewing his movements and monitoring them by telemanipulators. Indeed, telementoring, where the more experienced surgeon supervises from a distance and is able to intervene, is already happening in some hospitals.

Acknowledgements

The author wishes to thank the members of the 'Telemedicine and perinatal medicine' Group, Hospitals Division, Ministry of Labor and Social Affairs, for their contributions to the French guidelines for projects in telemedicine.

Bibliography

Bashshur, R. L. (1995). Telemedicine: cost, quality and access. *J. Med. Syst.*, **19**, 2

Casey, F., Brown, D., Craig, B. G. and Rogers, J. (1996). Diagnosis of neonatal congenital heart defects by remote consultation using a low cost telemedicine link. *J. Telemed. Telecare*, **2** (3), 165–9

Cunningham, T. and Bartlett, K. (1990). Integrated telematic support for paediatrics: a practical model. *Arch. Dis. Child.*, **65**, 238–40

Debra, N., Kundel, H. L., Arenson, R. L. and Seshadri, S. B. (1996). Effect of a digital imaging network on physician behavior in an intensive care unit. *J. Telemed. Telecare*, **2** (2), 71–80

Eichelberg, M., Hewett, A. and Jensch, P. (1996). Retain – an ATM pilot project for applications in health care. *J. Telemed. Telecare*, **2** (1), 13–16

Fisk, N. M. L., Sepulveda, W. and Drysdale, K. (1996). Fetal telemedicine: six months pilot of realtime ultrasound and video consultation between the Isle of Wight and London. *Br. J. Obstet. Gynaecol.*, **103**, 1092–5

Forbes-Dewey, C., Thomas, J. D., Murat, K. and Hunter, I. W. (1996). Prospects for telediagnosis using ultrasound. *J. Telemed. Telecare*, **2** (2), 87–90

Franken, E. and Berbaum, K. S. (1996). Subspeciality radiology consultation by interactive telemedicine. *J. Telemed. Telecare*, **2** (1), 35–41

Gardy, M. (1996). Telemedicine and economic realities. *J. Telemed. Telecare*, **2** (2) 83–6

Nesbitt, T. S. (1996). Rural maternity care: a new model of access. *Birth*, **23**, 161–5

Puskin, D. S. (1995). Opportunities and challenges to telemedicine in rural America. *J. Med. Syst.*, **19**, 1

Richardson, R. J., Goldberg, M. A., Sharif, H. S. and Matthew, D. (1996). Implementing global telemedicine: experience with 1097 cases from the Middle East to the USA. *J. Telemed. Telecare*, **2** (1), 79–81

Satava, R. M. and Jones, S. B. (1996). Virtual reality and telemedicine: exploring advanced concepts. *J. Telemed. Telecare*, **2** (3), 195–200

Smits, H. L. and Baum, A. (1995). Health care financing administration and reimbursement in telemedicine. *J. Med. Syst.*, **19**, 2

Tachakra, S., Mullett, S. T. H., Freij, R. and Sivakumar, A. (1996). Confidentiality and ethics in telemedicine. *J. Telemed. Telecare*, **2** (1), 68–71

New technology in gynecological endoscopy

11

M. A. Bruhat

Surgical endoscopy is a new technology, started in 1940 in Paris by Raoul Palmer. Conceived in the field of gynecology, it was destined to revolutionize surgery in general by introducing the concept of minimally invasive surgery. It is, moreover, an excellent example of the eruption of a new method of treatment in an area of classic therapeutic possibilities, with all the problems that implies.

New technology

Endoscopy provides a new way of looking at surgery: it is not just a different way of doing the same thing. It is a completely different approach for the following reasons:

(1) The new operating theatre is the pelvis, with all the constraints this brings, of course. The instruments are small in diameter, multiple ports are needed and the field of vision and movement is limited, requiring the use of gas or laparolifts. However, there are also advantages, such as the absence of any opening in the abdominal wall and no desiccation or air-borne contamination.

(2) The anatomy and physiology are respected thanks to the magnification afforded by the optics systems, the microinstruments which ensure precise surgical gestures and the necessity of adequate vision meaning that permanent hemostasis is required.

(3) Unexpected results, both from the point of view of organ reactions, such as spontaneous healing of the tube which was a surprise after the description of our method for treatment of ectopic preg-

nancy, or the effects on therapeutic strategy, underline the advantages of initial lymphadenectomy for cancer of the uterus.

(4) The therapeutic sequence during the same anesthesia is diagnosis, establishment of the prognosis and completion with surgical treatment.

However, the essential values of surgery must not be forgotten, because endoscopic surgery is a true surgery and, as such, must remain simple, elegant and sparing.

New surgery

Endoscopy now covers the whole field of gynecological surgery, including the following.

Adnexal surgery

Since we described the technique of surgical treatment in 1973, it has become the 'milestone' for treatment of tubal pregnancy. Tubal infertility caused by adhesions or obstruction is the favored application for operative endoscopy. The diagnosis and present-day treatment of ovarian cysts are founded on this surgical approach, but with one problem still remaining, i.e. peritoneal reactivity to physical and pathological aggression, which is the subject of clinical research. The diagnosis, pathogenesis and treatment of endometriosis have been revolutionized by this surgery. There are a number of other operative indications which have been completely changed by the endoscopic technique, such as adnexal torsion, pelvic inflammatory disease (PID) or pelvic pain.

Hysterectomy

Hysterectomy is such a symbolic operation for the gynecologist and still the subject of heated discussion, but our series of 1000 cases operated over the past 6 years using the technique of endoscopy should be noted.

Final frontiers

Cancer The second look for ovarian cancers was the first positive contribution of the technique to cancer surgery. Radical hysterectomy by laparoscopy was first carried out in 1989, and has shown just how radical the technique is. There is also the strategic advantage of lymphadenectomy which can even be proposed in the pretreatment work-up.

Prolapse This condition is now also treated by endoscopic surgery. Bladder-neck suspension using the Burch technique is now an everyday procedure with the same efficiency as other routes. However, all techniques of support or reinforcement of the vaginal walls (vaginal repair) must still be considered.

Taking into account these various positive effects, each major field of pathology can benefit from endoscopic surgery, whether for the operative technique or the strategic approach to treatment.

New assessment

This surgery must be subjected to a new assessment because its eruption into the field of traditional surgery means that all the aspects need to be evaluated in very little time.

Complications

These cannot be assessed by simply listing the possible complications; a large number of articles indeed have already been written. Sufficiently long series carried out by adequately trained teams are needed so that the complications specific to this technique can be recognized. However, problems which are due to insufficient knowledge of the method or faulty training are not complications.

Training

Laparoscopic surgery is a true surgery. Training is required and this cannot be achieved by simply watching a few videos or practicing for a few days on a pelvic trainer or animal tissues. Lengthy training is necessary to produce a team which knows the method and possesses all the other techniques of gynecological surgery.

Results

The results of this surgery need to be assessed by comparative series, without involving the approach to the pathology itself. For example, any study of ectopic pregnancy needs to integrate the means currently available for early diagnosis. In the field of infertility surgery, the place for endouterine means of assessment needs to be recognized. Surgery for endometriosis will need to take into account the current lack of knowledge concerning the physiopathology of this disease. Hysterectomies will need to be differentiated into hysterectomies on large uteri and those on normal uteri, and into hysterectomies with and hysterectomies without prolapse. Cancer surgery study will need to draw the distinction between what should be classed as endoscopic surgery and what is oncology itself. The extent of lymphadenectomy must be made clearer before the advantages of laparoscopy can be discussed. And finally, any study of prolapse surgery needs to take into account the physiopathology of prolapse.

The costs

A clear distinction should be made between the cost of the endoscopic surgery itself with the acquisition of the basic equipment needed to carry it out, and the optional cost of sophisticated instruments which are often associated with this surgery: the purchase of lasers is expensive, of course; automatic tools (stapler, clip) also increase the cost of this surgery. They are not, perhaps, always needed. Bipolar coagualtion, for example, is good enough for hemostasis in a great many cases.

Assessment of this surgery from the point of view of efficiency, cost and training must be based on what truly is required and other, more circumstantial aspects should be disregarded.

New techniques help evolution

Endoscopic surgery must always obey the rules, but it will certainly evolve considerably with all the progress made in technology. Its recent history has shown this, and the future will provide further confirmation.

Importance of imaging

Imaging is important whether the images concerned are sensitized images using fluorescence and certain wavelengths for neoplastic metastases, or images of endometriosis on the peritoneum, for example. Enhanced reality uses images made earlier to help during actual surgery. Virtual reality will make it possible to try out various surgical hypotheses or develop training on machines using robotics and the computer. This technique also makes remote operations or assistance with operations possible.

Microendoscopy

This technique, using diameters of 2 mm or less, will enable the diagnostic part of endoscopy to be reviewed and perhaps permit its use without anesthesia but simple sedation instead.

Multi-purpose instruments

These will reduce the number of trocars and avoid over-frequent insertion and removal of the surgeon's instruments during operations.

Gas

The study of gas and the peritoneal environment will bring new knowledge concerning modifications of temperature, pH, lighting and peritoneal reactivity to these physical aggressions.

Anesthetics

The new anesthetic techniques take into account modifications of the internal environment due to the eruption of pneumoperitoneal gases or the uterine dilation liquids such as glycine; modifications in cardiovascular, thoracic or circulatory pressures explain incidents of oliguria in certain long anesthesias; the new gases may perhaps avoid modifications of the internal environment and hypercapnia.

In summary, it appears that a revolution in treatments has only just started to develop.

Intracytoplasmic sperm injection

12

A. De Vos and A. Van Steirteghem

Introduction

In 1992, our group reported the first pregnancies and births to result from replacement of embryos generated by a novel procedure of assisted fertilization, known as intracytoplasmic sperm injection (ICSI), which involves injection of a single spermatozoon through the zona pellucida directly into the oocyte[1]. Soon after this report, it became obvious that ICSI resulted in higher fertilization rates and more embryos with higher implantation rates than did subzonal insemination (SUZI), in which several motile spermatozoa are injected through the zona pellucida into the perivitelline space[2,3]. Since then, ICSI has been introduced into clinical practice to treat couples with severe male-factor infertility, who cannot be helped with conventional *in vitro* fertilization (IVF) because they have an insufficient number of progressively motile spermatozoa with normal morphology available to achieve successful fertilization[4–7]. The procedure of ICSI is also the technique of choice when epididymal or testicular sperm is surgically obtained from patients with obstructive or non-obstructive azoospermia[8–13].

This review reports the results of 6 years of ICSI practice (1991–96) with ejaculated, epididymal and testicular sperm at the Brussels Free University Center for Reproductive Medicine. Patient selection, ovarian stimulation and oocyte handling, semen evaluation and preparation, the ICSI procedure and its assessment as regards oocyte damage, pronuclear status after ICSI, embryo development, transfer and freezing, and results of obstetrical outcome will be outlined.

Evaluation of 6 years of clinical use of ICSI

Between January 1991 and December 1996, almost 6200 ICSI cycles involving almost 64 000 metaphase-II oocytes were carried out and evaluated in our center.

A total of 6353 ICSI cycles were scheduled in couples with long-standing infertility. The ICSI procedure could not be carried out in 185 cycles (2.9%) because there were no cumulus–oocyte complexes or metaphase-II oocytes (81 cycles), or because no spermatozoa were available for the microinjection procedure (104 cycles). The latter condition occurred in patients with non-obstructive azoospermia who were scheduled for ICSI with testicular spermatozoa. The ICSI procedure was carried out, therefore, in 6168 treatment cycles.

The ICSI procedure was performed with spermatozoa from the ejaculate in 5391 (87%) cycles for couples who had had no, or only poor, fertilization in one or more cycles of conventional IVF. It was also performed in couples with semen values too impaired to be accepted for conventional IVF, i.e. fewer than 500 000 progressively motile spermatozoa with normal morphology were present in the total ejaculate after semen preparation.

The procedure was also performed with spermatozoa retrieved from the epididymis for men with azoospermia caused by congenital or acquired obstruction; ICSI was carried out with freshly collected epididymal spermatozoa in 158 cycles (3%) and with frozen-thawed epididymal spermatozoa in 116 cycles (2%).

Using testicular spermatozoa obtained from testicular biopsy specimens, ICSI was performed in 503 cycles (8%), for patients with obstructive azoospermia where motile epididymal spermatozoa could not be found and for some patients with non-obstructive azoospermia.

Ovarian stimulation was performed with gonadotropin-releasing hormone (GnRH) agonists, human menopausal gonadotropin (hMG) and human chorionic gonadotropin (hCG) as previously described elsewhere[14]. When the serum estradiol level exceeded 1000 pg/ml (3670 pmol/l), and when at least three follicles of 18 mm or more in diameter were found on ultrasound examination, ovulation was induced with 10 000 IU of hCG. Oocyte retrieval was performed 36 h after hCG administration by means of ultrasound-guided transvaginal aspiration.

Our experience is based on a total of 79 731 cumulus–oocyte complexes retrieved during 6353 cycles, which represents a mean of 12.6 complexes per cycle. In most cases, the cumulus and the corona cells were well dispersed. Cumulus and corona cells were removed by means of a combination of enzymatic and mechanical procedures as previously described elsewhere[15]. A recent study performed in our laboratory has indicated that enzymatic denudation is also feasible with only 10 IU of hyaluronidase, and this lower concentration is currently being used in order to avoid the exposure of the oocytes to relatively large amounts of hyaluronidase. Denuded oocytes are observed under an inverted microscope at × 200 magnification. Observations include assessment of the zona pellucida and the oocyte, and the presence or absence of a germinal vesicle or a first polar body[16]. Of the 79 731 cumulus–oocyte complexes presently studied, 95% contained an oocyte with intact zona pellucida: 81% contained metaphase-II oocytes that had extruded the first polar body, 10% contained germinal-vesicle-stage oocytes and 4% contained metaphase-I oocytes that had undergone breakdown of the germinal vesicle but had not yet extruded the first polar body. The distribution of oocytes with different nuclear maturity was quite variable from patient to patient. Since only metaphase-II oocytes have reached the haploid

state and, thus, can be fertilized normally, ICSI is only carried out on such oocytes. However, in a few rare cases, where too few, or no, metaphase-II oocytes were available or remained unfertilized after ICSI, *in vitro* matured germinal-vesicle-stage oocytes were injected the day after oocyte pick-up. For this, germinal-vesicle-stage oocytes are matured *in vitro* for 24 h in either Ménézo B$_2$ medium or in a coculture system with Vero cells[17]. Only one pregnancy and birth resulting from this procedure has been reported to date[18].

Patients selected for ICSI with ejaculated semen undergo a preliminary semen assessment prior to the treatment cycle, in order to verify whether enough, preferably motile, spermatozoa are present to perform ICSI. In our laboratory, semen assessment is performed according to the recommendations of the World Health Organization (WHO)[19], except for sperm morphology, which is assessed by the strict criteria of Kruger and colleagues[20]. Semen values are considered normal if the volume of the ejaculate is at least 2 ml, sperm concentration is at least 20×10^6/ml, progressive sperm motility is at least 40% and normal sperm morphology is at least 14%. The distribution of characteristics of the freshly ejaculated semen used in 5215 ICSI cycles is such that all three semen values were abnormal in 43% of the cycles, two semen values were abnormal in 30% of the cycles, one semen value was abnormal in 19% of the cycles and all three semen values were normal in 8% of the cycles. Most of the couples with normal semen values had previously undergone conventional IVF treatments without success.

Only a minority of our sperm samples for ICSI (~15%) are of sufficient quality to allow a swim-up procedure. The other ejaculated sperm samples for ICSI are prepared by centrifugation using a discontinuous Percoll gradient[21].

Epididymal sperm is usually recovered from the most proximal part of the caput of the epididymis in a microsurgical procedure[8,10]. During microsurgical epididymal sperm aspiration, several sperm fractions are collected into separate tubes. Sperm fractions with similar concentration and motility are pooled and then treated in the same way as ejaculated semen. Whenever possible, some of the freshly recovered sperm should be frozen for later use, to avoid surgical procedures in subsequent cycles[8].

Testicular spermatozoa are isolated from a testicular biopsy specimen, which is usually obtained by means of surgical excisional biopsy performed under general anesthesia[11]. The testicular biopsy specimen is transferred to a Petri dish with HEPES-buffered Earle's medium, and shredded into small pieces with sterile microscope slides on the heated stage of a stereomicroscope. The presence of spermatozoa is assessed on the inverted microscope. The pieces of the biopsy tissue are removed, and the medium is centrifuged at 300 g for 5 min. The pellet is then resuspended for the ICSI procedure.

Microtool preparation and the actual microinjection procedure have been described elsewhere[16]. A single, living, immobilized spermatozoon is aspirated tail-first into the injection pipette. The oocyte is fixed with the holding pipette; care is taken that the polar body is situated at the 6 o'clock position. The injection pipette is pushed through the zona pellucida and into the cytoplasm at the 3 o'clock position, and the sperm is delivered with the smallest possible amount of medium[22]. Orienting the oocyte in this way minimizes the risk that the injection pipette will damage the metaphase plate. It is useful to aspirate the cytoplasm gently into the injection pipette before the sperm injection, to be certain that the tip of the pipette has penetrated the oolemma rather than simply indenting it.

Sixteen to 18 h after ICSI, oocytes are inspected for intactness and fertilization. The number and aspect of polar bodies and pronuclei are recorded. Oocytes are considered to be normally fertilized when two individualized or fragmented polar bodies are present together with two clearly visible pronuclei that contain nucleoli. In total, ICSI was performed in 6168 cycles on 63 698 metaphase-II oocytes (a mean of 10.3 oocytes per cycle). The number of intact oocytes was 57 506 (90.3% of the oocytes that had received injections), i.e. a damage rate of approximately 10% of the injected oocytes. The mean number of successfully injected oocytes here was 9.3 per treatment. Normally fertilized oocytes resulted from nearly 71.8% of the successfully injected oocytes, 64.8% of the injected metaphase-II oocytes and 51.8% of the retrieved cumulus–oocyte complexes. Abnormal fertilization occurred as one-pronuclear (PN) oocytes in 2.9% (1819) of the injected metaphase-II oocytes, and 3.9% (2467) of the injected metaphase-II oocytes revealed three pronuclei. If such abnormally fertilized 1-PN oocytes cleave, they are not transferred, because they are likely to be parthenogenetically activated as a result of mechanical or chemical factors. The occasional finding of three-pronuclear oocytes after injection of a single spermatozoon into the ooplasm is probably caused by non-extrusion of the second polar body at the time of fertilization. Neither type of embryo resulting from 3-PN oocytes is transferred to the patients.

Damage and pronuclear status after ICSI were analyzed for all four types of sperm (ejaculated, fresh and frozen-thawed epididymal, and testicular) used in performing ICSI (Table 1). The percentage of oocytes that remained intact after ICSI varied between 89.6 and 91.7% and was similar for the four different types of spermatozoa. The percentage of oocytes fertilized normally (two pronuclei) varied between 55.9 and 66.1%. The normal fertilization rate for ICSI was higher when ejaculated sperm was used than when other types of sperm were used. The percentage of oocytes with one pronucleus after ICSI varied between 2.7 and 4.3%. The percentage of oocytes with three pronuclei after ICSI varied between 3.5 and 5.0%. Abnormal fertilization occurred to a similar extent in the four different groups of spermatozoa.

The exceptional circumstances by which no injected oocytes fertilize normally are associated with only very few metaphase-II oocytes being available for ICSI, only totally immotile spermatozoa being available for the injection, gross abnormalities present in the oocytes, round-headed spermatozoa being injected or all oocytes being damaged in the injection procedure.

In this case, most of the patients involved achieve fertilization in a subsequent cycle[23].

After a further 24 h of *in vitro* culture, embryo cleavage is evaluated. The cleaving embryos are scored according to equality of size of the blastomeres and proportion of anucleate fragments[24]. Three categories according to the percentage of anucleate fragments are distinguished: excellent, type-A embryos (no anucleate fragments); good-quality, type-B embryos (between 1 and 20% of the volume filled with anucleate fragments); and fair-quality, type-C embryos (between 21 and 50% of the volume filled with anucleate fragments). Cleaved embryos with less than one-half of their volume filled with anucleate fragments are eligible for transfer. Supernumerary embryos with less than 20% anucleate fragments are cryopreserved on day 2 or day 3 after oocyte retrieval by means of a slow-freezing protocol with dimethylsulfoxide[25].

The total number of embryos of sufficient quality to be transferred, i.e. those with less than 50% anucleate fragments, was 32 786: 79.4% of the two-pronuclear oocytes, 57.0% of the

successfully injected oocytes, 51.5% of the injected metaphase-II ooytes and 41.1% of the retrieved cumulus–oocyte complexes.

The percentages of two-pronuclear oocytes developing into excellent, good-quality and fair-quality embryos for the different types of spermatozoa used for ICSI are summarized in Table 2. A higher percentage of good-quality embryos was obtained in the group of ejaculated spermatozoa. The percentages of embryos actually transferred or frozen as supernumerary embryos was similar for the four types of spermatozoa and varied between 59.1 and 65.2% of the 2-PN oocytes.

Embryo replacement of at least one embryo was possible in 5714 of the 6168 treatment cycles with ICSI (92.6%). This may be considered a high transfer rate because it represents couples with previous fertilization failure in conventional IVF, ejaculated sperm too poor to be included in IVF or men with obstructive or non-obstructive azoospermia. As indicated in Table 3, the percentage of transfers was similar across the four groups of sperm used for ICSI; the transfer rate varied from 85.3 to 93.0%. Of the

Table 1 Sperm origin, oocyte damage and pronuclear status after intracytoplasmic sperm injection (ICSI)

	Ejaculated semen	Epididymal Fresh	Epididymal Frozen-thawed	Testis
No. of cycles	5 391	158	116	503
No. of oocytes that received ICSI	54 792	1850	1244	5812
Percentage of intact oocytes	90.3	89.6	91.7	90.1
Percentage of injected oocytes with				
one pronucleus	2.7	4.1	3.3	4.3
two pronuclei	66.1	59.4	55.9	56.3
three or more pronuclei	3.9	5.0	5.0	3.5

Table 2 Sperm origin and embryo development after intracytoplasmic sperm injection (ICSI)

	Ejaculated semen	Epididymal Fresh	Epididymal Frozen-thawed	Testis
No. of two-pronuclear oocytes	36 236	1098	696	3272
Percentage of excellent embryos	6.7	7.7	3.4	5.1
Percentage of good-quality embryos	58.1	48.9	41.4	47.2
Percentage of fair-quality embryos	15.8	14.9	18.5	20.3
Percentage of transferred or frozen embryos	65.2	64.2	59.1	60.8

Table 3 Sperm origin and outcome of embryo transfers after intracytoplasmic sperm injection (ICSI)

| | Ejaculated semen | Epididymal | | Testis |
		Fresh	Frozen-thawed	
1991–1996				
No. of cycles	5391	158	116	503
No. of transfers	5011	146	99	458
Transfer rate (%)	93.0	92.4	85.3	91.1
No. of pregnancies	1803	64	31	148
Pregnancy rate per transfer* (%)	36.4	44.1	33.0	33.0
one embryo	12.2	25.0	16.7	10.3
two embryos	24.7	30.0	18.8	29.0
two embryos (elective)	42.6	33.3	50.0	28.6
three embryos	38.6	47.7	30.8	33.3
three embryos (elective)	45.4	59.4	50.0	40.3
more than three embryos	35.3	41.7	35.7	40.2
Pregnancy rate per cycle* (%)	33.8	40.8	27.9	30.0
1991–1995				
No. of transfers with known outcome (until delivery)	3680	131	65	277
No. of deliveries	986	40	19	62
Delivery rate per transfer (%)	26.8	30.5	29.2	22.4

*With known serum human chorionic gonadotropin (hCG) outcome

5714 embryo replacements, 5637 transfers were with known serum hCG outcome; for the other 77 transfers (62 in the ejaculated semen group, one in the freshly collected epididymal spermatozoa group, five in the frozen-thawed epididymal spermatozoa group and nine in the testicular spermatozoa group), the serum hCG outcome was unknown. The overall pregnancy rate per transfer with known serum hCG outcome and the pregnancy rate per number of embryos transferred were similar for the four types of spermatozoa. Especially high pregnancy rates were observed when elective transfer of two or three embryos was performed[26]. The pregnancy rate per cycle with known serum hCG outcome varied from 27.9 to 40.8%. Delivery rates per transfer with known outcome until delivery were calculated for the ICSI treatment cycles performed from 1991 to 1995. All but 26 (20 in the ejaculated semen group, two in the freshly collected epididymal spermatozoa group and four in the testicular spermatozoa group) embryo replacements with positive serum hCG resulted in a known pregnancy outcome. Delivery rates per transfer with known pregnancy outcome varied from 22.4 to 30.5%.

Owing to the novelty of the ICSI procedure and possible unknown aspects of the outcome, couples were counseled and agreed to participate in a prospective follow-up study of the pregnancies and the children born after ICSI[27–33]. To date, the results indicate that there is a slight increase in *de novo* chromosomal aberrations (~1%), which probably reflects the characteristics of the infertile men treated rather than the ICSI technique itself. A slightly higher frequency of transmitted structural chromosomal aberrations of ~1% is a result of transmitted aberration from the fathers. Major malformations are found in an expected range of 2.5% of the children, comparable with the figures from other studies after assisted reproduction treatment or in general population registries. These observations should be completed further by others and by collaborative efforts. In the meantime, patients should be counseled, before deciding on any treatment, about available data, including details of the higher risk of transmitted chromosomal aberrations, the risk of *de novo*, mainly sex-chromosomal aberrations, and the risk of transmitting fertility problems to the offspring. They should also be reassured that there seems to be no higher incidence of congenital malformations in children born after ICSI.

Summary

In the past 6 years, ICSI has been developed to alleviate long-standing infertility in couples with severe andrological infertility who could not be accepted for IVF because too few motile and morphologically normal spermatozoa were present in the ejaculate. The ICSI procedure can also be carried out with epididymal and testicular spermatozoa in patients with azoospermia. The practice of 6 years of ICSI (1991–1996) has been reviewed in this chapter. The procedure was carried out in 97% of the 6353 planned treatment cycles. About 10% of the injected metaphase-II oocytes were damaged after ICSI, 72% of the intact oocytes had two pronuclei and about two-thirds of these normally fertilized oocytes developed into embryos, which were transferred or cryopreserved. After transfer of fresh embryos, the percentage of cycles with positive serum hCG was 31%. From 1991 to 1995, 27% of the treatment cycles with known pregnancy outcome resulted in delivery. The procedure of ICSI can be considered a breakthrough in the management of male-factor infertility. The follow-up of ICSI children is indicated so that future parents may receive thorough counseling.

Acknowledgements

The expert assistance of the clinical, scientific, nursing and technical staff of the Center for Reproductive Medicine and the Center for Medical Genetics is kindly acknowledged. Frank Winter of the VUB Language Education Center corrected the manuscript. The work was supported by grants from the University Research Council and the Belgian Fund for Medical Research, and by an unrestricted educational grant from Organon International.

References

1. Palermo, G., Joris, H., Devroey, P. and Van Steirteghem, A. C. (1992). Pregnancies after intracytoplasmic injection of single spermatozoon into an oocyte. *Lancet*, **340**, 17–18
2. Palermo, G., Joris, H., Derde, M.-P., Camus, M., Devroey, P. and Van Steirteghem, A. C. (1993). Sperm characteristics and outcome of human assisted fertilization by subzonal insemination and intracytoplasmic sperm injection. *Fertil. Steril.*, **59**, 826–35
3. Van Steirteghem, A. C., Liu, J., Joris, H., Nagy, Z., Janssenswillen, C., Tournaye, H., Derde, M.-P., Van Assche, E. and Devroey, P. (1993). Higher success rate by intracytoplasmic sperm injection than by subzonal insemination. Report of a second series of 300 consecutive treatment cycles. *Hum. Reprod.*, **8**, 1055–60
4. Van Steirteghem, A. C., Nagy, Z., Joris, H., Liu, J., Staessen, C., Smitz, J., Wisanto, A. and Devroey, P. (1993). High fertilization and implantation rates after intracytoplasmic sperm injection. *Hum. Reprod.*, **8**, 1061–6
5. Van Steirteghem, A., Liu, J., Nagy, Z., Joris, H., Tournaye, H., Liebaers, I. and Devroey, P. (1993). Use of assisted fertilization. *Hum. Reprod.*, **8**, 1784–5
6. Nagy, Z., Liu, J., Joris, H., Verheyen, G., Tournaye, H., Camus, M., Derde, M.-P., Devroey, P. and Van Steirteghem, A. C. (1995). The result of intracytoplasmic sperm injection is not related to any of the three basic sperm parameters. *Hum. Reprod.*, **10**, 1123–9
7. Van Steirteghem, A., Tournaye, H., Van der Elst, J., Verheyen, G., Liebaers, I. and Devroey, P. (1995). Intracytoplasmic sperm injection three years after the birth of the first ICSI child. *Hum. Reprod.*, **10**, 2527–8
8. Devroey, P., Silber, S., Nagy, Z., Liu, J., Tournaye, H., Joris, H., Verheyen, G. and Van Steirteghem, A. (1995). Ongoing pregnancies and birth after intracytoplasmic sperm injection with frozen–thawed epididymal spermatozoa. *Hum. Reprod.*, **10**, 903–6
9. Nagy, Z., Liu, J., Janssenswillen, C., Silber, S., Devroey, P. and Van Steirteghem, A. (1995).

Using ejaculated, fresh, and frozen-thawed epididymal and testicular spermatozoa gives rise to comparable results after intracytoplasmic sperm injection. *Fertil. Steril.*, **63**, 808–15

10. Silber, S. J., Nagy, Z., Liu, J., Tournaye, H., Lissens, W., Ferec, C., Liebaers, I., Devroey, P. and Van Steirteghem, A. (1995). The use of epididymal and testicular spermatozoa for intracytoplasmic sperm injection: the genetic implications for male infertility. *Hum. Reprod.*, **10**, 2031–43

11. Silber, S. J., Van Steirteghem, A., Liu, J., Nagy, Z., Tournaye, H. and Devroey, P. (1995). High fertilization and pregnancy rate after intracytoplasmic sperm injection with spermatozoa obtained from testicle biopsy. *Hum. Reprod.*, **10**, 148–52

12. Devroey, P., Nagy, Z., Tournaye, H., Liu, J., Silber, S. and Van Steirteghem, A. (1996). Outcome of intracytoplasmic sperm injection with testicular spermatozoa in obstructive and non-obstructive azoospermia. *Hum. Reprod.*, **11**, 1015–18

13. Silber, S. J., Van Steirteghem, A., Nagy, Z., Liu, J., Tournaye, H. and Devroey, P. (1996). Normal pregnancies resulting from testicular sperm extraction and intracytoplasmic sperm injection for azoospermia use to maturation arrest. *Fertil. Steril.*, **66**, 110–17

14. Smitz, J., Devroey, P., Camus, M., Deschacht, J., Khan, I., Staessen, C., Van Waesberghe, L., Wisanto, A. and Van Steirteghem, A. (1988). The luteal phase and early pregnancy after combined GnRH-agonist/hMG treatment for superovulation in IVF or GIFT. *Hum. Reprod.*, **3**, 585–90

15. Van de Velde, H., Nagy, Z. P., Joris, H., De Vos, A. and Van Steirteghem, A. (1997). The effects of different hyaluronidase concentrations and mechanical procedures for cumulus-corona cell removal on the outcome of ICSI. *Hum. Reprod.*, **12**, 2246–50

16. Van Steirteghem, A. C., Joris. H., Liu, J., Nagy, Z., Bocken, G., Vankelecom, A., Desmet, B., Van Ranst, H. and Franceus, N. (1995). Protocol for intracytoplasmic sperm injection. *Hum. Reprod. Update*, 1(3), CD-ROM

17. Janssenswillen, C., Nagy, Z. P. and Van Steirteghem, A. (1995). Maturation of human cumulus-free germinal vesicle-stage oocytes to metaphase II by coculture with monolayer Vero cells. *Hum. Reprod.*, **10**, 375–8

18. Nagy, Z. P., Janssenswillen, C., Liu, J., Loccufier, A., Devroey, P. and Van Steirteghem, A. (1996). Pregnancy and birth after intracytoplasmic sperm injection of *in vitro* matured germinal vesicle-stage oocytes: case report. *Fertil. Steril.*, **65**, 1047–50

19. World Health Organization (1992). *WHO Laboratory Manual for the Examination of Human Semen and Sperm-Cervical Mucus Interaction.* (Cambridge: Cambridge University Press)

20. Kruger, T. F., Menkveld, R., Stander, F. S. H., Lombard, C. J., Van der Merwe, J. P., Van Zeyl, J. A. and Smith, K. (1986). Sperm morphologic features as a prognostic factor in *in vitro* fertilization. *Fertil. Steril.*, **46**, 1118–23

21. Liu, J., Nagy, Z. P., Joris, H., Tournaye, H., Devroey, P. and Van Steirteghem, A. C. (1994). Intracytoplasmic sperm injection does not require special treatment of the spermatozoa. *Hum. Reprod.*, **9**, 1127–30

22. Nagy, Z. P., Liu, J., Joris, H., Bocken, G., Desmet, B., Van Ranst, H., Vankelecom, A., Devroey, P. and Van Steirteghem, A. C. (1995). The influence of the site of sperm deposition and mode of oolemma breakage at intracytoplasmic sperm injection on fertilization and embryo development rates. *Hum. Reprod.*, **10**, 3171–7

23. Liu, J., Nagy, Z., Joris, H., Tournaye, H., Smitz, J., Camus, M., Devroey, P. and Van Steirteghem, A. (1995). Analysis of 76 total fertilization failure cycles out of 2732 intracytoplasmic sperm injection cycles. *Hum. Reprod.*, **10**, 2630–6

24. Staessen, C., Camus, M., Khan, I., Smitz, J., Van Waesberghe, L., Wisanto, A., Devroey, P. and Van Steirteghem, A. (1989). An 18-month survey of infertility treatment by *in vitro* fertilization, gamete and zygote intrafallopian transfer, and replacement of frozen-thawed embryos. *J. In Vitro Fertil. Embryo Transfer*, **6**, 22–9

25. Van Steirteghem, A. C., Van der Elst, J., Van den Abbeel, E., Joris, H., Camus, M. and Devroey, P. (1994). Cryopreservation of supernumerary multicellular human embryos obtained after intracytoplasmic sperm injection. *Fertil. Steril.*, **62**, 775–80

26. Staessen, C., Nagy, Z. P., Liu, J., Janssenswillen, C., Camus, M., Devroey, P. and Van Steirteghem, A. C. (1995). One year's experience with elective transfer of two good quality embryos in the human *in-vitro* fertilization and intracytoplasmic sperm injection programmes. *Hum. Reprod.*, **10**, 3305–12

27. Bonduelle, M., Desmyttere, S., Buysse, A., Van Assche, E., Schiettecatte, J., Devroey, P., Van Steirteghem, A. C. and Liebaers, I. (1994). Prospective follow-up study of 55 children born after subzonal insemination and intracytoplasmic sperm injection. *Hum. Reprod.*, **9**, 1765–9

28. Bonduelle, M., Legein, J., Derde, M.-P., Buysse, A., Schiettecatte, J., Wisanto, A., Devroey, P., Van Steirteghem, A. and Liebaers, I. (1995). Comparative follow-up study of 130 children born after intracytoplasmic sperm injection and 130

children born after *in-vitro* fertilization. *Hum. Reprod.*, **10**, 3327–31

29. Liebaers, I., Bonduelle, M., Van Assche, E., Devroey, P. and Van Steirteghem, A. (1995). Sex chromosome abnormalities after intracytoplasmic sperm injection. *Lancet*, **346**, 1095

30. Wisanto, A., Magnus, M., Bonduelle, M., Liu, J., Camus, M., Tournaye, H., Liebaers, I., Van Steirteghem, A. C. and Devroey, P. (1995). Obstetric outcome of 424 pregnancies after intracytoplasmic sperm injection. *Hum. Reprod.*, **10**, 2713–18

31. Bonduelle, M., Legein, J., Buysse, A., Van Assche, E., Wisanto, A., Devroey, P., Van Steirteghem, A. C. and Liebaers, I. (1996). Prospective follow-up study of 423 children born after intra-

cytoplasmic sperm injection. *Hum. Reprod.*, **11**, 1558–64

32. Wisanto, A., Bonduelle, M., Camus, M., Tournaye, H., Magnus, M., Liebaers, I. and Van Steirteghem, A. C. (1996). Obstetric outcome of 904 pregnancies after intracytoplasmic sperm injection. In *Genetics and Assisted Human Conception*, Suppl. 4 to *Hum. Reprod.*, **11**, 121–30

33. Bonduelle, M., Wilikens, A., Buysse, A., Van Assche, E., Wisanto, A., Devroey, P., Van Steirteghem, A. and Liebaers, I. (1996). Prospective follow-up study of 877 children born after intracytoplasmic sperm injection (ICSI), with ejaculated epididymal and testicular spermatozoa and after replacement of cryopreserved embryos obtained after ICSI. In *Genetics and Assisted Human Conception*, Suppl. 4 to *Hum. Reprod.*, **11**, 131–59

Genetic counseling: recent advances   13

Z. Papp, E. Tóth-Pál and Cs. Papp

Basis of genetic counseling

One of the first definitions of genetic counseling was provided by the American Society of Human Genetics in 1974[1]. Genetic counseling involves the complex interactions of medical, psychological and social factors, its goal being to convey relevant genetic facts and reproductive options to families who are, or who might be, affected by a genetic disorder[2]. In other words, genetic counseling is the process by which patients or relatives at risk of a disorder that may be hereditary are advised of the consequences of the disorder, the probability of developing or transmitting it and of the ways in which this may be prevented or ameliorated. Within the past few years, there has been considerable progress in medical genetics, especially in molecular genetics, and therefore genetic counseling has also been changing[3].

Progress of genetic counseling

Classical genetic counseling aimed to help families with emotional support and by disclosing and discussing the causes of certain 'genetic' problems, the risks of recurrence and the possibilities for prevention or other options. In many situations no reliable figures for recurrence risk were available.

Subsequently, a number of diagnostic techniques applicable to pregnancy became available, together with a much better understanding of genetically determined disease at many levels. The classic options in many cases included contraception, sterilization, adoption or heterologous insemination by donor.

Now, in many disorders, one can suggest undertaking further pregnancies, with the offer of prenatal genetic counseling: the fetal phenotype may be examined (ultrasound for malformations or growth retardation; biochemical tests for metabolic disorders), or the fetal genotype may be examined (cytogenetic analysis for chromosome disorders; DNA tests for direct or indirect identification of mutant genes). There remain disorders for which no diagnosis is available, or for which one can offer no more than 'classical genetics', but it is likely that many disorders at present of unknown cause will soon be understood at the biochemical or gene level, and that many presently 'unmapped' genes will be mapped within the next few years. The Human Genome Project plans to sequence the whole human genome by 2005, and after identification of the whole sequence the search for disease-causing genes should be easier[4]. The increased availability of prenatal diagnosis (available in more centers, for more patients, for more disorders) has stimulated the development of screening for genetic disease. Subpopulations at particular risk may be easily identified (e.g. older mothers), or identified only after specific testing (e.g. for thalassemia, hemoglobinopathies, Tay–Sachs disease and cystic fibrosis). The screening process may take place before or during an actual pregnancy, e.g. maternal serum alpha-fetoprotein (MSAFP), ultrasound, fetal echocardiography during pregnancy or biochemical screening and DNA tests of parents before conception in order to identify couples at risk for a specific disorder.

Main elements of genetic counseling

Diagnosis

Diagnosis of the affected individual is the foundation of genetic counseling. An initial part of genetic counseling must therefore be to confirm whatever genetic disorder is under consideration. This may involve a direct clinical assessment of the affected individual, but frequently will depend on the quality of hospital records[5].

Confirmation of an exact diagnosis may be difficult. Obtaining old or recent medical records, pedigree analysis[6], clinical examination of relatives, special laboratory tests and other investigations (maybe involving referral to other special departments) can all be relevant or necessary procedures.

Disease, whether genetic or non-genetic, may be due to a variety of factors. Genetic disease is particularly likely to be heterogeneous in this respect. For example, muscular dystrophy may result from a number of mutant genes. It should be noted that there are diseases which do not usually manifest until adulthood (e.g. Huntington's disease, facioscapulohumeral muscular dystrophy), and that in connection with certain diseases of recessive (autosomal or X-linked) inheritance heterozygotes may also show clinical symptoms.

In some cases, medical documents may be incomplete or unobtainable; certain tests, that are now considered essential for the diagnosis, may not have been carried out or have been available at that time. There may be no histological information, no post-mortem report, no roentgenograms, no photographs and no biochemical or molecular genetic results. Genetic counseling cannot be based on a diagnosis like 'mental retardation', 'growth disorder' or 'degenerative disease'. Sometimes an exact diagnosis, like 'achondroplasia', may be clearly misleading. To make a correct diagnosis, with a few exceptions, requires detailed and correct information.

Nowadays, molecular genetics may help to clarify the exact diagnosis even after the affected patient's death. For example, the Guthrie card of a newborn can be examined for the presence of specific mutations in some monogenic and polygenic disorders. This possibility is a great advance of both medical genetics and genetic counseling. Therefore, the role of a genetic counselor is more complex than previously.

Sometimes the genetic counselor has subsequently to manage the diagnostic process in a specific disorder.

Risk estimation

This is the second element of genetic counselling and, therefore, the knowledge of basic genetics is essential so that patterns of single-gene inheritance, as well as non-Mendelian patterns, can be correctly recognized. Before risks can be estimated, family details must be collected. Risk estimation does not only consider the primary genetic risk data obtained from family details, but has to relate them to other information which may be the results of laboratory tests, or information relating to the genotype of other family members. As a result of progress in carrier screening programs in some monogenic disorders, the risk can be estimated before even the first pregnancy (e.g. cystic fibrosis)[7].

There is also a general population risk. Many couples have no idea at all of general population risks. They may imagine that it is extremely unusual to abort spontaneously, bear a baby with an anomaly or have a child with mental retardation[8,9]. They cannot understand how such things can happen, if they are not in the family already. They do not understand why a particular disaster happened to them, as they had done nothing to deserve or provoke it[10]. The general population risks for a few commonplace situations are given in Table 1.

All genetic counseling has to be given, and understood, against this general 'background' risk. For example, a couple may be horrified to

Table 1 General population risks

Condition	Risk
Fetal loss	
in first trimester	1/6
in second and third trimesters	1/30–1/100
Neonatal death	1/100
Malformation detectable at birth	1/33
Mental retardation	1/50
Chronic disease in adulthood	1/5

be told there is a 1% recurrence risk for a certain anomaly. It may help couples realize that an additional risk of 1% for an anomaly is not so enormous when compared with the starting risk of 3–5%.

In some counseling situations, couples may be at increased risk for one or a number of problems compared with general population risks, yet one is not talking of a 'recurrence risk': the condition provoking anxiety and the request for counseling has not yet happened. In these situations the actual risk still may not be very high, even if it is much above the general population level. For example, a woman of age 40 has a risk of bearing a live-born with Down's syndrome that is 20-fold the risk she ran when she was only age 20, yet the actual risk is only 1/100.

Very high levels of risk, for a problem that has not yet appeared within the family, will seldom be met except in connection with specific screening programs, for example detection of Tay-Sachs heterozygotes in Ashkenazi Jews, of thalassemia carriers in Mediterranean populations and detection of cystic fibrosis carriers in Caucasian populations. In these situations, when both parents are heterozygotes, the risk of an affected child is 25%. In virtually all of these very high-risk situations identified by screening, a prenatal test can be offered, but this would not be acceptable to all couples.

When a disorder has already appeared within a family, recurrence risks may be high (> 1/10), intermediate (1/10–1/100) or low (< 1/100).

Most congenital anomalies are multifactorially determined. After having a child with an isolated exomphalos, or tracheo-esophageal malformation, recurrence risks may be only 1–2%; although this represents a 20–40-fold increase over the general population level it is still not a very daunting risk. After having a child with congenital heart disease, recurrence risks are usually 2–5% (depending on the malformation type); the background rate, for congenital heart disease, is nearly 1% (8/1000). When dealing with a congenital anomaly problem the counselor must be sure that it really is isolated and not part of a syndrome (that may be monogenic), for example, an occipital encephalocele

alone might suggest a recurrence risk of about 3%. If the encephalocele was accompanied by cystic kidneys or polydactyly, the Meckel syndrome would probably be diagnosed, with a recurrence risk of 25%.

The background general population risk is not identical with the risk within a given family (specific risk), nor with the risk calculated for a given pregnancy (actual risk). For example, the background risk (in Hungary) for a healthy subject of being heterozygous for cystic fibrosis is 1/25, and the risk of his/her child being affected by the disease is 1/2500. However, the situation will change completely if it is revealed that the couple already have a child suffering from cystic fibrosis. In this case, the specific risk of a further child being affected is 1/4. If the couple undertake a pregnancy and the prenatal tests give normal results, the actual risk of having an affected child will fall to a very low value. To talk about 100% reliability of a biochemical or molecular prenatal diagnosis is, in practice, nonsense. The counselor[11] should not use words like 'never' or 'always'.

Communication

In addition to diagnosis and risk estimation the communication[12] is an important element of genetic counseling. It is, however, the element that is likely to be most neglected by practicing clinicians, and most complaints from patients about previous information which they had been given concerned not errors, but the manner of communication. Some people are better communicators than others, but factors which are relevant include: sufficient time, the timing of counseling, ability to listen and privacy.

Prognosis and therapy

Without a correct diagnosis the genetic counselor[13] cannot tell the parents whether there is a high or low risk of recurrence within the family, whether tests can be carried out to detect those persons/couples at high risk of having an affected child, whether prenatal diagnosis is possible (and if so, how, where and when), whether the disease is in any way treatable, whether the severity is highly variable within a family, whether there are other (as yet undiscussed) serious implications or whether other 'reproductive options' are available.

Although much genetic disease remains untreatable, the counselor must know the possibilities for the disease in question. He/she must be up-to-date and informed about surgical procedures and appliances (e.g. neonatal or prenatal surgery, transplantation), about medical treatment and about what is available within the community (e.g. help from social services, financial help for parents with handicapped children, institutional care). He/she must be able to discuss more remote possibilities, such as 'gene therapy', within a realistic perspective. He/she must be able to talk to the parents in a way, and at a level, that is appropriate to their pre-existing knowledge and education, and their degree of anxiety or depth of grief. He/she must be prepared to educate them further.

Prenatal diagnosis

In many counseling situations, the specific recurrence risk is so low that, apart from a general screening for malformations, further tests are superfluous. A simple reassurance may disappoint certain couples if they feel that their problem has been oversimplified[14,15].

For most couples running a higher than average risk/recurrence risk one can offer prenatal diagnosis. Cases require individual assessment. The reliability and the safety of the diagnostic procedures should be discussed with the parents. These should be carefully weighed, bearing in mind the nature and severity of the disease/disorder prompting the desire for diagnosis/termination. It should be explained that the test(s) will be for one problem only, or a limited range of disorders, and normal results will not guarantee a child normal in every way.

The final decision, to accept or reject the offer of prenatal diagnosis, is for the couple to make[16]. Their decision will reflect their attitude to the disorder in question, and also their feelings regarding termination of pregnancy, should the test show an 'affected' fetus. They should not be required to give any consent in advance regarding abortion, in this latter eventuality.

Decision-making

The couple decide whether or not to undertake pregnancy, and they decide whether or not to accept an offer of prenatal diagnosis. However, prenatal testing is time-consuming, laborious and expensive, and uses human resources and materials that are, as a result, not available to others. It involves certain risks for the mother and fetus. If a couple are convinced that they would not terminate pregnancy in any event (an 'affected' fetus) they will probably also be convinced that the risks, to mother and pregnancy, are not worth taking[17,18].

In some situations prenatal diagnosis is, at present, impossible, even though the genetic risk is high. Recently, the number of disorders in which prenatal diagnosis is impossible has been reduced significantly.

Progress in genetic counseling and prenatal diagnosis of spina bifida

Neural tube defects including severe spina bifida are usually incompatible with human life. Therefore, there is parental demand to prevent these anomalies. Spina bifida results from defective neural tube closure along some or all the length of the vertebral column. There are several forms of spina bifida. When no tissue is extruded through the defect, and it is covered by normal skin, it is termed spina bifida occulta. When the defect forms a protruding sac, the term spina bifida cystica is used. It is this latter form that is ordinarily meant by the simple designation 'spina bifida'. This group can also be subdivided.

It is important to determine the risk of recurrence of spina bifida in the practice of genetic counseling, so that, even with prenatal diagnosis, the parents are able to determine the probability of an affected fetus or the decision against pregnancy. The risk of recurrence of spina bifida is influenced by the severity of the previous anomaly, by the number of the affected members in the family, by the degree of relationship and environmental factors as well[19].

Based on data obtained from nearly 30 000 genetic counselings collected from our genetic register (Table 2), the risk of recurrence in isolated spina bifida is 2.9%, but it is 6.8% when it is associated with hydrocephalus. These are valuable data for genetic counseling. If we know the severity of the defect of the proband and the degree of relationship, we can calculate the risk of recurrence more exactly. In classical genetic counseling only the recurrence risk could be estimated in spina bifida. In the past few decades we have also been able to offer prenatal screening and prenatal diagnosis of spina bifida.

General population screening for neural tube defects using maternal serum alpha-fetoprotein (AFP) was previously the most widely performed test world-wide. If an elevated level of maternal serum AFP was found, amniocentesis was performed in order to rule out neural tube defects.

Recently a combined screening program, using maternal AFP and ultrasound, has been extended to cover larger populations in most countries. Despite the fact that maternal serum AFP is a good biochemical marker for neural tube defects, the ultrasound examination alone can provide prenatal diagnosis of spina bifida in the fetus[20].

Some publications have documented the decreasing trend of spina bifida in newborn infants over the past two decades. Due to improvements in screening methods and to their widespread use, the birth prevalence of neural tube defects including spina bifida decreased from 3 to 1 per 1000 in Hungary. Some authors also believe in the role of vitamin and folate supplementation in prevention of neural tube defects[21]. Probably the decrease of birth prevalence of spina bifida is due to the improvement of welfare in Hungary and also in other countries, and not only to vitamin supplementation.

It has recently been shown that a common mutation, 677C→T, which has been detected in the methylenetetrahydrofolate reductase (MTHFR) gene, results in an elevated serum homocysteinic acid concentration in the serum of the affected person, and by this route it seems to be a genetic risk factor for spina bifida[22]. First observations suggested a correlation between the mutation and spina bifida. Several studies have been published since then, with differing results. In the Hungarian population, an elevated mutation frequency could be detected among fetuses with spina bifida and also in their mothers (21.4% in fetuses with spina bifida, 19.6% in their mothers, 14.9% among healthy controls). Many years ago we could only calculate the recurrence risk of spina bifida; however, we can presently offer maternal serum AFP measurement, ultrasound examination, amniocentesis for detecting the level of some biochemical markers and molecular genetic investigation of some risk factors like 677C→T mutation of MTHFR (Table 3).

Table 2 Risk of recurrence of fetal neural-tube defects in Hungarian families

Family history	Recurrence risk (%)
Pregnant woman or partner is affected	2.5
One sibling or one parent is affected	2.9
One distant relative is affected	3.2
One child is affected	3.5
One child and one relative are affected	4.2
Two relatives are affected	5.0
Three or more members of family are affected	9.1
Two children are affected	14.8
Spina bifida with hydrocephalus	6.8

Table 3 Advances in genetic counseling and prenatal screening of spina bifida

Risk estimation of recurrence
Maternal serum AFP screening
Amniotic fluid examination (AFP, AChE)
Ultrasound examination combined with MSAFP
Determination of genetic risk factors for spina bifida by molecular genetic methods

AFP, alpha-fetoprotein; AChE, acetylcholinesterase; MSAFP, maternal serum alpha-fetoprotein

Advances in genetic counseling and prenatal diagnosis of cystic fibrosis

Cystic fibrosis (CF) is the most common auto-somal recessive disease in the Caucasian population. The association of pancreatic disease and lung disease was described in the 1930s, and the high-chloride sweat in the early 1950s. Although present treatment cannot completely cure the disease, substantial improvements in life-expectancy have been achieved. Despite improving prospects, many parents of affected children seek prenatal diagnosis for subsequent pregnancies, and also many couples would like to participate in heterozygote screening programs[7,23].

The mode of inheritance of cystic fibrosis is autosomal recessive. The carrier rate is 1/20 to 1/25 in most European populations, corresponding to a birth prevalence of 1/1600 to 1/2500. The carrier frequency in the Hungarian population is 1/25[24].

In the early 1960s we could only calculate the recurrence risk of CF in families already having an affected child. In the 1970s, attention turned to the microvillar enzymes which are secreted directly into the gut lumen. The low activity of these enzymes in the amniotic fluid may be of value in the diagnosis of intestinal obstruction. It was shown that at 16–20 weeks of gestation, the amniotic-fluid activity of some microvillar enzymes was low in some pregnancies involving a CF fetus. Despite the improvement in prenatal diagnosis of CF there were several false-positive and false-negative results using this method.

Ultrasound examination combined with the detection of microvillar enzymes in amniotic fluid could improve the reliability of prenatal diagnosis. In a fetus with CF, dense mucus may form meconium plugs already *in utero* and may be visualized by ultrasound examination.

In 1985 the gene responsible for cystic fibrosis was mapped to chromosome 7, and a large number of linked probes were available for linkage analysis. These permitted prenatal diagnosis

Table 4 History of cystic fibrosis (CF)

First observation of meconium ileus	1905
First exact description of disease	1938
Description of mode of inheritance	1952
Sweat test	1953
Newborn screening by immunoreactive trypsin	1979
Prenatal diagnosis using microvillar enzymes	1983
Mapping of CF gene to chromosome 7	1985
Prenatal diagnosis by linkage analysis	1986
Identification of CFTR gene	1989
Prenatal diagnosis using direct mutation detection	1989
Heterozygote screening in cystic fibrosis	1989
First trials of gene therapy in cystic fibrosis	1990
Identified mutation in CFTR gene is more than 600	1997

CFTR, cystic fibrosis transmembrane regulator

in almost all couples with a previous living CF child. The analysis was done on a fetal DNA sample obtained by chorionic villus sampling (CVS) using the restriction fragment length polymorphism (RFLP) technique.

In 1989 the CF gene was cloned and the most frequent mutations were identified. This raised the hope that heterozygote detection would lead to a definite answer about the carrier status of any arbitrary individual. Unfortunately, at present, more than 600 mutations have been detected and it makes the wide heterozygote screening of CF very difficult. The main steps in the history of CF are given in Table 4.

At present, a genetic counselor can offer prenatal diagnosis of CF for every family having an affected child, either by direct or indirect DNA analysis of a fetal DNA sample[25]. He/she can also offer a heterozygote screening test for the most frequent CF mutations before the first pregnancy, in order to define the specific risk of the couple. We hope that with the help of heterozygote screening programs and prenatal diagnoses the birth prevalence of cystic fibrosis can be decreased as in the case of spina bifida.

References

1. Fraser, F. C. (1974). Genetic counselling. *Am. J. Hum. Genet.*, **26**, 636–59

2. Herrmann, J. and Opitz, J. M. (1980). Genetic counselling. *Posgrad. Med.*, **67**, 233–43

3. Abramovsky, I., Godmilow, L., Hirschhorn, K. and Smith, H. (1980). Analysis of a follow-up study of genetic counselling. *Clin. Genet.*, **17**, 1–12

4. Collins, F. S. (1997). Sequencing the human genome. *Hosp. Pract.*, **32**, 35–53

5. Harper, P. S. (1983). Genetic counselling and prenatal diagnosis. *Br. Med. Bull.*, **39**, 302–9

6. Gelehrter, T. D. (1983). The family history and genetic counseling. *Genet. Dis.*, **73**, 119–26

7. Brock, D. J. H. (1994). Carrier screening for cystic fibrosis. *Prenat. Diag.*, **14**, 1243–52

8. Jones, R. J. (1982). Genetic counseling and prevention of birth defects. *J. Am. Med. Assoc.*, **248**, 221–4

9. Lloyd, J. and Laurence, K. M. (1985). Sequelae and support after termination of pregnancy for fetal malformation. *Br. Med. J. Clin. Res. Ed.*, **290**, 907–9

10. Simpson, J. L., Elias, S., Gatlin, M. and Martin, A. O. (1981). Genetic counseling and genetic services in obstetrics and gynecology: implications for educational goals and clinical practice. *Am. J. Obstet. Gynecol.*, **140**, 70–80

11. Kessler, S. (1980). Genetic associates/counselors in genetic services. *Am. J. Med. Genet.*, **7**, 323–34

12. Hof, J. O. and Kopinsky, S. M. (1982). Communication in genetic counselling. *S. Afr. Med. J.*, **62**, 758–64

13. Wertz, D. C. and Fletcher, J. C. (1988). Attitudes of genetic counselors. A multinational survey. *Am. J. Hum. Genet.*, **42**, 592–600

14. Holzgreve, B,. Holzgreve, W. and Golbus, M. S. (1983). The relevance of pre-amniocentesis pedigree analysis and genetic counselling. *Clin. Genet.*, **24**, 429–33

15. Lorenz, R. P., Willard, D. and Botti, J. J. (1986). Role of prenatal genetic counseling before amniocentesis. A survey of genetics centers. *J. Reprod. Med.*, **31**, 1–3

16. Sorenson, J. R., Scotch, N. A., Swazey, J. P., Wertz, D. C. and Heeren, T. C. (1987). Reproductive plans of genetic counseling clients not eligible for prenatal diagnosis. *Am. J. Med. Genet.*, **28**, 345–52

17. Weaver, D. D. (1988). A survey of prenatally diagnosed disorders. *Clin. Obstet. Gynecol.*, **31**, 253–69

18. Wertz, D. C. and Sorenson, J. R. (1986). Client reactions to genetic counselling. Self-reports or influence. *Clin. Genet.*, **30**, 494–502

19. Hall, J. G., Friedmann, J. M. and Kenna, B. A. (1988). Clinical, genetic, and epidemiological factors in neural tube defects. *Am. J. Hum. Genet.*, **43**, 827–37

20. Papp, Z., Tóth, Z. and Török, O. (1987). Prenatal diagnosis policy without routine amniocentesis in pregnancies with a positive family history for neural tube defects. *Am. J. Med. Genet.*, **26**, 103–10

21. MRC Vitamin Study Research Group (1991). Prevention of neural-tube defects: results of the Medical Research Council Vitamin Study. *Lancet*, **338**, 131–7

22. van der Put, N. M. J., Steegers-Theunissen, R. P. M,. Frosst, P., Trijbels, F. J. M., Eskes, T. K. A. B., van der Heuvel, L. P., Mariman, E. C. M., den Heyer, M., Rozen, R. and Blom, H. J. (1995). Mutated methylenetetrahydrofolate reductase as a risk for spina bifida. *Lancet*, **346**, 1070–1

23. Colten, H. R. (1990). Screening for cystic fibrosis. *N. Engl. J. Med.*, **322**, 328–9

24. Németi, M., Louie, E., Papp, Z. and Johnson, J. P. (1991). Molecular analysis of cystic fibrosis in the Hungarian population. *Hum. Genet.*, **87**, 511–12

25. Papp, Z. (1990). *Obstetric Genetics.* (Budapest: Academic Press)

Possibilities of prenatal therapy

14

A. E. Dastur and N. A. Dastur

---

*'In times to come
the people will not judge us by
the creed we profess or
the label we wear or
the slogans we shout but
by our work, industry,
sacrifice,
honesty and purity of
Character.'*

Mahatma Gandhi

The modern world is a technological marvel: telephone that used to rest on the kitchen wall now fit in a shirt pocket; computers that used to fill a medium-sized gymnasium now sit snugly on the palm; photograph albums that used to gather dust in the family room can now be converted into a compact disc and transmitted on television.

From the wheel to the magnetic train, calligraphy to computer language, the flintlock to the hydrogen bomb and the stethoscope to *in vitro* fertilization, this is the story of invention; this is the core of technology: science, machinery and people.

Looking ahead to the horizon of the 21st century, the new millenium, it can be visualized that biotechnology, molecular biology, genetic engineering and virtual reality surgery will totally recast, restyle, remodel, reorganize, reform, revolutionize and redefine health-care. So it is with prenatal diagnosis and therapy.

Physicians follow the dictum, '*Primum, noli nocere*', meaning: first do no harm. The risks, benefits, costs, weaknesses and strengths of the tried and true conventional methods must be weighed against newer techniques.

To progress in a true and meaningful fashion, a balanced approach to the acquisition of new knowledge is needed. At the end of the day, the wonder of knowing must be weighed against the actual benefit of these newer concepts to the fetal patient.

Embryoscopy

Embryoscopy is an invasive procedure performed early in pregnancy, and entails direct visualization of the embryo by introducing a high-quality, narrow-diameter scope transvaginally, through the patent cervical canal, perforating the chorion to enter the extracelomic space. This is carried out under ultrasound guidance. Chorionic puncture is performed by using a sharp stab, trying to avoid the placenta. The combination of wide-angle lens and small embryo size means that total body visualization is possible in 75–90% of the procedures.

A number of embryonic abnormalities have been visualized using this technique, and its scope for first-trimester diagnosis and therapy is promising[1].

Access to the embryonic yolk-sac circulation is possible because the vessels on the yolk-sac are accessible in the extra-embryonic space. However, the full scope of embryonic blood sampling is yet to be explored. Actual embryo biopsy by embryoscopy would necessitate rupture of the amnion and, hence, currently is not feasible.

Complications of embryoscopy include placental separation, amniotic rupture and fetal demise.

Recently, early high-resolution endovaginal ultrasound with color flow imaging has shown to be useful in detecting early embryonic yolk-sac abnormalities between 5 and 10 weeks of gestation.

Future applications for embryoscopy include first-trimester prenatal diagnosis and therapeutic interventions, such as gene or cell therapy, at a time when the embryo is immunologically tolerant[2,3].

Fetoscopy

Fetoscopy is indicated for fetal visualization during biopsy procedures when fetal imaging by high-resolution ultrasound is not ideal. Examples are lesion-specific skin biopsy, muscle biopsy and soft-tissue biopsy. As more expertise is gained in performing skin, liver and other biopsy procedures under direct ultrasound control, fetoscopy procedures for such biopsies may take a back seat.

Unfortunately, ultrasound technology continues to advance at a tremendous pace, whereas fetoscopic technology is not the direct focus of much technological innovation. With the current surge in the development of endoscopy techniques, if a little attention be diverted to the refinement in instrumentation for operative fetoscopy, it is feasible that certain disorders could be treated with intrauterine surgery. Current instrumentation for operative fetoscopy during tissue biopsy permits continued visualization of the target only as a maximum diameter of nearly 3 mm. To negate the drawbacks of this relatively big incision, multiple-entry fetoscopy techniques with ultrasound guidance and monitoring would be more feasible.

Thin-gauge fetoscopy

Although high-resolution transvaginal ultrasound, color flow imaging and biochemical studies are playing an important role in diagnosing congenital anomalies in early pregnancies, a number of conditions may still escape early detection. Thin-gauge fetoscopy is a minimally invasive procedure, performed with telescopes of a diameter of 1 mm or less, and allows visualization of the external anatomy of the fetus after 12–14 weeks' gestation.

With the advanced lens system, wide-angle lens and fiberoptic illumination, the resolution surpasses that of ultrasound. In selected cases it is of use to confirm or to exclude the suspicion of a congenital anomaly from 12 weeks of pregnancy onwards[3–6].

In the management of birth defects, a thin-gauge fetoscope is used for visualization, and a separate entry port (or ports) of 1–1.5 mm diameter is employed for biopsy, shunt placements, needle aspirations, laser applications, etc. Surgery is performed under ultrasound guidance. Because of the very small size of the entry port, with instruments used for operative fetoscopy, the disturbance of the pregnancy is kept to a minimum. Hence, the risk of pregnancy loss, bleeding, leaking membranes and other maternal complications is very low. Depending upon the skill of the operating surgeon and his team, regional, local or general anesthesia may be used.

A thin-gauge fetoscope with flexible distal ends may enhance the overall scope of fetal and placental visualization, leaving no recess or corner of the pregnancy inaccessible[5]. Fetoscopy is not a dying art but one with scope and vision.

Fetal lower urinary-tract obstruction

The incidence of obstruction of the lower portion of the urinary tract of the fetus is 1:5000–8000 male babies. As the pregnancy advances, the blockage to the outflow of urine may lead to back pressure and severe damage to the fetal kidneys. Fetal death may occur *in utero* or shortly after birth if the obstruction is not treated promptly. On ultrasound examination of the fetus, the fetal bladder is markedly distended and is not seen to empty out, and marked distention of the ureter and the pelvicalyceal system is noted. There is accompanying oligohydramnios with low amniotic-fluid index. The treatment lies in relieving the obstruction by placing a vesicoamniotic shunt either directed by ultrasound or, more accurately, by a combination of operative fetoscopy under ultrasound guidance[7]. Recently, intrauterine fetal cystoscopy has been performed by Dr Quintero and his team from the Florida Institute for fetal diagnosis and therapy at the St Joseph's Women's Hospital, Tampa, Florida[5]. This technique allows visualization of the inside of the fetal bladder using an endoscope with a needle. The needles are not too dissimilar from those used in the evaluation of renal function of the fetus. The endoscopic visualization of the inside of the bladder allows better understanding of the obstruction. In some cases, it also allows elimination of the obstruction altogether.

Twin-to-twin transfusion syndrome

Twin-to-twin transfusion syndrome is a condition in which an unbalanced sharing of blood occurs between two fetuses through vascular communications that are present in a common placenta. It has a mortality rate close to 100% if not treated. The cause of death may be from cardiac overload in the recipient twin, exsanguination of the donor twin or preterm labor from polyhydramnios.

Laser photocoagulation of the abnormally communicating vessels consists of identifying the placental vessels that pass between the fetuses and interrupting them with laser energy. According to Dr Quintero and colleagues[5], a 0.1-in incision is performed on the maternal abdomen and the working instrument is inserted under ultrasound guidance. Identification and successful coagulation of the vessels is carried out endoscopically. The success rate for this procedure is approximately 66–75% for at least one fetus surviving. The disadvantages of this technique include non-availability in many centers, requirement of special equipment and skills and requirement of anesthesia[5].

Fetal-wound healing

Wound healing in the fetus fundamentally differs from healing in the adult. It has been shown that the fetus appears to heal without the inflammation, fibrosis and scar formation that can compromise wound healing in the adult[8].

In the fetus, acute inflammation is almost always absent; fibroblast proliferation and abundant collagen are frequently lacking; thus, scarring is not seen. As such, there are some similarities between fetal 'healing' and regeneration, notably the lack of aggressive acute inflammation, of fibroplasia and of a collagen matrix. Instead, an extracellular matrix (ECM) that is rich in hyaluranic acid (HA) is deposited. In several models, open wounds do not contract. Experimental manipulations suggest a possible role for amniotic fluid in the inhibition of fetal-wound contraction[9,10].

The unique qualities of fetal-wound healing may be attributed to its unique ECM, an entirely different profile of macromolecular structural constituents when compared with the adult ECM. The fetal ECM is richer in glycosaminoglycans, particularly HA[11,12].

Prospects of gene therapy

Genetic engineering in humans (i.e. the insertion of one or more genes into cells of the human body) could, theoretically, be accomplished for a variety of purposes. By using somatic-cell gene therapy (SCGT), the new genetic information would be introduced only into the somatic (non-reproductive) cells of a patient to correct a genetic disease. Germ-line gene therapy also has the goal of treating a disease, but this type of therapy involves introducing the new genetic information into the reproductive cells so that the defect would be corrected not only in the patient but also in his or her future offspring[13].

Somatic gene therapy is a new form of medical research that may lead to powerful treatments for a wide range of diseases. In the future, somatic gene therapy could treat cystic fibrosis, Duchenne's muscular dystrophy (DMD), certain autoimmune conditions such as severe combined immune deficiency (SCID), some forms of cancer, diabetes and even coronary heart disease.

Gene therapy techniques will introduce copies of the 'healthy' gene into those cells (called target cells) in the body that are affected by the faulty gene. Ideally, no other cells in the body should accept these genes and there are a number of proposed methods for inserting human genes into target cells. Much research is being concentrated on gene transfer into hematopoietic stem cells which divide to form white blood cells. Stem cells are found in the bone marrow of children and adults. The first condition to be treated by gene therapy was the immune condition SCID.

When stem cells divide, T-cells are formed. Stem cells can be removed from the bone marrow and working copies of the adenosine deaminase (ADA) gene inserted into them. The modified cells can be returned to the patient, where they will divide to produce white blood cells.

A virus can penetrate a cell, inserting its genes into the nucleus. The genes are then expressed using the host cell's genetic machinery. Viruses that infect human cells can offer a powerful way of delivering therapy genes into the nuclei of a particular type of human cell. Viruses must be altered before they are used for gene therapy. Modified adenoviruses are an important approach to gene therapy for cystic fibrosis.

The genes of a virus that enable it to infect new cells are removed from the viral genome, and the therapy gene is added. The virus is called a vector because it carries genes into target cells. The long-term aim is that the therapy genes be routinely incorporated into the genome, so that they are replicated whenever the cell divides. It is possible that the insertion of a therapy gene into a critical gene sequence might cause unforeseen problems. Some genes that cause cancer can become active in this way.

Alternative methods of delivering genes into cells are being developed. Therapy genes can be added to a plasmid and enclosed in a coating of liposomes. Liposomes can fuse with cell membranes, creating a passageway for the genes into the cell. Liposomes are a potentially safer method of delivering genes than modified viruses, but have the problem of easily delivering genes to non-target cells.

Proposals for new gene-therapy projects have to be considered very carefully by many different expert committees before they can begin. The safety of the therapy has to be considered, both for the patient and the general public. The anticipated benefit to the patient has to be balanced against the risk.

Transplantation of fetal cells

Cellular transplantation has long been considered as a possible alternative to whole-organ transplantation for a variety of tissues. In experimental systems, encouraging results have been seen with transplantation of hematopoietic stem cells (HSCs), pancreatic islet cells and hepatocytes.

For individuals with inherited defects in bone marrow-produced cell lines that can be diagnosed by chorionic villus sampling (e.g. hemoglobinopathies, immunodeficiencies), reconstitution with a normal cell line early in gestation has many theoretical advantages and considerable clinical appeal.

The fetus should be the ideal donor of HSCs for transplantation. During human gestation, HSCs are first found in the yolk-sac at about the fourth week of gestation. From here, the liver (sixth week of gestation) and spleen (seventh week of gestation) are seeded. From about the 14th to the 20th week of gestation, hematopoiesis finally switches to the bone marrow.

The fetus makes an ideal host for transplantation of HSCs, not only because of its ontological readiness for engraftment before 20 weeks' gestation, but also because the fetus is immunotolerant at a very early stage in gestation, and permits foreign grafts without rejection.

The concept of *in utero* transplantation of HSCs is so appealing that it has already been attempted clinically.

In the period before the 20th week of gestation, the human fetus not only has a depleted stromal environment, but it is also programmed for the reception of HSCs. Fetal immunotolerance and stromal preparedness obviate the need for host preparation with chemotherapy or irradiation, which is a significant disadvantage of postnatal bone-marrow transplantation.

In conclusion, cellular transplantation may provide a method for replacing absent or defective cells without the need for a solid-organ transplant. The fetus may be an ideal donor for these cells in several situations because of its unique immunological and functional attributes. By the same token, the fetus makes an ideal recipient for HSCs and, potentially, for many other cellular transplants. Experimental work using fetal HSCs, islet cells and dopaminergic cells suggests that the fetus may soon play an important role in the field of cellular transplantation[14].

References

1. Rotmensch, S., Reece, E. A. and Hobbins, J. C. (1992). Embryoscopy and fetoscopy. In Iffy, L., Apuzzio, J. J. and Vintzileos, A. M. (eds.) *Operative Obstetrics*, 2nd edn, Vol. 11, pp. 114–23. (New York: McGraw-Hill)
2. Reece, E. A. (1992). Embryoscopy: new development in prenatal medicine. *Curr. Opin. Obstet. Gynecol.*, **4**, 447–55
3. Reece, E. A., Honko, C., Goldestein, I. and Witznitzer, A. (1995). Toward fetal therapy using needle embryofetoscopy. *Ultrasound Obstet. Gynecol.*, **5**, 281–5
4. Reece, E. A., Goldestein, I., Chatwani, A., Brown, R., Honko, C. and Witznitzer, A. (1994). Transabdominal needle embryoscopy: a new technique paving the way for early fetal therapy. *Obstet. Gynecol.*, **84**, 634–6
5. Quintero, R., Munoz, H., Hasbun, J. *et al.* (1995). Fetal endoscopic surgery in a case of twin pregnancy complicated by reversed arterial perfusion sequence (TRAP sequence). *Rev. Chile. Obstet. Gynecol.*, **60**, 112–27
6. Estes, J. M., MacGillivery, T. E., Hedrick, M. H., Adzick, N. S. and Harrison, M. R. (1992). Fetoscopic surgery for treatment for congenital anomalies. *J. Pediatr. Surg.*, **27**, 950–4
7. Estes, J. M. and Harrison, M. R. (1993). Fetal obstructive uropathy. *Semin. Petiatr. Surg.*, **2**, 129–35
8. Krummel, M. T. and Longaker, T. M. (1991). Fetal wound healing. In Harrison, M. R., Golbus, M. S. and Filly, R. A. (eds.) *The Unborn Patient – Prenatal Diagnosis and Therapy*, 2nd edn, pp. 526–36. (London, Montreal, Philadelphia: W. B. Saunders)
9. Gross, R. H. (1969). *Principles of Regeneration*. (New York: Academic Press)
10. Gross, R. H. (1987). Why mammals do not regenerate – or do they? *News Physiol. Sci.*, **2**, 112
11. Depalma, R. L., Krummel, T. M., Nelson, J. M. *et al.* (1978). Fetal wound matrix is composed of proteoglycan rather than collagen. *Surg. Forum*, **38**, 626
12. Krummel, T. M., Nelson, J. M., Diegelmann, R. F. *et al.* (1986). Wound healing in the fetal and neonatal rabbit. *Surg. Forum*, **37**, 595
13. Karson, E. M. and Anderson, W. F. (1991). Prospects of gene therapy. In Harrison, M. R., Golbus, M. S. and Filly, R. A. (eds.) *The Unborn Patient – Prenatal Diagnosis and Therapy*, 2nd edn, p. 481. (London, Montreal, Philadelphia: W. B. Saunders)
14. Crombleholme, T. M., Zanjane, E. D., Langer, J. C. and Harrison, M. R. (1991). Transplantation of fetal cells. In Harrison, M. R., Golbus, M. S. and Filly, R. A. (eds.) *The Unborn Patient – Prenatal Diagnosis and Therapy*, 2nd edn, pp. 495–6, 505. (London, Montreal, Philadelphia: W. B. Saunders)

In utero surfactant for prophylaxis of idiopathic respiratory distress syndrome

15

E. V. Cosmi

Introduction

Neonatal respiratory distress syndrome (NRDS) remains a major cause of mortality and morbidity in preterm newborn infants. Prenatal corticosteroids 'prophylaxis', although beneficial, are not a panacea, and remain problematic for several reasons: (1) about 10% of neonates so treated are still affected by NRDS; and (2) their efficacy before 28 weeks' gestation on both the incidence and severity of NRDS still remains to be defined albeit a beneficial impact on neonatal mortality and on the reduction of intraventricular hemorrhage (IVH) have been suggested[1]. Administration of supplementary surfactant (SS) to neonates affected by NRDS has become a common method of treatment. However, tracheal intubation and repeated doses of SS are often required to facilitate its uniform distribution within the lung. It seems logical, therefore, that the most rational approach would be the prevention rather than treatment of NRDS and that the most natural way would be to instill SS into the fetal pulmonary liquid (FPL) compartment (1) at birth before the first breath; (2) after endotracheal intubation of the extracted head from the vagina or from the uterine muscle during Cesarean section (CS); or (3) as we have found, *in utero* by direct injection into amniotic fluid (IAF) close to the fetal mouth and nostrils so that uniform distribution within the FPL is enhanced.

The scientific basis for this 'prophylactic' IAF administration of SS spans three decades of research on the fluid dynamics and related biochemistry of FPL and amniotic fluid (AF)

compartments. Three lines of research have paved the way. Adams and colleagues[2,3] provided the first detailed and systematic studies of FPL. They defined organic and inorganic composition, surface activity, fluid movement and comparison with other liquid compartments of the maternal–fetal complex. Gluck and co-workers[4,5] presented meticulous studies of the chemical development of FPL and fetal pulmonary tissue. Scarpelli[6,7] proved the metabolic origin of FPL surfactant from pulmonary tissue and defined the lipid and protein gradients between FPL and AF. From these data, Scarpelli suggested that AF phospholipids may be used to diagnose fetal lung maturity (FLM); Gluck and colleagues[8] later proved this to be correct. Collectively, these studies had established the fluid and chemical interrelationships between FPL and AF. Two additional findings have reinforced our appreciation of the importance of FPL surfactants to successful transition to airbreathing at birth: (1) FPL surfactants are the principal substrate for formation of intraalveolar bubbles from FPL at the onset of airbreathing at birth[9]. Surfactants form the ultrathin films of bubbles that carry air to the alveoli ('saccules') and establish normal gas exchange and alveolar stability; (2) even after therapeutic intratracheal instillation of surfactant to the postnatal infant, first reported in the pioneering study of Fujiwara and associates[10], significant clinical intervention is required. For example, multiple doses of SS may be needed and the positions of the neonate must be regularly changed to facilitate an even distribution of SS into the lungs. In addition, the untoward effects of endotracheal intubation and postnatal instillation of SS must be considered, including the associated hypoxia, bradycardia and barotrauma.

Intra-amniotic delivery of surfactant is subject both to immediate dilution at the instillation site and to fetal swallowing, so that SS may not enter the FPL compartment in sufficient concentrations[11,12]. Our observation on fetal sheep shows that there is no net flow of FPL out of the lungs in the absence of fetal breathing movements (FBMs)[13,14]. On the other hand, we have found in pregnant sheep and rabbits that aminophylline given to the mother induces and/or increases FBMs[15]. This observation has prompted us to combine antenatal administration of aminophylline to the mother with IAF administration of natural SS. We anticipated that, during FBMs, SS would enter the FPL and, hence, be distributed to the peripheral airways of the fetus[13,14]. Most of the data presented below have been reported in previous publications[16-19].

Materials and methods

Table 1 summarizes maternal conditions of the study group. Four fetuses were affected by severe intrauterine growth retardation (IUGR); two mothers had presented with HELLP syndrome (hemolysis, elevated liver enzymes, low platelets). The indications for CS in nine cases was the rapid deterioration of the fetal condition. The sixth case was affected by vaginal bleeding which contraindicated further treatment with ritodrine. Because labor proceeded rapidly without signs of fetal distress and the presentation was cephalic, it was decided to deliver the fetus vaginally.

After obtaining informed consent from all patients, amniocentesis was performed under ultrasound guidance to collect AF for testing FLM; the needle was directed near the fetal nares and mouth and was kept in place. Fetal lung maturity was assessed by a rapid test, the shake test, and later on by lecithin/sphingomyelin (L/S) determination and phosphatidylglycerol measurement using the method of

Table 1 Summary of cases treated with intra-amniotic supplementary natural surfactant

Case	Gestational age (weeks)	Diagnosis	CTG	Doppler flow analysis[†]	Pre-surfactant Shake test	L/S	PG
1	28	IUGR	non-reactive	RED	neg.	1.8	abs.
2	32	IUGR	reactive	AED	neg.	2.0	abs.
3	32	HELLP	reactive	> RI of uterine arteries	neg.	1.9	abs.
4	28	IUGR	non-reactive	RED	neg.	NA	NA
5	28	HELLP	reactive	> PI umbilical artery	neg.	2.0	abs.
6	24	preterm labor, uncontroll- able vaginal bleeding	reactive	normal	neg.	10	abs.
7*	33	Sjögren syndrome–IUGR < 5 centile	non-reactive	ARED	NA NA	NA	
8	27	placenta previa, uncon- trollable bleeding	reactive	normal	neg.	2.0	abs.
9	28	PIH	non-reactive	AED	neg.	1.0	abs.
10	32	PIH, polyhydramnios	non-reactive	normal		2.4	abs.

*In spite of aminophylline to mother at high dosage, it was impossible to elicit fetal breathing movements (FBMs); [†]umbilical artery; CTG, cardiotocography; L/S lecithin/sphingomyelin; PG, phosphatidylglycerol; IUGR, intrauterine growth retardation; HELLP, hemolysis–elevated liver enzymes–low platelets; PIH, pregnancy induced hypertension; RED, reversed end-diastolic flow; AED, absent end-diastolic flow; RI, resistance index; PI, pulsatility index; ARED, absent and/or reversed blood flow; neg., negative; abs., absent; NA, not analyzed

Gluck and colleagues[8]. If the shake test indicated fetal lung immaturity, a bolus of 240 mg of aminophylline was administered over 10 min to the mother followed by intravenous infusion at the rate of 0.02–0.1 mg/kg/min. The fetus was continuously monitored with Doppler velocimetry and intermittently with external cardiotocography (CTG). Five to fifteen minutes after the bolus dose of aminophylline, FBMs first appeared as vortexes of nasal fluid waveforms through the fetal nares, then began at a rate of 10–12/min as documented both by chest wall movements and inspiratory and expiratory flows of liquid through the nares. This activity was recorded continuously with color Doppler equipment. Natural surfactant (Curosurf; Chiesi Farmaceutici, Parma, Italy), 80–120 mg in 1 ml normal saline solution, was then instilled through the amniocentesis needle directed towards the fetal mouth and nares. In nine cases, CS was performed under epidural anesthesia, 60–150 min after the administration of surfactant. Before the incision of amniotic membranes, a sample of AF was collected for further analysis of FLM.

Results

After IAS injection, entry of the surfactant was seen by ultrasound as a sonolucent material that moved down the trachea and upper airways during FBMs, which, from 10–12/min had increased in depth and frequency to 88/min during aminophylline infusion. Some of the SS was swallowed by the fetus. Following aminophylline infusion to the mother, the fetal heart rate increased by 10–15 beats/min. Treatment with SS resulted in a significant increase of the L/S ratio. Phosphatidylglycerol was also identified in the AF samples taken at CS. Time to sustained respiration, Apgar score at 1 and 5 min, sex and weight are given in Table 2. The neonates were transferred to the neonatal ward. Seven of the infants followed an uneventful clinical course to the time of discharge from the hospital. Case 5 showed radiological signs of mild RDS and, at 3 h after birth received a dose of 120 mg of Curosurf. He was extubated 72 h later. Case 6 (birth weight 630 g) was born at 24 weeks' gestation in good condition and was administered a prophylactic dose of 120 mg of Curosurf, in accordance with the protocol in use

Table 2 Outcome of cases treated with intra-amniotic supplementary natural surfactant

| Case | Mode of delivery | Post-surfactant at CS | | | Weight (g) | Sex | TSR (s) | Apgar at 1/5 min | Clinical outcome |
		Shake test	L/S	PG					
1	CS	pos.	5.0	pres.	1035	M	30	8/10	uneventful
2	CS	pos.	3.5	pres.	1650	M	25	8/9	uneventful
3	CS	pos.	2.5	pres.	1700	M	45	8/10	uneventful
4	CS	pos.	NA	NA	1095	M	30	7/10	uneventful
5	CS	pos.	2.4	pres.	970	M	20	5/8	mild RDS*
6	VD	NA	NA	NA	630	F	35	6/9	uneventful[†]
7	CS	NA	NA	NA	675	F	45	6/9	uneventful
8	CS	NA	NA	NA	950	F	35	6/9	uneventful
9	CS	pos.	2.0	pres.	1228	M	40	6/9	RDS[‡]
10	CS	pos.	3.0	pres.	1950	M	50	7/7	pulmonary hypoplasia**

*Treated at birth with one dose of supplementary natural surfactant and extubated after 72 h; [†]same as case 5, extubated after 13 days: died at 35 days of life following blood-borne cytomegolovirus (CMV) infection; [‡]mother did not receive aminophylline because of fetal gasping: at birth he was treated with two additional doses of supplementary surfactant (SS), complete recovery followed; **neonate died 12 h after birth of severe pulmonary hypoplasia, after second dose of intra-amniotic surfactant (IAS) before delivery; L/S, lecithin/sphingomyelin; PG, phosphatidylglycerol; TSR, time to sustained respiration (normal value ≤ 60 s); CS, Cesarean section; VD, vaginal delivery; pos., positive; pres., present; NA, not analyzed; M, male; F, female; RDS, respiratory distress syndrome

in our Neonatology Department for all babies weighing less than 900 g. Because of the above protocol, she was artificially ventilated for 13 days and then extubated. At 35 days of life she died because of a disseminated cytomegalovirus (CMV) infection acquired following a blood transfusion for the treatment of anemia of prematurity. Because case 9, whose mother was suffering from pregnancy induced hypertension (PIH), was gasping *in utero*, we decided not to give aminophylline to the mother. At birth, he showed some signs of respiratory distress and required two doses of SS in the neonatal period. Case 10 was born to a mother affected by hypertension and polyhydramnios; in this case, even after a second dose of intra-amniotic surfactant (IAS) before delivery, the neonate died 12 h after birth at 32 + 4 weeks' gestation because of severe pulmonary hypoplasia.

Table 3 summarizes laboratory and clinical data of two neonates whose mothers refused IAS therapy. The first was born by emergency CS from a mother affected by HELLP and developed signs of RDS; for this reason she was given four doses of SS after birth. The infant developed interstitial emphysema and died 36 h following delivery. The other neonate was delivered vaginally because of bleeding that contraindicated further tocolytic therapy. He was treated for RDS with two doses of SS, with high-frequency ventilation for 48 h and continuous positive airway pressure for 4 weeks. He died at 8 months of age of severe bronchopulmonary dysplasia.

Discussion

The present study follows our previous reports[16–19] and shows a successful outcome following prenatal administration of natural surfactant to the human fetus. Whereas definitive demonstration of distribution of surfactant into distal airways was not expected, several lines of evidence suggest that effective intrapulmonary distribution was achieved:

(1) The surfactant was injected at the level of the mouth and nares of the fetus and was seen to be distributed into the upper airways;

(2) FBMs induced by the intravenous administration of aminophylline to the mother were sustained and deep and increased in frequency to 88/min;

(3) At the beginning, nasal fluid waveforms were synchronous with chest wall breathing movements as documented by ultrasound and color Doppler. Entry of surfactant into and distribution by diffusion throughout all potential airspaces are promoted by the agitation produced by FBMs[13,14]: this is analogous to the mixing of added substrates in lamb fetal lungs[13];

(4) It is also possible that smooth muscle relaxation induced by aminophylline may lower the resistance to the movement of SS through the airways;

(5) Some of the SS was seen to be swallowed by the fetus which was expected particularly as gastric fluid at birth often reflects surfactant content of the lung;

(6) Continued FBMs favor rapid dispersion and uniform distribution of the surfactant into the smallest airways and saccules as suggested by our studies in the sheep fetus and also by Adams and colleagues[2,3];

(7) Consequently, the previously surfactant-poor FPL had been enriched by the prophylactic surfactant at sites required for successful adaptation to air-breathing at birth;

(8) The uneventful clinical course of the newborn infants in our study is consistent with the known role of FPL as the first substrate for normal surfactant function at birth[9]. Studies in baboons[11,12] indicate that antenatal intra-amniotic instillation of surfactant can be an effective prophylactic therapy;

(9) IAF administration of Curosurf with a suspension of microparticles of coal in pregnant rabbits is followed by inhalation

Table 3 Characteristics of patients who refused treatment with intra-amniotic surfactant

Case	Gestational age (weeks)	Diagnosis	CTG	Doppler flow analysis	L/S	PG	Mode of delivery	Weight (g)	Sex	TSR (s)	Apgar at 1/5 min	Clinical outcome
1	26	HELLP	react.	AED	1.0	abs.	CS	630	F	120	1/6	4 doses of SS to neonate, interstitial emphysema, died 36 h after birth
2	26	PROM/ bleeding	react.	AED	ND	ND	VD	960	M	50	6/8	2 doses of SS to neonate, 48 h under HFV, CPAP for 4 weeks; severe BPD, died at 8 months of age

CTG, cardiotocography; L/S, lecithin/sphingomyelin; PG, phosphatidylglycerol; TSR, time to sustained respiration; HELLP, hemolysis–elevated liver enzymes–low platelets; PROM, premature rupture of membranes; react., reactive; AED, absent end-diastolic flow; ND, not determined; abs., absent; CS, Cesarean section; VD, vaginal delivery; F, female; M, male; SS, supplementary surfactant; HFV, high-frequency ventilation; CPAP, continuous positive airway pressure; BPD, bronchopulmonary dysplasia

of the surfactant into the peripheral airways as documented at birth[20];

(10) Petrikovsky and colleagues[21] have also shown the feasibility of intrauterine administration of surfactant. However, in their study, SS was injected into the mouth of the human fetus under direct vision through a fiberoptic endoscope, which had been passed through the cervical canal during active preterm labor after spontaneous rupture of the membranes. The authors found no fetal, maternal or neonatal complications in the three cases reported.

If we rephrase the National Institutes of Health (NIH) Consensus Development Conference[22], intra-amniotic surfactant is particularly useful in pregnancies where delivery is expected to be imminent and there is no time for corticosteroids to elicit their effect. However, because the placenta is rich in 11β-ol-hydroxy-steroid dehydrogenase, which converts active steroids into inactive 11-keto-steroids, the question has been posed as to whether certain corticosteroids administered to the mother reach the fetus in sufficient quantities to elicit their biological effect, e.g. acceleration of FLM[23]. Betamethasone crosses the placenta to the extent that fetal concentrations are about 33% of those in the maternal circulation[24]. In any event, direct prenatal administration of SS appears to be a potentially powerful and unambiguous clinical approach. In one of our cases (9), the mother was affected by severe PIH with absent end diastolic flow and non-reactive CTG. Because the fetus was gasping, we did not administer aminophylline to the mother. This fetus was delivered by CS, weighed 1228 g, had a time to sustained respiration of 40 s and Apgar scores of 6 at 1 min and 9 at 5 min, but showed signs of respiratory distress. Thus, after birth, he received two additional doses of SS, which were followed by full recovery after 14 days of intubation and continuous positive airway pressure. Whereas fetal gasping may favor the influx of SS into the potential airspaces of the fetus, some of it may be extruded following a subsequent grunt. We speculate further, therefore, that administration of aminophylline or of another analeptic drug may be essential to induce the vortexes and regular FBMs, and thereby favor the influx of SS into the fetal lung.

Acknowledgement

This work was supported in part by the Italian National Research Council (CNR), Italy.

References

1. Crowley, P., Chalmers, I. and Keirse, M. J. N. (1990). The effects of corticosteroid administration before preterm delivery: an overview of the evidence from controlled trials. *Br. J. Obstet. Gynaecol.*, **97**, 11–25
2. Adams, F. H. and Fujiwara, T. 1963). Surfactant in the fetal lamb's tracheal fluid. *J. Pediatr.*, **63**, 537–42
3. Adams, F. H., Fujiwara, T. and Rowshan, G. (1963). The nature and origin of the fluid in the fetal lamb lung. *J. Pediatr.*, **63**, 881–8
4. Gluck, L., Motoyama, E. K., Smits, H. L. and Kulovich, M. V. (1967). The biochemical development of surface activity in mammalian lung. I. *Pediatr. Res.*, **1**, 237–46
5. Gluck, L., Scribney, M. and Kulovich, M. V. (1967). The biochemical development of surface activity in the mammalian lung. II. *Pediatr. Res.*, **1**, 247–65
6. Scarpelli, E. M. (1967). The lung tracheal fluid, and lipid metabolism of the fetus. *Pediatrics*, **40**, 951–61
7. Scarpelli, E. M. (1968). *The Surfactant System of the Lung*. (Philadelphia: Lea & Febiger)
8. Gluck, L., Kulovich, M. V., Borer, R. C. Jr, Brenner, P. H., Anderson, G. G. and Spellacy, W. N. (1971). Diagnosis of respiratory distress syndrome by amniocentesis. *Am. J. Obstet. Gynecol.*, **109**, 440–5

9. Scarpelli, E. M. (1978). Intrapulmonary foam at birth: an adaptional phenomenon. *Pediatr. Res.,* **12**, 1070–80

10. Fujiwara, T., Chida, S., Watabe, Y., Maeta, H., Morita, T. and Abe, T. (1980). Artificial surfactant therapy in hyaline membrane disease. *Lancet,* **1**, 155–9

11. Galan, H. L., Cipriani, C., Coulson, J. J., Bean, J. D., Collier, G. and Kuehl, T. J. (1993). Surfactant replacement therapy *in utero* for the prevention of hyaline membrane disease in the preterm baboon. *Am. J. Obstet. Gynecol.,* **169**, 817–24

12. Galan, H. L., Cipriani, C., Coalson, J. J., Bean-Lijewski, J. D., Collier, G. and Kuhel, T. J. (1996). Hyaline membrane disease surfactant prophylaxis in the preterm baboon: a comparison of postpartum versus *in utero* therapy. *Prenat. Neonat. Med.,* **1**, 122–30

13. Scarpelli, E. M., Condorelli, S. and Cosmi, E. V. (1975). Fetal pulmonary fluid. I. Validation and significance of method for determination of volume and volume change. *Pediatr. Res.,* **9**, 190–5

14. Scarpelli, E. M., Condorelli, S. and Cosmi, E. V. (1975). Lamb fetal pulmonary fluid. II. Fate of phosphatidylcholine. *Pediatr. Res.,* **9**, 195–201

15. Cosmi, E. V., Felli, F., Grossmann, G., Lachmann, B. and Robertson, B. (1979). Improved survival in the premature rabbit neonate following antenatal treatment with aminophylline. *IRCS Med. Sci.,* **7**, 115–22

16. Cosmi, E. V., La Torre, R., Di Iorio, R. and Anceschi, M. M. (1996). A novel treatment of fetal lung immaturity. Society for Perinatal Obstetricians, 16th Annual Meeting. *Am. J. Obstet. Gynecol.,* **174**, 487 (abstr. 653)

17. Cosmi, E. V., La Torre, R., Di Iorio, R. and Anceschi, M. M. (1996). Surfactant administration to the human fetus *in utero*: a new approach to prevention of neonatal respiratory distress syndrome (IRDS). *J. Perinat. Med.,* **24**, 191–3

18. Cosmi, E. V., La Torre, R. and Di Iorio, R. (1996). Intraamniotic instillation of surfactant for prevention of neonatal respiratory distress syndrome (IRDS): a preliminary report. *Appl. Cardiopulm. Pathophysiol.,* **6**, 3–5

19. Cosmi, E. V. (1996). Prenatal administration of surfactant. *Prenat. Neonat. Med.,* **1**, 109–11

20. Tannuri, U., Maksoud, F., Diniz, E. M. A., Santos, M. M., Tannuari, A. C. A., Rodrigues, C. J. and Rodrigues, E. V., Jr. (1997). Intraamniotically infused surfactant is aspirated by the fetus and improves functional and morphometric parameters in an animal model of congenital diaphragmatic hernia (CDH). Presented at *12th International Workshop on Surfactant Replacement,* Stockholm, May–June

21. Petrikovsky, B. M., Lysikiewicz, A., Markin, L. B. and Slomko, Z. (1995). *In utero* administration to preterm human fetuses by endoscopy. *Fetal Diag. Ther.,* **10**, 127–30

22. National Institutes of Health (1995). Consensus Development Conference Statement. Effect of corticosteroids for fetal maturation on perinatal outcomes. *Am. J. Obstet. Gynecol.,* **173**, 246–52

23. Cosmi, E. V. (ed.) (1980). *Obstetric Anesthesia and Perinatology,* Ch. 7, Part I. (New York: Appleton-Century-Crofts)

24. Marinoni, E., Korebrits, C., Di Iorio, R., Cosmi, E. V. and Challis, J. R. G. (1997). Effect of betamethasone *in vivo* on placental corticotropin-releasing hormone (CRH) in human pregnancy, in press

In utero fetal steroid or surfactant treatment and perinatal outcome

16

I. Szabó, T. Ertl, M. Vizer, A. Arany and E. Gács

Introduction

Respiratory distress syndrome (RDS) is one of the most common causes of neonatal mortality in premature infants. Different therapeutic approaches have been attempted to prevent this condition[1]. Among agents investigated for beneficial effects on lung maturation, antenatal glucocorticoid is the most effective single strategy for reducing the adverse consequences of preterm birth[2]. Meta-analysis of randomized controlled trials of maternal corticosteroid therapy has provided evidence of efficacy and safety of antenatal corticosteroid therapy[3].

A single direct fetal injection of corticosteroids alone or in combination with thyroid hormones has been shown to improve ventilatory and cardiovascular functions and augment postnatal metabolic adaptive responses in prematurely delivered animals[4–6]. It is technically feasible to accomplish fetal intramuscular injection in the human; however, steroids have never yet been administered by this route.

The outcomes for infants with RDS have been significantly improved by the use of exogenously administered surfactant to treat RDS[7]. It has been suggested that the combined use of prenatal maternal corticosteroids and postnatal surfactant on the lungs is synergetic[8]. Studies in animal models have shown that for the prevention of RDS, antenatal intra-amniotic instillation of surfactant is as effective as post-delivery intratracheal administration[9,10]. Moreover, Cosmi and colleagues have successfully developed a novel method for intra-amniotic fluid administration of surfactant in human pregnancies complicated with intrauterine growth retardation (IUGR) and the perinatal outcome was favorable[11,12]. Petrikovsky and his co-workers have reported on the feasibility of *in utero* administration of surfactant to preterm human fetuses by endoscopy[13].

Patients and methods

Our department has recently changed the protocol for the conservative management of preterm premature rupture of membranes (PPROM). If there is no clinical and laboratory evidence of intrauterine infection, and sonography reveals a four-quadrant amniotic-fluid index (AFI) of 4 cm or less, intra-amniotic saline infusion is used instead of labor induction. Conservative management of PPROM and the introduction of amnioinfusion in selected cases may improve functional lung maturity and perinatal outcome by advancing gestational age[14].

The study cohort consisted of 16 patients whose pregnancies were complicated with PPROM or pre-eclampsia, IUGR and severe oligohydramnios. The research protocol was approved by the local ethical committee of the university. Mothers were informed and written consent had been obtained prior to the procedure. Criteria for enrollment included singleton pregnancy, normal fetal-heart rate tracing and AFI of 4 cm or less. Exclusion criteria included fetal heart rate abnormalities, fetal malformations and clinical chorioamnionitis. Before the intervention had been started a complete transabdominal ultrasound (U/S) examination was carried out including fetal biometry, biophysical profile, umbilical artery flow-velocimetry, AFI measurement, and evaluation

116

of fetal and placental position to determine the correct puncture site. A stable peripheral intravenous catheter was inserted, and 0.25 mg of terbutaline was given subcutaneously to the mother for uterine quiescence. Complying with sterile conditions, patients underwent amniocentesis with a 20 gauge spinal needle under continuous U/S guidance, and amniotic-fluid samples were sent for culture as well as assayed for fetal lung maturity tests. The needle was left in place and, before an attempt for amniotic fluid replacement was made, the fetuses of the 10 patients in the first group were given betamethasone intramuscularly (Celestone, 0.5 mg/kg estimated fetal weight) for the prevention of RDS.

In the second group of six patients, we prophylactically instilled surfactant (Survanta, 100 mg/kg estimated fetal weight) near the fetal nose and mouth through the amniocentesis needle, when fetal breathing movements induced by maternal intravenous aminophylline were sustained. During the procedure, blood pressure and heart rate were measured every 5 min. In all cases, immediate and serial daily non-stress tests (Oxford Sonicaid-System 8000 Oxford Sonicaid Ltd., Chichester, England), biophysical profile, umbilical artery flow-velocimetry and assessment of AFI were performed, as well as recording of clinical and laboratory signs of infection, from after the procedure until delivery, for fetal surveillance. Fetuses were delivered by Cesarean section under spinal anesthesia for fetal or combined fetal/maternal indications.

In order to evaluate the effects of direct fetal steroid therapy on the perinatal outcome, we carried out a retrospective analysis of premature infants born at less than 32 weeks of gestation in our department. During the same study period, 25 patients were admitted in the advanced stage of labor who were subsequently delivered without any steroid prophylaxis (NS), and 38 infants were born whose mothers received complete steroid prophylaxis before delivery (MS). To correct for gestational age and birth weight, two patients were excluded from the original fetal steroid cohort (FS; $n = 8$).

For statistical analysis, Student's t-test and relative risk (RR) with the corresponding 95% confidence interval (CI) were computed.

Results

No evidence of clinical infection was documented. All but one of the amniotic-fluid culture results were negative. All samples assayed for fetal lung maturity showed immature indices. Following each procedure, cardiotocographic findings demonstrated normal placental reserve capacity, and flowmetry results and AFI values were within normal range until labor induction. Table 1 summarizes clinical data of all patients treated either with *in utero* steroid or surfactant. Table 2 lists in detail clinical characteristics of eight fetuses born at less than

Table 1 Direct fetal steroid or surfactant treatment. Data are expressed as absolute values or mean (range)

	Steroid	*Surfactant*
Cases (*n*)	10	6
Gestational age at admission (weeks)	27.5 (25–31)	26.8 (25–32)
PPROM/intact membranes	6/4	2/4
Gestational age at delivery (weeks)	29.6 (26–35)	27.5 (26–32)
Interval, procedure–delivery (days)	10.6 (0.1–52)	1.1 (0.1–3.5)
Birth weight (g)	1250 (640–2030)	912 (770–1100)
Apgar score (5-min)	8.5 (7–10)	8.8 (8–10)
Severe RDS (*n*)	2	2
Postnatal surfactant needed (*n*)	6	4
28-day survival (*n*)	9	5

PPROM, preterm premature rupture of membranes; RDS, respiratory distress syndrome

Table 2 Direct fetal steroid treatment

	Case 1	Case 2	Case 3	Case 4	Case 5	Case 6	Case 7	Case 8
Gestational age at delivery (weeks)	31	28	31	26	30	30	27	26
PPROM	yes	yes	yes	no	no	no	no	yes
Amniotic fluid	minimal	minimal	minimal	severe oligo	normal	severe oligo	normal	minimal
Presentation	cephalic	breech	cephalic	cephalic	transverse	breech	breech	breech
Amnioinfusion	yes	yes	no	no	no	no	no	yes
Interval, procedure–delivery (days)	11	5	2	1	0.1	2.5	1.2	1.6
Mode of delivery	C/S	C/S	C/S	C/S	C/S	C/S	C/S	C/S
Indication	fetal	fetal	fetal	combined	combined	combined	fetal	fetal
Birth weight (g)	1570	950	1820	670	1050	1040	890	640
Apgar score (5-min)	9	9	7	8	7	9	9	8
RDS	+	+	+	++++	++	++	+	+
Postnatal surfactant	no	yes	no	yes	yes	yes	yes	yes
28-day survival	yes	yes	yes	no	yes	yes	yes	yes

PPROM, preterm premature rupture of membranes; C/S, Cesarean section; RDS, respiratory distress syndrome

32 weeks of gestation and exposed to direct intramuscular betamethasone. Table 3 gives the respective data of prophylactic intra-amniotic fluid surfactant therapy.

The gestational age at delivery and birth weight of NS, MS and FS groups were 28 ± 2.0, 28.6 ± 1.7 and 29.1 ± 2.0 weeks, and 1209 ± 482, 1261 ± 360 and 1228 ± 449 g, respectively (mean $\pm$ SD). The prevalence of severe RDS and intraventricular hemorrhage (IVH) tended to decrease both after fetal (FS) and maternal steroid treatment (MS). Moreover, the duration of mechanical ventilation was significantly shorter in the FS group compared with the need for ventilatory support of either the MS or NS group ($p < 0.05$). The survival rates of FS vs. NS (RR 1.56, CI 1.01–2.41) and MS vs. NS (RR 1.46, CI 1.01–2.13) groups were significantly higher (Table 4).

One neonate from the FS group had severe RDS and IVH and on the sixth day of life the newborn died as a consequence of pulmonary hemorrhage. We lost 11 infants from the NS and 7 from the MS group.

The perinatal outcome of those infants who were prophylactically treated *in utero* with surfactant was also favorable (gestational age 27.5 ± 2.3 weeks, birth weight 912 ± 152 g, survival rate 83%). There was no maternal complication as a result of the procedure.

Table 3 Intra-amniotic surfactant treatment

	Case 1	Case 2	Case 3	Case 4	Case 5	Case 6
Gestational age at delivery (weeks)	26	32	27	26	27	27
PPROM	no	no	yes	no	yes	no
Amniotic fluid	minimal	severe oligo	minimal	normal	minimal	severe oligo
Presentation	breech	breech	cephalic	breech	cephalic	cephalic
Amnioinfusion	yes	no	yes	no	no	no
Interval, procedure–delivery (h)	84	3	36	4	21	4
Mode of delivery	C/S	C/S	C/S	C/S	C/S	C/S
Indication	fetal	fetal	combined	combined	combined	combined
Birth weight (g)	780	1050	990	770	1100	780
Apgar score (5-min)	10	10	8	9	8	8
RDS	++	+	+	+++	+	++
Postnatal surfactant	yes	no	yes	yes	no	yes
28-day survival	yes	yes	yes	yes	yes	no

PPROM, preterm premature rupture of membranes; C/S, Cesarean section; RDS, respiratory distress syndrome

Table 4 Perinatal outcome of premature infants born at less than 32 weeks of gestation in 1996, Department of Obstetrics and Gynecology, University Medical School of Pécs, Hungary. Data are expressed as absolute values or mean $\pm$ SD

	No steroid	Maternal steroid	Fetal steroid
Cases (n)	25	38	8
Gestational age at delivery (weeks)	28 ± 2.0	28.6 ± 1.7	29.1 ± 2.0
Birth weight (g)	1209 ± 482	1261 ± 360	1228 ± 449
Severe RDS (n)	15 (60%)	16 (42%)	2 (25%)
Time on ventilator (days)	4.5 ± 2.9	4.4 ± 3.2	$1.7 \pm 1.4*$
Severe IVH (n)	6 (24%)	7 (18%)	1 (13%)
28-day survival (n)	14 (56%)	31 (82%)	7 (88%)
RR	—	MS vs. NS 1.46	FS vs. NS 1.56
95% CI	—	1.01–2.13	1.01–2.41

RDS, respiratory distress syndrome; IVH intraventricular hemorrhage; MS, maternal steroid treatment more than 24 h before delivery; NS, no steroid; FS, fetal steroid; RR, relative risk; CI, confidence interval; $*p < 0.05$

Discussion

To our best knowledge, this is the first report with regard to intramuscular corticosteroid therapy of the human fetus for the antenatal prevention of RDS.

In fetal lambs, markedly improved postnatal lung function was demonstrated 24–48 h after a single dose of betamethasone. Compliance increased and efficiency of ventilation and maximal lung volumes improved[5]. The minimal interval from fetal exposure to corticosteroids to delivery for improved postnatal lung function was between 8 and 15 h. Corticosteroid effects on pulmonary edema and blood pressure occurred within 8 h[15]. Two doses of betamethasone administered 1 week apart in the same animal model did not further enhance postnatal pulmonary function, although retreatment augmented surfactant protein B mRNA levels[16].

In the fetal sheep model, significant augmentation in cardiovascular function at birth was seen after fetal corticosteroid treatment. Corticosteroid-induced improvements in cardiovascular function (hemodynamic stability and normotension) may be involved in the reduction in incidence or severity of IVH, periventricular leukomalacia, necrotizing enterocolitis and patent ductus arteriosus. Antenatal glucocorticoid injection in the fetal lamb resulted in a brisk increase in plasma glucose and free fatty acid levels, which is important for metabolic adaptations to postnatal life[6].

Exposure of preterm lambs to a single injection of corticosteroids was associated with lower cortisol levels 24 h after betamethasone exposure, suggesting some degree of feedback inhibition of the pituitary–adrenal axis. Fetal treatment with betamethasone significantly increased triiodothyronine levels in cord blood and postnatally[5].

With regard to adverse consequences of fetal intramuscular corticosteroid treatment, pulmonary interstitial emphysema should be considered with 2 mg/kg betamethasone, but with a lower dose of 0.5 mg/kg it may be avoided[5].

Our preliminary results suggest that fetal intramuscular administration of corticosteroids may be indicated if: (1) clinical signs of fetal distress and/or severe maternal complications require termination of pregnancy at less than 32 weeks of gestation; (2) maternal steroid prophylaxis should be avoided; (3) as a consequence of severe oligo-anhydramnios, amnioinfusion is recommended and preterm delivery is threatening. The direct fetal route of administration seems to be more effective than maternal treatment, since the action does not depend on placental transfer, the dosage is more exact and rapid fetal response can be anticipated. If an extremely low birth-weight fetus is at high risk and subject to imminent delivery within hours, he/she may gain more benefit from prophylactic intra-amniotic surfactant instillation. Our main goal with fetal corticosteroid injection or antenatal surfactant treatment is to promote lung maturation and transition to air-breathing at the impending preterm birth, whereas the aim of amnioinfusion is to attempt to manage these pregnancies conservatively. Despite the fact that our study has a number of shortcomings (e.g. low number of cases, combined use of different therapeutic approaches), we believe that as early as the 25th week of gestation, U/S-guided single direct fetal intramuscular glucocorticoid or intra-amniotic fluid surfactant treatment combined with transabdominal amnioinfusion has great potential for becoming a clinically relevant approach for improvement of fetal lung maturation in selected cases of pregnancies complicated with severe oligohydramnios. Although in our study RDS developed in several cases, the fetal betamethasone or surfactant treatment followed by postnatal surfactant therapy reduced the severity of clinical symptoms and the duration and side-effects of mechanical ventilation, and provided favorable outcome in these very low birth-weight premature infants. Further investigation is needed to evaluate physiological and adverse effects, dosage, efficacy and safety of both fetal corticosteroid and surfactant therapy in human pregnancies.

References

1. Ballard, R. A. and Ballard, P. L. (1995). Lung maturation in prenatal preparation of the fetus. In Reed, G. B., Claireaux, A. E. and Cockburn, F. (eds.) *Diseases of the Fetus and Newborn,* 2nd edn, pp. 1337–43. (London: Chapman and Hall)

2. Liggins, G. C. and Howie, R. N. (1972). A controlled trial of antepartum glucocorticoid treatment for prevention of the RDS in premature infants. *Pediatrics,* **50**, 515–25

3. Crowley, P. A. (1995). Antenatal corticosteroid therapy: a meta-analysis of the randomized trials, 1972 to 1994. *Am. J. Obstet. Gynecol.,* **173**, 322–35

4. Jobe, A. H., Polk, D. H., Ikegami, M., Newnham, J., Sly, P., Kohen, R. and Kelly, R. (1993). Lung responses to ultrasound-guided fetal treatments with corticosteroids in preterm lambs. *J. Appl. Physiol.,* **75**, 2099–105

5. Polk, D. H., Ikegami, M., Jobe, A. H., Newnham, J., Sly, P., Kohen, R. and Kelly, R. (1995). Postnatal lung function in preterm lambs: effects of a single exposure to betamethasone and thyroid hormones. *Am. J. Obstet. Gynecol.,* **172**, 872–81

6. Padbury, J. F., Polk, D. H., Ervin, M. G., Berry, L. M., Ikegami, M. and Jobe, A. H. (1995). Postnatal cardiovascular and metabolic responses to a single intramuscular dose of betamethasone in fetal sheep born prematurely by cesarean section. *Pediatr. Res.,* **38**, 709–14

7. Fujiwara, T., Chida, S., Watabe, Y., Maeta, H., Morita, T. and Abe, T. (1980). Artificial surfactant therapy in hyalin membrane disease. *Lancet,* **1**, 55–9

8. Jobe, A. H., Mitchell, B. R. and Gunkel, J. H. (1993). Beneficial effects of the combined use of prenatal corticosteroids and postnatal surfactant on preterm infants. *Am. J. Obstet. Gynecol.,* **168**, 508–13

9. Galan, H. L., Cipriani, C., Coalson, J. J., Bean, J. D., Collier, G. and Kuehl, T. J. (1993). Surfactant replacement therapy *in utero* for prevention of hyaline membrane disease in the preterm baboon. *Am. J. Obstet. Gynecol.,* **169**, 817–24

10. Galan, H. L., Cipriani, C., Coalson, J. J., Bean-Lijewski, J. D., Collier, G. and Kuehl, T. J. (1996). Hyaline membrane disease surfactant prophylaxis in the preterm baboon: a comparison of postpartum versus *in utero* therapy. *Prenat. Neonat. Med.,* **1**, 122–30

11. Cosmi, E. V., La Torre, R., Di Iorio, R. and Anceschi, M. M. (1996). Surfactant administration to the human fetus *in utero*: a new approach to prevention of neonatal respiratory distress syndrome (RDS). *J. Perinat. Med.,* **24**, 191–3

12. Cosmi, E. V. (1996). Prenatal administration of surfactant. (Editorial). *Prenat. Neonat. Med.,* **1**, 109–11

13. Petrikovsky, B. M., Lysikiewicz, A., Markin, L. B. and Slomko, Z. (1995). *In utero* surfactant administration to preterm human fetuses by endoscopy. *Fetal Diagn. Ther.,* **10**, 127–30

14. Szabó, I., Szilágyi, A., Gács, E. and Székely, J. (1993). Amnioinfusion for management of preterm prelabour rupture of membranes. *Lancet,* **341**, 443–4

15. Ikegami, M., Polk, D. H. and Jobe, A. H. (1996). Minimum interval from fetal betamethasone treatment to postnatal lung responses in preterm lambs. *Am. J. Obstet. Gynecol.,* **174**, 1408–13

16. Polk, D. H., Ikegami, M., Jobe, A. H. Sly, P., Kohan, R. and Newnham, J. (1997). Preterm lung function after retreatment with antenatal betamethasone in preterm lambs. *Am. J. Obstet. Gynecol.,* **176**, 308–15

The scientific evaluation of the content of antenatal care: what is left?

17

P. Bergsjø

Background

The most recent estimate of maternal mortality from the World Health Organization (WHO) approaches 600 000 deaths in the world annually[1]. This is more than previously thought, indicating a substantial underestimation of maternal mortality in the past. The fact that 99% of these deaths occur in developing countries is even more frightening. While fewer than ten mothers die per 100 000 live births in the most affluent countries, the corresponding ratio in eastern and western Africa, south of the Sahara, is about 1000 per 100 000, or 100 times higher than in the rich countries.

The global figures for perinatal deaths are even more staggering. It is estimated that there are more than 7.6 million perinatal deaths worldwide, 98% of which take place in developing countries[2]. The ratios range from more than 100 per 1000 births in some African countries to 5 per 1000 in some northern and western countries in Europe.

Clearly, a substantial number of mothers and children could be saved by appropriate action. An audit of perinatal deaths in Norway in 1980 revealed that 30% of the cases were possibly avoidable[3], and the reports on confidential inquiries into maternal deaths in the United Kingdom[4] regularly mention instances where appropriate action might have saved lives. How much higher is the potential for benefit in the developing countries, even in the absence of high technology tools?

Philosophy and content of antenatal care

Antenatal care is one of the four pillars of the Safe Motherhood Programme. It has been called a perfect example of prophylactic medicine. But today's plea is for 'evidence-based medicine', and in that light the antenatal care programs fall short, being based on tradition rather than evidence.

Antenatal care, as we know it today, originates from models developed in the early decades of this century in Europe. The original objective was to prevent eclampsia by testing urine for protein and to take appropriate measures when it was detected. A memorandum from the Ministry of Health of the British Commonwealth in 1929 described antenatal clinics, their conduct and scope. The contents and timing of the visits described in this memorandum are essentially the same as we practice today. The principles of antenatal care were:

(1) To ensure that a difficult labor should be foreseen as far as this can be done by efficient examination. Interestingly, the home conditions of the patient were to be investigated as part of this endeavor;

(2) To ensure the early detection and treatment of toxemia;

(3) To include measures directed against infection (for example, dental care, the treatment of infection of the cervix, and measures to detect and treat venereal diseases).

We might say that most of the measures apply equally today, with possibly less emphasis on dental care.

Most of the early measures required little technological equipment, and the programs continued without much change for about 40 years. Then, during the 1970s and 1980s ultrasound increasingly came to dominate the programs, at least in places where money was not a major concern – and in some where it was. Other tests were added according to temporal or geographical needs, sometimes haphazardly. For example, since 1987, all pregnant women in Norway and Sweden have been tested (after consent) for HIV antibodies without much concern for cost and effectiveness.

Since the inception of antenatal care, the visits have followed a schedule of increasingly shorter intervals. The typical program starts well before week 12, to continue with 12–13 visits before term, regardless of age or parity. Although in some countries official recommendations may be for fewer visits in low-risk cases, the care providers appear to stick to the old rules, in the belief that more visits will reap higher benefits. For example, in 1989 an Expert Panel on the Content of Prenatal Care in the USA recommended a new schedule for healthy, low-risk women, combining visits for risk assessment and health promotion into fewer visits than previously recommended[5]. These recommendations were largely ignored, the physicians preferring to rely on the 14 visits for low-risk women

advocated by the American College of Obstetricians and Gynecologists.

From time to time, we are presented with a very clear correlation between the number of visits and reduced perinatal mortality, which fall short of being evidence for a causal relationship. Although it may be true for very high-risk women that many visits are beneficial, I feel that the majority of low-risk women can manage with many fewer visits. When the above-mentioned recommendations from the US Expert Panel on the Content of Prenatal Care were tested in a randomized controlled trial among low-risk women, it turned out that good perinatal outcomes and patient satisfaction were maintained when the schedule with fewer perinatal visits was observed[6].

Globally, the antenatal care programs are basically similar, with only slight variation according to prevalence of region-specific diseases. However, attendance rates and compliance with the schedule vary greatly (Figure 1). In developed countries, 98% of pregnant women attend the programs, most of them from the first trimester onward. The situation is

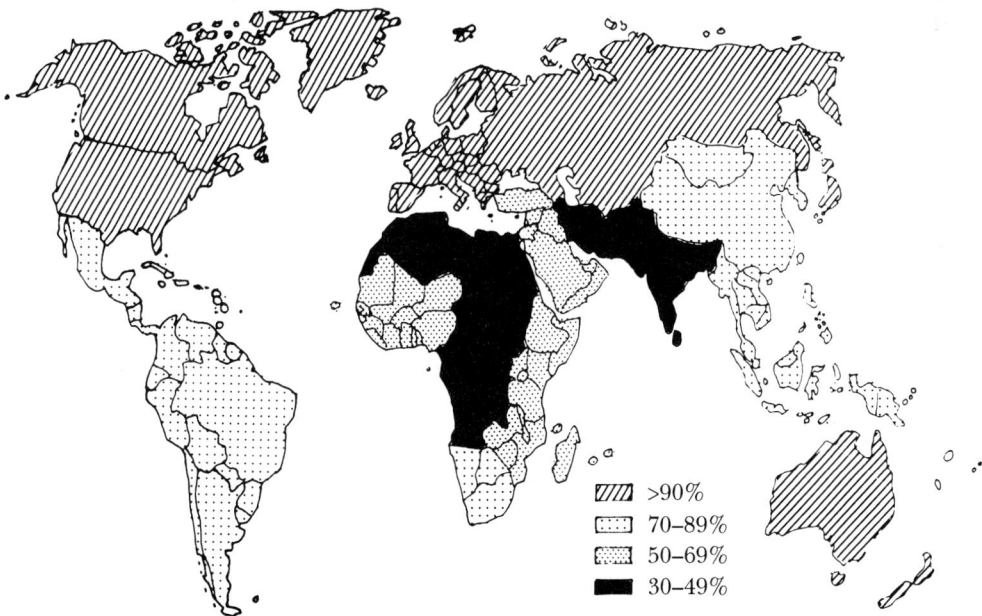

Figure 1 Regional estimates of proportion of births for which the women received prenatal care (around 1993). Source: World Health Organization[7]

different in developing countries. While Europe and all of the former Soviet Union, North America, Australia and New Zealand have over 90% coverage, Latin America, Southern Africa, China, Mongolia, and other Far Eastern countries have 70–89% coverage, while in the Middle East and the rest of Africa less than 70% of pregnant women receive some form of antenatal care. According to these estimates, presented by the World Health Organization, some North African and Central African countries are least provided for. 'Coverage' means any sort of care. In the poorest countries, many women attend only once or twice, although the traditional number of visits is prescribed. This is often due to late initiation of antenatal care rather than non-adherence to the recommended standards. In some instances, social and cultural constraints may be an obstacle to attendance, but the main reasons for non-attendance are lack of resources among the care providers and lack of money and opportunity among the care receivers.

Ideally, all pregnant women should have the same right and opportunity to attend antenatal care. This ideal is constrained by poverty and by living in remote rural districts. In industrialized countries, services are in theory available to all pregnant women, either through private or public systems. In England and Wales, and in France, various effects of social inequality have been demonstrated, and in the USA there are several barriers to utilization of services by women with low socioeconomic status.

With changing emphasis on the different aspects of antenatal care programs, I suggest the following as a common set of objectives of antenatal care. Care providers should:

(1) Offer parents help and guidance on pregnancy and child care;

(2) Ensure that pregnancy and delivery follow a natural course by securing the mother's physical, social and mental well-being;

(3) Monitor the health of the fetus so that it will be born alive without avoidable disease or injury;

(4) Detect and treat illness and other threats to the mother's health, to avoid ill effects to her and the child;

(5) Give advice and counsel the mother on place of birth.

What, then, is the evidence that antenatal care programs as practised today attain these goals?

Critique of ritualistic antenatal care

The core content of antenatal care programs comprises the mother's height, weight, weight gain, blood pressure, tests for protein and glucose in the urine, presence of edema, and growth of the uterus and the fetus, and detection of the fetal heart beat. Most of these are repeated at every visit, more as a ritual than with a purpose. For example, in most Scandinavian centers, hemoglobin is measured at every visit and the mothers reassured that a slight increase within the normal range means improvement. In some poor countries, severe anemia of pregnancy may be life-threatening, but measuring hemoglobin more than once will be considered a luxury. As most of the adverse events of pregnancy occur during delivery, one aim of antenatal care is to identify risk factors and special conditions which may threaten a safe spontaneous birth. Thus, planning of place and type of delivery becomes an important part of the program.

Considering all the well-intended tests and interventions, surprisingly little is known about the effectiveness of modern antenatal care in reducing maternal morbidity and mortality. Table 1 lists the main reasons why mothers die from obstetric complications worldwide, with figures derived from the Maternal Health and Safe Motherhood Programme of WHO. Hemorrhage, sepsis and unsafe abortion are the major causes of both sickness and death among mothers. Eclampsia has the highest mortality rate; of 100 stricken, six die.

What can antenatal care providers do to prevent or alleviate the consequences of the

Table 1 Estimated global incidence and mortality from the main obstetric complications worldwide (1993). Source: World Health Organization

Obstetric complications	Incidence (%)	Number of cases (thousands)	Number of deaths (thousands)	% of all maternal deaths
Hemorrhage	10.0	14 000	127	25
Sepsis	8.0	12 000	76	15
Hypertensive disorders of pregnancy	4.5	6 400	22	4
Eclampsia	0.5	700	43	8
Obstructed labor	5.0	7 000	38	8
Unsafe abortion		20 000	67	13
Other direct causes	3.0	4 000	39	8
Indirect causes	9.0	13 500	100	20
Total		77 600	510	100

complications listed in Table 1? There is little we can do to prevent hemorrhage, but it is possible to do something to reduce its impact. A number of cases of sepsis may be prevented through educational programs on cleanliness and detection and treatment of genital infections. Hypertensive disorders can be detected and referred to higher level for care, thereby reducing the risk of complications. Obstructed labor can in some cases be foreseen and the necessary precautions taken. The events leading to unsafe abortion are, as a rule, not part of the antenatal care programs.

hookworm disease in endemic areas. Anemia itself is dangerous only at very low levels of hemoglobin concentration, but may aggravate the dangers of bleeding. As most women in developing countries are iron-deficient, iron tablets should be given to all, with folate added to prevent neural tube defects. Only in symptomatic or suspected severe cases is hemoglobin determination essential, in some cases and places supplemented by a search for malaria parasites or intestinal worms. Other measures, such as intramuscular iron or transfusions, are seldom required.

Effective antenatal care: what is left?

We all agree that it is possible to reduce the number of maternal complications and deaths through the antenatal care program, but there may be disagreement about the effectiveness of each individual test and intervention. Indeed, a list of interventions known to be effective turns out to be fairly brief. There are effective interventions against three threats to mother and child: anemia, hypertensive disorders including eclampsia, and a few specific infections.

The case of anemia

Anemia is firstly and foremost caused by iron deficiency, secondly by malaria and thirdly by

The case of pre-eclampsia

The incidence of pregnancy hypertension varies between countries and populations, for reasons which are poorly understood. Pregnancy-induced hypertension without proteinuria carries little added risk for mother or fetus, but progression of the condition to pre-eclampsia is unpredictable. The most dreaded complication of hypertension in pregnancy is eclampsia, which may occur at any time during the latter half of pregnancy and in the puerperium; it has a high mortality rate, especially if not properly treated. The means of detection of hypertension in pregnancy are simple: measurement of blood pressure and analysis of the urine for protein. Women with severe pre-eclampsia should be transferred to higher referral level for expert care. It has been demonstrated that improved detection and care of women with hypertensive disease of pregnancy leads to better outcomes, and that some women who die of this condition have had substandard antenatal care. It is, however, questionable whether specific medications will improve the outcome. There is no convincing data that treatment of mild disease with antihypertensive drugs will prevent more severe disease, nor that low-dose aspirin will prevent pre-eclampsia or perinatal mortality, but two trials have demonstrated the protective effect of 2 g of calcium supplementation in primiparous women[8,9]. In cases of eclampsia, immediate measures may save life. The problem is that most attacks occur at home, long before any qualified help can be given.

The case of sepsis

As to infection, including sepsis, three measures have been shown to be effective:

(1) Serological screening for syphilis, with consequent treatment;

(2) Screening for gonorrhea with consequent treatment;

(3) Screening for bacteriuria with further culture of urine for urinary tract infection and consequent treatment.

Tetanus can be prevented through prophylactic immunization during pregnancy.

All the tests and interventions described are relatively cheap and simple and can therefore be employed universally. By adding malaria prophylaxis in endemic areas and employing the measures consistently, and if there is an efficient system for referral of high-risk cases, I foresee a substantial reduction in maternal suffering and child death and disability. All of this can be achieved without the help of ultrasound. The US Expert Panel in 1989 made no mention of ultrasound in its recommendations for a reduced antenatal care package[5].

Testing the schedule of antenatal care

A ritual which has lasted almost a century needs to be critically reviewed. Several elements of antenatal care, and their timing, are applied routinely without much reflection about their true value. The number of visits is high up on the scale of diminishing returns.

In recent years, there have been attempts to assess the system and to test alternative programs, in the Netherlands, Scotland, the USA and elsewhere. The emphasis is variously put on fewer visits for low-risk cases, on social and psychological aspects, and on midwives partly replacing doctors as care providers. In a recent article, we reviewed randomized controlled trials evaluating, on the one hand, the effect of enhanced prenatal care by relatively broad-based interventions, and on the other, more simplified programs with fewer visits for low-risk women, compared with traditional schedules[10]. The overall result in each of these trials was that there was no significant difference in birth weight, preterm delivery, frequency of Cesarean section or any of the other outcome variables that were tested. These trials had different designs, and hence different test hypotheses, but neither the more nor the less intensive care packages yielded better outcomes than the traditional one. This supports the claim that similar outcomes are achieved with simpler antenatal care packages, although one trial indicated that the new schedules may not meet women's current expectations in developed countries. Also, there was little evidence to support a stronger emphasis on psychosocial support during pregnancy on biological outcome or mother's well-being and satisfaction.

It may be argued that, although fewer routine visits in low-risk cases may be acceptable in rich countries, frequent visits may still be beneficial in poor countries with high rates of maternal and infant morbidity and mortality. This hypothesis is refuted by a randomized controlled trial of a reduced-visits program of antenatal care in Harare, Zimbabwe, in which preterm delivery was actually lower for women on the new program. This was the only significant difference between the two programs in the major indices of pregnancy outcome[11].

Testing a new package of antenatal care

Almost 20 years ago, the World Health Organization introduced the 'Risk Approach' without much success. Then, in 1992, the Human Reproduction Programme and Maternal Health and Safe Motherhood, Division of Family Health, convened a group of experts to develop a new antenatal care model.

The basic principles of this model are as radical as they are simple: we should aim for a set of tests and prophylactic measures which are known to be beneficial; each of these elements should be applied at the most appropriate time, that is, when an abnormal test result requires intervention, and examinations should not be repeated unnecessarily. Sufficient time for listening to and counselling the woman is emphasized. The system should be universally applicable, with due consideration of local needs.

Based on these considerations, the new model consists of four antenatal visits and one visit postpartum, with reasoned justification for each element of tests and interventions (Table 2). It is envisaged that the scheme is sufficient for the majority of pregnant women. While most current risk scales have liberal rules for referral, the new model prescribes referral to higher levels of care only when the higher level care

Table 2 Content of the basic components of the antenatal care program currently being tested in a multi-center international trial

Activity	First*	Second (26 weeks)	Third (32 weeks)	Fourth (38 weeks)	At discharge
Pregnancy test	❑†	✗	✗	✗	✗
Medical/obstetric history (risk evaluation)	■	✗	✗	✗	✗
Question of rhesus immunization with fetal/newborn disease in previous pregnancy	❑‡	✗	✗	✗	✗
Complete clinical examination	■	✗	✗	✗	■
Clinical examination for severe anemia	■	■	■	■	■
Obstetric examination**		■	■	■	✗
Gynecological examination/detection of symptomatic sexually transmitted disease	■††				
Maternal weight/height	■	✗	✗	✗	■
Maternal weight (follow up)	✗	❑	❑	❑	✗
Uterine height	■	■	■	■	■
Gestational age assessment	■	■	■	■	✗
Blood pressure	■	■	■	■	✗
Blood type/rhesus	■	✗	✗	✗	✗
Hemoglobin	❑	❑	■	✗	✗
Syphilis	■	✗	✗	✗	✗
Urine test	■‡‡	❑	❑	❑	✗
Tetanus toxoid	■	✗	■	✗	■
Folic acid/iron supplement	■	■	■	■	❑
Fetal heart rate	❑	❑	❑	❑	✗

■, All women; ❑, Only in some cases: (a) proteinuria: nulliparous or with previous pre-eclampsia or hypertension; (b) fetal heart rate: only if requested or no fetal movements seen or reported; (c) maternal weight: only those with low weight/height at first visit or obese women; (d) anemia: only if signs of severe anemia; ✗, Not necessary; *For all women at first contact with clinic, regardless of gestational age; †Only if required at first trimester and no clinical evidence of pregnancy; ‡Multiparous; **Number of fetuses, fetal situation and presentation; ††Could be postponed to second or third visit; ‡‡Multiple dipstick provision can reduce the risk or alter the outcome. The four visits are scheduled:

(1) Before or around week 12;

(2) In the 26th week;

(3) In the 32nd week;

(4) Between weeks 36 and 38. Details about the program will be published in a forthcoming Supplement to *Journal of Paediatric and Perinatal Epidemiology*.

This new model is presently being tested in a randomized, multi-center controlled trial in different parts of the world, namely Argentina, Cuba, Saudi Arabia and Thailand. The basic hypothesis is that the new model of antenatal care is equal to the traditional package with regard to specified maternal and perinatal endpoints, among singleton pregnancies, and is not more expensive. Results are expected to appear in 1999.

Meanwhile, let us try to increase the early attendance rates by whatever means we can, apply the prophylactic measures known to be effective[10,12] and try to convince those at obvious risk that hospital birth is safer than home birth.

References

1. World Health Organization (1996). *Revised 1990 estimates of maternal mortality. A new approach by WHO and UNICEF.* (Geneva: World Health Organization)
2. World Health Organization (1996). *Perinatal mortality. A listing of available information. Maternal Health and Safe Motherhood Programme.* (Geneva: World Health Organization, Family and Reproductive Health
3. Larssen, K. E., Bakketeig, L. S., Bergsjø, P., Finne, P. H., Laurini, R., Knoff, H., Holt, J., Vogt, H. and Hapnes, C. (1982). Vurdering av perinatal service i Norge 1980. Perinatal audit in Norway 1980. *Norsk institutt for sykehusforskning. Norwegian Institute for Hospital Research, NIS-rapport 7/82*
4. Department of Health, Welsh Office, Scottish Home and Health Department, Department of Health and Social Services, Northern Ireland (1991). *Report on Confidential Enquiries into Maternal Deaths in the United Kingdom 1985–87.* Department of Health, Welsh Office, Scottish Home and Health Department, Department of Health and Social Services, Northern Ireland. (London: Her Majesty's Stationery Office)
5. Public Health Service, Department of Health and Human Services (1989). *Caring for Our Future: The Content of Prenatal Care. A Report of the Public Health Service Expert Panel on the Content of Prenatal Care.* (Washington, DC: Public Health Service, Department of Health and Human Services)
6. McDuffie, R. S., Beck, A., Bischoff, K., Cross, J. and Orleans, M. (1996). Effects of frequency of prenatal care visits on perinatal outcome among low-risk women. A randomized controlled trial. *J. Am. Med. Assoc.*, **275**, 847–51
7. Maternal Health and Safe Motherhood Programme (1993). *Coverage of Maternity Care. A Tabulation of Available Information*, 3rd edn. (Geneva: World Health Organization, Division of Family Health)
8. Belizan, J. M., Villar, J., Pineda, O. *et al.* (1983). Blood pressure reduction in young adults with calcium supplementation: a randomized trial. *J. Am. Med. Assoc.*, **249**, 1161
9. Villar, J., Repke, J., Belizan, J. M. and Pareja, G. (1987). Calcium supplementation reduces blood pressure during pregnancy: results of a randomized controlled clinical trial. *Obstet. Gynecol.*, **70**, 17–22
10. Villar, J. and Bergsjø, P. (1997). Scientific basis for the content of routine antenatal care. I. Philosophy, recent studies, and power to eliminate or alleviate adverse maternal outcomes. *Acta Obstet. Gynecol. Scand.*, **76**, 1–14
11. Munjanja, S. P., Lindmark, G. and Nyström, L. (1996). Randomized controlled trial of a reduced-visits programme of antenatal care in Harare, Zimbabwe. *Lancet*, **348**, 364–9
12. Bergsjø, P. and Villar, J. (1997). Scientific basis for the content of routine antenatal care. II. Power to eliminate or alleviate adverse newborn outcomes; some special conditions and examinations. *Acta Obstet. Gynecol. Scand.*, **76**, 15–25

World Health Organization randomized antenatal care trial

18

H. Ba'aqeel, for the WHO Antenatal Care Trial Research Group*

Introduction

Antenatal care programs, as currently practiced, originate from models developed in the early decades of this century in Europe, notably the United Kingdom. The core of these early models remains practically unchanged and unevaluated although, as medical knowledge and technology have evolved, new technologies for screening for disease and primary and secondary preventive activities have been added to routine antenatal care mostly in developed countries. Unfortunately, these new components, and the timing of visits, have most often been introduced without proper scientific evaluation[1], and only a few attempts have been made recently to evaluate the number of visits[2–4].

The traditional models for antenatal care contain a substantial number of visits for the mothers (as many as 16) with little or no distinction between high- and low-risk mothers. Recently, cost-benefit aspects of antenatal care have been addressed in several countries, and attempts are being made to reduce costs for clients and the health-care services[1]. To a large extent, developing countries have adopted in theory the antenatal programs of the developed countries with only minor adjustments. However, the care often consists of irregularly spaced visits with long waiting time and poor feedback to mothers, and there is little communication between the antenatal care clinics and the obstetric departments and maternity units.

The validity of the content and the rationale for the frequency and timing of visits need to be evaluated. This was earlier recognized by Cochrane[5] when he stated 'By some curious chance, antenatal care has escaped the critical assessment to which most screening procedures have been subjected.' More recently, the US Public Health Service Expert Panel on the Content of Prenatal Care noted in its review that 'the literature on prenatal care activities was often limited, and many studies were conducted without maximal scientific rigor'[1]. Similar conclusions were arrived at by a European panel[6].

The need for randomized controlled trials on procedures and examinations included in currently practiced antenatal care has been identified[7], as well as the evaluation of the content, number and timing of prenatal care visits for women with differing medical and social risk. Such trials can establish minimal levels of care for women at low risk through comparison of less frequent or less intense prenatal care with standard care[8–10].

By means of a randomized controlled trial, the UNDP/UNFPA/WHO/World Bank Special Programme of Research, Development and Research Training in Human Reproduction and the Safe Motherhood Initiative of the World Health Organization (WHO), in close collaboration with research institutions in developing countries, are evaluating whether a program of antenatal care which emphasizes essential elements of care that have been demonstrated to affect pregnancy outcome is more effective than a traditional 'Western' type of antenatal care in preventing maternal and fetal morbidity.

---

*Other members of the 'WHO Antenatal Care Trial Research Group' are listed in the Appendix

The relative cost of the two programs, and women's satisfaction with the new intervention, will also be assessed. The trial includes random allocation of antenatal care clinic clusters to either a traditional program of care (i.e. the Western model as currently in place) or to a rationally designed program focusing on the essential elements of proven efficacy.

Methods

Trial organization

This trial is co-ordinated by a Steering Committee and a Co-ordinating Unit whose members are the principal investigator(s) of each participating center, a group of internationally recognized experts in this field and WHO staff. They are supported by a Data Co-ordinating Unit and two specialized groups on health economics and quality of care–women's satisfaction evaluation. An independent Data-Monitoring Committee was organized; it periodically reviews incoming data and is monthly informed of all severe adverse events by trial arm (maternal deaths, eclampsia and fetal death), recruitment rates and percentage of high-risk women that are not eligible for the basic component of the intervention.

Trial design

A randomized controlled trial is necessary for the evaluation of the effect of antenatal care on pregnancy outcome, specifically to control for the bias in patient selection that can occur in observational studies[11]. The study currently under way is a multicenter randomized trial of two different models of antenatal care. A new model of care will be compared with the traditional Western model as it is presently implemented in the selected sites. Antenatal care clinics serving well-defined geographical areas are randomized (cluster randomization) to the two arms of the study within each of four study sites. The clinics are stratified by site (Table 1). The sites selected for the trial include: the province of Khon Kaen, Thailand; and the cities of

Rosario, Argentina; Havana, Cuba; Jeddah, Saudi Arabia.

The rationale for choosing clinics as the unit of randomization is to reduce the risk of treatment contamination, to encourage participation and to facilitate administrative and logistic convenience in the implementation of the intervention. This design has been used previously by other investigators in the perinatal field[12–15].

Trial entry

The population attending the clinics in each country is expected to be similar with regard to sociodemographic factors, and have study-relevant mortality and morbidity rates of the same order of magnitude. An antenatal care program following traditional standards delivered through the public sector is already available to pregnant women. Each clinic or cluster is expected to ideally manage between 450 and 500 new antenatal care patients during the study period. However, as the number of clusters has a greater impact on statistical power than the sizes of the clusters, smaller antenatal

Table 1 Allocation of clinics across sites

| Stratum | Arm | | Total |
	Intervention	Control	
Argentina			
Hospitals	1	1	2
Clinics	8	7	15
Cuba			
Clinics	6	6	12
Saudi Arabia			
Medium clinics	2	2	4
Small clinics	4	4	8
Thailand			
Large hospitals	1	1	2
Medium hospitals	3	3	6
Small hospitals	2	2	4
All strata	27	26	53

Stratum, definition based on number of new patients/year, type of clinic (free-standing/hospital-associated) and health-care system to which they belong

clinics, supplying as few as 300 patients are accepted.

All patients attending prenatal care for the first time after the start of the study at one of the selected clinics, regardless of their gestational age, medical or obstetrical characteristics or previous antenatal care, will be included for follow-up. Those enrolled for prenatal care at the control clinics will follow the standard procedure and be referred for delivery at the usual referral hospitals. Women enrolled in the clinics belonging to the intervention group will receive the new prenatal care program and any other treatments medically required, and be referred to the routine place of delivery for these clinics. At the first antenatal visit to intervention clinics, patients will be classified by a simple risk classification form as to whether or not they require special care, e.g. referral to a high-risk clinic.

All women attending the study clinics will be included in the assessment of trial outcomes (intention to treat) and followed until discharge from the hospital postpartum, including those who refuse to participate or discontinue the new program because of either medical or personal situations. Women who refuse to initiate or continue the new antenatal care program will be offered the 'traditional' antenatal care at the same clinic or referred to an alternative clinic if it is located nearby and does not represent any inconvenience for the patient. The proportion of patients refusing the new program (transfer rate) will be regarded as a process outcome.

Intervention

The trial involves a direct comparison of two programs of antenatal care. One is the standard antenatal care presently offered in the selected sites which follow the 'traditional' model. A detailed description of baseline antenatal care was obtained before the randomization (see 'Baseline survey' section below). The new program includes scientifically evaluated objective-oriented activities[16,17].

Activities to be included in the new program are within three general areas:

(1) Screening actions for health conditions likely to increase the risk of specific adverse outcomes of pregnancy;

(2) Therapeutic interventions known to affect these outcomes beneficially;

(3) Sensitizing pregnant women to potential health problems, especially emergencies, and instructing them on appropriate responses.

Therapeutic interventions known to have a positive effect on pregnancy outcomes were selected from an extensive literature review of randomized controlled trials[16,17].

It is inevitable in a multinational trial such as this that the actual implementation of the intervention will vary somewhat from site to site, depending on resources available, historical patterns and cultural factors. This may be regarded as a design strength from the point of view of external validity, but will undoubtedly create difficulties in any attempt to disentangle the effects of individual components of the intervention. However, in order to standardize the intervention, all study sites use a 'manual of clinical activities' and a clinical activities 'checklist' that is translated into the local language and added to all medical records in the intervention clinics, and completed at each antenatal care visit.

Outcome measures

Antenatal care is a complex set of activities (basically a multiphasic screening procedure) aimed at reducing maternal and perinatal morbidity and mortality. It is clear that if only maternal mortality and pre-labor fetal death are considered (the ideal outcomes), the sample size required would be extremely large and unrealistic; thus, surrogate measures and/or an index will be used to measure outcome.

Trials that are expected to have modest improvements or no improvements on relatively rare outcomes can use a combined index (e.g. maternal morbidity index) or surrogate measures to the ideal outcomes. The rate of a 'maternal morbidity indicator index' was chosen as the primary outcome of the trial in relation to maternal conditions. This is defined as the presence of at least one of the following severe conditions for which antenatal care is likely to be relevant: (1) proteinuric pre-eclampsia or eclampsia during pregnancy or within 24 h of delivery; (2) postpartum anemia (< 90 g/l of hemoglobin); and (3) severe urinary tract infection/pyelonephritis, defined as an episode requiring antibiotic treatment or hospitalization. Each of these conditions will be explored independently as secondary outcomes.

The primary outcome in relation to fetal conditions will be the rate of low birth weight (< 2500 g), as a surrogate measure to perinatal mortality. It is considered very unlikely that antenatal care will influence perinatal mortality without changing the rate of low birth weight. Secondary outcome variables include other maternal and perinatal events such as the rate of incomplete tetanus immunization, breech presentation at birth, the rate of treated syphilis or a postpartum hospital stay of 1 week or more (Table 2).

Sample size

The determination of the sample size required for the trial corresponds to the stratified cluster randomization design described above, and applies to both the low birth weight outcome and the morbidity index, both expected to be in the region of 10%. The calculation takes into account that the design involves five sites, with clinics within each site randomly assigned to intervention or control. Further stratification by clinic size, done principally to ensure balanced allocation of subjects across intervention groups, is expected to impact conservatively on power, and is therefore ignored for this purpose. A procedure for estimating sample size requirements for stratified cluster randomization designs is provided by Donner[18]. The results of applying the above procedure show that 19 161 patients recruited in five study sites will provide a power of 90% for detecting an

Table 2 Outcomes of WHO antenatal care randomized controlled trial

Primary outcomes
Rate of maternal morbidity indicator index (see text)
Rate of low birth weight (< 2500 g)

Secondary outcomes
Maternal
  Rate of treated syphilis and any other STDs during pregnancy
  Rate of postpartum positive syphilis test among women without treatment during pregnancy
  Rate of incomplete tetanus immunization
  Rate of postpartum hospital stay ≥ 7 days for maternal complications

Newborn
  Rate of intrauterine growth retardation
  Rate of preterm delivery (< 37 weeks)
  Rate of spontaneous preterm premature rupture of the membranes
    < 35 weeks
    35–36 weeks
  Rate of breech presentation at birth
  Rate of medically indicated preterm delivery
    < 35 weeks
    35–36 weeks
  Rate of very low birth weight (< 1500 g)
  Rate of Apgar score < 5 at 5 min
  Rate of intensive care unit stay > 2 days
  Rate of fetal death
  Rate of predischarge neonatal death

3rd, Process outcomes
Rate of antenatal hospital admission, total and by cause
Rate of Cesarean sections

4th, Cost of antenatal care
To health service
To patient

5th, Satisfaction and perceived quality of care (only in random sample)
By health workers
By patient

intervention odds ratio of 1.2 in a two-sided test at the 5% significance level. The value 1.2 was chosen as the maximum value of the odds ratio that would be regarded as consistent with the conclusion that the new program is as 'equally effective' as the standard program, taking into account the increased costs and logistics associated with the latter.

Masking of intervention

Considerable efforts will be made to mask treatment status for delivery and neonatal care providers (as this is an unmasked trial), as well as those responsible for data collection after birth. However, it is possible that they will know the treatment status and perhaps act differently based on their belief of antenatal care effect. The primary outcomes are little influenced by intrapartum care, however, and it is expected that this effect will be minimal. We will nevertheless attempt to evaluate this effect, if present, using two mechanisms:

(1) Information on intrapartum events partially unrelated to antepartum care, e.g. emergency Cesarean section, forceps delivery, will be collected. Comparisons will be made between the two treatment groups.

(2) Trends will be observed in perinatal events at all participating hospitals irrespective of whether patients are participating in the antenatal care study.

Data quality control

In a trial of this magnitude, one of the first priorities is to maintain uniformity in data collection, as well as careful documentation of data quality. An internal system for monitoring the quality of the data will be instituted; this will include a series of small studies aimed at monitoring data reliability and agreement among observers in each site.

Statistical analysis

Data entry and preliminary checks for error and internal validity will be done at each study site, with statistical analyses conducted at a central level. All principal analyses will be based on the clusters as allocated in the randomization ('intention to treat'). Baseline tables will be created comparing the intervention groups with respect to both cluster-level and individual-level risk factors.

Since sample size calculations were conducted using the standard Mantel–Haenszel statistic modified to adjust for the cluster design, the main analytical technique used to assess the effect of intervention will be an application of the Mantel–Haenszel test adapted to the cluster randomization design[15]. Secondary analyses will explore the relationship between maternal baseline characteristics and various binary outcomes. Continuous outcome variables, such as measured levels of hemoglobin, will be analyzed using mixed model regression. Secondary analyses will also be conducted to explore the possibility of an interaction effect between intervention and clinic size, although it is recognized that the power for detecting such an intervention effect will be low. Given the equivalence nature of the trial it will be particularly important to calculate confidence limits for the intervention effect that are consistent with the observed data.

Baseline survey

A formal survey describing antenatal care practices was implemented in all eligible clinics immediately before randomization to obtain a detailed description of clinic and services characteristics before the interventions; it will be repeated within the last 3 months of patient recruitment. There are two components of this antenatal care survey: clinic level and patient level. At the clinic level, one form was completed for each clinic participating in the study in each country.

The patient component of the survey was also conducted before randomization and after completing the 'clinic level' form. A minimum of 64 consecutive women visits were recorded for each clinic (cluster). A total of 2800 medical records of pregnant women were reviewed.

Ethical issues

This trial has been approved by the Scientific and Ethical Review Group of the UNDP/UNFPA/WHO/World Bank Special

Programme on Research, Development and Research Training in Human Reproduction, the WHO Ethical Review Committee and the Institution–Review Boards of the individual participating centers and the corresponding health authorities of the regions where the trial was implemented.

Discussion

This large, complex, randomized community trial is implemented with the assistance of collaborating centers in developing countries and a selected group of international scientists acting as advisers. It is the unanimous opinion of all concerned that this rigorous evaluation is long overdue[5].

The new antenatal care package represents a major departure from the present recommended form of care, which is strongly incorporated into the obstetric culture. If the results of the study demonstrate that the new model is similar or even better than the traditional model, this randomized controlled design would be basic to the acceptance of the proposed new program. None the less, there are disturbing reports that results of randomized trials showing clear beneficial effects have not been incorporated into practice long after the formal publication of the trials[19].

One concern of a trial such as this is whether or not clinicians are complying with the new model of antenatal care. Obviously, if the two groups receive more or less the same type of care the trial will be of limited value. This can be as a result of the intervention group being provided with extra care or the staff of the control group adopting the – new – model (therapeutic contamination). Actually, this could be ob-

served as several obstetricians were disappointed to learn that they were in the control group. There is a trial evaluating the routine use of episiotomy that has encountered this problem[20]. The following mechanisms are in place in the WHO trial to reduce or evaluate treatment compliance: extensive initial training with trial protocol; continuous monitoring by visiting the clinics at least every 2 weeks; frequent visits to the study sites by trial co-ordinators; random sampling for evaluation of the 'antenatal care check list' which was included in the medical records of all women enrolled in the intervention group.

Randomized controlled trials evaluating drugs and non-drugs forms of medical care are particularly important for developing countries where the scarce resources allocated to health have to be utilized for the implementation of effective forms of care. Randomized controlled trials also represent the best 'defense mechanism' against the transfer of ineffective treatment or diagnostic modalities from north to south. Furthermore, results of randomized controlled trials conducted recently in developing countries have also influenced practice in industrialized regions[21–23]. In both settings, multicentered randomized controlled trials would have avoided the widespread use of perinatal technologies of dubious effectiveness[16,17].

There is now clear evidence that priority health interventions can be evaluated by developing-country researchers in a large randomized controlled trial and results published in leading journals[2,22–25]. Despite these success stories, conducting large-scale, cutting-edge, health-service research in developing countries is a formidable task.

Appendix

WHO Antenatal Care Trial Research Group

Co-ordinating Unit
José Villar, Trial Co-ordinator
Dina Khan, Research Associate
Olav Meirik, Epidemiologist
Rick Guidotti, Gynecologist–Epidemiologist

Data Co-ordinating Unit
Gilda Piaggio, Statistician
Alain Pinol, Systems Analyst
Milena Vucurevic, Statistical Assistant
Allan Donner, Consultant Statistician

Steering Committee
Yagob Al-Mazrou, Investigator, Saudi Arabia
Hassan Ba'aqeel, Investigator, Saudi Arabia
Leiv Bakketeig, Public Health Obstetrician, Norway
José M. Belizan, Investigator, Argentina
Heinz Berendes, Epidemiologist, USA (Chairman)
Guillermo Carroli, Investigator, Argentina
Ubaldo Farnot, Investigator, Cuba
Pisake Lumbiganon, Investigator, Thailand

Vivian Wong, Obstetrician/Gynecologist, Hong Kong
Gunilla Lindmark, Obstetrician/Epidemiologist, Sweden

Health Economic Group
Miranda Mugford, Health Economist, UK
Guy Hutton, Health Economics Researcher, UK
Julia Fox-Rushby, Health Economist, UK

Quality of Care Group
Ana Langer, Pediatric Epidemiologist, Mexico
Gustavo Nigenda, Public Health Specialist, Mexico

Data and Safety Monitoring Committee
Per Bergsjø, Obstetrician/Epidemiologist, Norway (Chairman)
Gerard Breart, Epidemiologist, France
Alfredo Morabia, Biostatistician/Epidemiologist, Switzerland
Heinz Berendes, Epidemiologist, USA (ex officio)
Gilda Piaggio, Statistician, WHO (ex officio)
José Villar, Obstetrician/Epidemiologist, WHO (ex officio)

References

1. Rosen, M., Merkatz, I. and Hill, J. (1991). Caring for our future: a report by the expert panel on the content of prenatal care. *Obstet. Gynecol.*, **77**, 782–7
2. Munjanja, S., Lindmark, G. and Nyström, L. (1996). Randomised controlled trial of a reduced visits programme of antenatal care in Harare, Zimbabwe. *Lancet*, **348**, 364–9
3. McDuffie, R., Beck, A., Bischoff, K., Cross, J. and Orlans, M. (1996). Effects of frequency of antenatal care visits on perinatal outcome among low-risk women. *J. Am. Med. Assoc.*, **275**, 847–51
4. Sikorski, J., Wilson, J., Clement, S., Das, S. and Smeeton, N. (1996). A randomised controlled trial comparing two schedules of antenatal visits: the antenatal care project. *Br. Med. J.*, **312**, 546–53
5. Cochrane, A. L. (1989). *Effectiveness and Efficiency – Random Reflections on Health Services*, pp. 45–66. (Cambridge, UK: Cambridge University Press)
6. Lindmark, G. and Crattingius, S. (1991). The scientific basis of antenatal care. Report from a state of the art conference. *Acta Obstet. Gynecol. Scand.*, **70**, 105–9
7. Steer, P. (1993). Rituals in antenatal care – do we need them? *Br. Med. J.*, **307**, 697–8
8. Fiscella, K. (1995). Does prenatal care improve birth outcome? A critical review. *Obstet. Gynecol.*, **85**, 468–79
9. Tucker, J., Hall, M., Howie, P. W., Reid, M., Barbour, R., Florey, C du V and McIlwine, G. (1996). Should obstetricians see women with normal pregnancies? A multicentre randomised controlled trial of routine antenatal care by general practitioners and midwives compared

with shared care led by obstetricians. *Br. Med. J.*, **312**, 554–9

10. Bakketeig, L. S. (1992). Methodological problems and possible endpoints in the evaluation of antenatal care. *Int. J. Tech. Assess. Health Care*, **8** (Suppl. 1), 33–9

11. Villar, J. and Carroli, G. (1996). Methodological issues of randomised controlled trials for the evaluation of reproductive health interventions. *Prevent. Med.*, **25**, 365–75

12. Grant, A., Elbourne, D., Valentin, L. and Alexander, S. (1989). Routine formal fetal movement counting and risk of antepartum late death in normally formed singletons. *Lancet*, **2**, 345–9

13. Bullough, C., Msuku, R. and Karonde, L. (1989). Early suckling and postpartum haemorrhage: controlled trial in deliveries by traditional birth attendants. *Lancet*, **2**, 522–5

14. Kendrick, J. S., Zahniser, S. C. and Miller, N. (1995). Integrating smoking cessation into routine public prenatal care: the smoking cessation in pregnancy project. *Am. J. Publ. Health*, **85**, 217–22

15. Donner, A. and Klar, N. (1994). Cluster randomisation trials in epidemiology: theory and application. *J. Stat. Plann. Inference*, **40**, 1–20

16. Villar, J. and Bergsjø, P. (1997). Scientific basis for the content of routine antenatal care: I. Philosophy, recent studies, and power to eliminate or alleviate adverse maternal outcomes. *Acta Obstet. Gynecol. Scand.*, **76**, 1–14

17. Bergsjø, P. and Villar, J. (1997). Scientific basis for the content of routine antenatal care: II. Power to eliminate or alleviate adverse newborn outcomes; some special conditions and examinations. *Acta Obstet. Gynecol. Scand.*, **76**, 15–25

18. Donner, A. (1992). Sample size requirements for stratified cluster randomisation designs. *Stat. Med.*, **1**, 743–50

19. Anon (1993). Clinical trials and clinical practice. *Lancet*, **342**, 877–8

20. Schulz, K. F. (1995). Unbiased research and the human spirit: the challenges of randomised controlled trials. *Can. Med. Assoc. J.*, **153**, 783–6

21. Mabey, D. (1996). Importance of clinical trials in developing countries. *Lancet*, **348**, 11–13

22. Eclampsia trial collaborative group (1995). Which anticonvulsant for women with eclampsia? Evidence from the collaborative eclampsia trial. *Lancet*, **345**, 1455–63

23. Argentine episiotomy trial collaborative group (1993). Routine *vs.* selective episiotomy controlled trial. *Lancet*, **342**, 151–8

24. Villar, J., Farnot, U., Barros, F., Victora, C., Langer, A. and Belizan, J. M. (1992). A randomized trial of psychosocial support during high-risk pregnancies. *N. Engl. J. Med.*, **327**, 1266–71

25. Belizan, J. M., Villar, J., Gonzalez, G., Compodomico, L. and Bergel, E. (1991). Calcium supplementation to prevent hypertensive disorders of pregnancy. *N. Engl. J. Med.*, **325**, 1399–1405

Women's rights and women's health 19

R. J. Cook

Introduction

The International Federation of Gynecology and Obstetrics' 1994 World Report on Women's Health concluded that improvements in women's health need more than improved science and health care[1]. They require state action, long overdue, to correct injustices to women. Women's health is often compromised, not because of lack of medical knowledge, but because of infringements on women's human rights.

The use of human rights to advance reproductive health and self-determination has gained momentum through recent United Nations (UN) conferences, particularly the 1994 International Conference on Population and Development, held in Cairo, and the 1995 Fourth World Conference on Women, held in Beijing[2]. The Programme of Action adopted by 184 UN Member States in Cairo (the Cairo Programme)[3] recognizes the importance of human rights in protection and promotion of reproductive health. The Declaration and Platform for Action adopted by 187 UN Member States in Beijing (the Beijing Declaration and the Beijing Platform, respectively)[4] reaffirm the Cairo Programme but extend women's wider interests to social justice. Key to this new approach is empowering women within their families and communities, and protecting their human rights, particularly those relevant to reproductive health.

This chapter will address the evolution of reproductive rights under international human rights law. It will explain how the meaning of reproductive rights is evolving through three evolutionary stages, and how the documents produced by the UN Conferences held in Cairo in 1994 and in Beijing in 1995 contribute to these stages. It will explain some of the decisions of national, regional and international courts to advance reproductive rights. It will survey the mechanisms which hold governments and their agents accountable for violations of reproductive rights. Finally, it will address what professional associations, such as medical associations, are doing and could do to ensure respect for reproductive rights.

Three evolutionary models

The modern history of the protection of reproductive rights has developed through three evolutionary states of family planning, reproductive health and women's empowerment[5]. An understanding of the evolutionary process helps us to understand where we are now, and how different actors in the area of women's human rights and protection of reproductive rights relate to each other. The advancement of one strategy need not preclude respect and pursuit of the others, and commitment to one strategy does not necessarily imply commitment to the others.

The international human rights regime

The three evolutionary stages have each been inspired in varying ways by respect for individual human rights that have become progressively defined upon the foundation established in 1948 by the Universal Declaration of Human Rights[6]. The Declaration itself was not proposed as a legally enforceable instrument, but it has gained legal acceptance and legal enforceability through a series of international human rights conventions. The primary modern human rights treaty concerning women's rights is the Convention on the Elimination of All Forms of Discrimination Against Women (the Women's

Convention)[7]. This gives expression to the values implicit in the Universal Declaration of Human Rights, and reinforces the Declaration's two initial implementing Covenants, the International Covenant on Civil and Political Rights (the Political Covenant)[8] and the International Covenant on Economic, Social and Cultural Rights (the Economic Covenant)[9]. Similarly derived from the Universal Declaration are regional human rights conventions, including the European Convention for the Protection of Human Rights and Fundamental Freedoms (the European Convention)[10], the American Convention on Human Rights (the American Convention)[11] and the African Charter on Human and Peoples' Rights (the African Charter)[12].

Through membership in these international human rights conventions, states commit themselves to report regularly to committees established under each convention to monitor state compliance or violation. Monitoring committees receive non-governmental reports or comments on state performance on treaty obligations, such as eliminating discrimination regarding women's health, submitted by national and international non-governmental organizations, such as FIGO or national societies of obstetrics and gynecology.

Mechanisms exist under some conventions, such as the European Convention on Human Rights and the International Covenant on Civil and Political Rights, that enable private persons from consenting countries to bring individual complaints against them for violations. The individual petitions mechanism is currently under consideration for the Women's Convention.

To assist countries in their reporting obligations, monitoring committees have developed a series of General Recommendations[13]. These Recommendations develop the content and meaning of human rights, and are somewhat akin to regulations developed by administrative agencies under statute law. Several interesting symposiums have begun to focus on the factors that might be considered in developing a General Recommendation on a woman's right to health[14]. The formulation of these rights is a significant opportunity to develop the multi-dimensional nature of a woman's right to health.

An increasingly important mechanism for developing the accountability for reproductive rights is the 'Concluding Observations' by monitoring committees of the reports submitted by state parties.

Emerging analyses of state responsibility for violations of human rights assess governmental neglect of preventable causes of women's mortality and morbidity as an affront to their human dignity and as part of a larger social phenomenon of systemic discrimination against women[15]. Laws that deny, obstruct or condition availability of, and access to, reproductive health services are being challenged as violating women's basic human rights protected by international human rights conventions. If international human rights law is to be truly universal, it has both to require states to take effective preventive and curative measures to protect women's reproductive health, and to afford women the capacity for reproductive self-determination. International human rights treaties require international and domestic application in order to secure women's rights to:

(1) Be free through their empowerment from all forms of discrimination and oppression;

(2) Achieve their rights to liberty and security, to marriage and foundation of families, to private family life and to information and education;

(3) Have access to health care and the benefits of scientific progress.

Women's reproductive self-determination under international human rights law is a composite right founded on these separate rights.

The family planning model

The family planning model remains the initial approach to women's reproductive rights and stresses the need to ensure access to all forms of contraceptive services. The unmet need for family planning services is immense. In developing countries, an estimated 350 million of the 747 million married women of reproductive age are not using contraceptives. Of these, 100 million would prefer to space timing of a next birth or not have more children. Worldwide, women would prefer to delay or avoid about 25% of all pregnancies that occur[16].

The family planning model strives to observe ethical duties of obtaining recipients' free and informed consent to services in form rather than substance. The Cairo Programme affirms that 'the principle of informed free choice is essential to the long-term success of family planning programmes [and that] any form of coercion has no part to play' (para. 7.12). This principle is reaffirmed in the Beijing Platform (paras. 106(g), 106(h), 107(e)). The Cairo Programme and the Beijing Platform reinforce women's autonomous and confidential choice in reproductive matters (Cairo paras. 7.3, 7.12, 7.17–7.20; Beijing paras. 103, 107(e), 108(m), 267). Claims by women to autonomous choices against their partners' attempted opposition have been consistently upheld by courts in all regions of the world[17].

The family planning model has established a number of traditions that are very worthy in themselves but that require periodic reconsideration for the purpose not so much of abandonment as of enrichment. For instance, routine informing and servicing of women's needs could be expanded to include the needs of men and unmarried women or adolescent girls[18]. A legal obstacle in the past has been the fact that preparing men for sexual activity with female partners who might be under the legal age of consent for sex could result in criminal charges. Preparing underage girls for sexual relations is legally defensible because of age of consent laws are designed to protect them and not criminalize them, so that services aimed at their protection are consistent with these laws and not a violation of them.

Courts have a tradition of holding that protection of health interests prevails over laws that seek to enforce moral imperatives. For instance, the European Court of Human Rights, established under the European Convention, held that compulsory sex education, 'conveyed in an objective, critical and pluralistic manner,' did not violate the rights of parents to ensure education of their children in conformity with their religious beliefs[19]. More recently, the same Court required the Republic of Ireland to accommodate the provision of information on access to abortion services in nearby countries[20].

Although the family planning movement has had to overcome laws that restrict its particular techniques and services, the movement has worked within social frameworks of women's status. The family planning model has not deliberately undertaken to reform or enlighten societies or women themselves concerning the greater role that women can play once they escape bondage to their biological functions in sexual relations. Further, because of historical origins in middle class services rendered to the poor and uneducated, the movement has followed rather than challenged the classical relationship between doctor and patient in supposing that the doctor knows best and that service recipients should be trained to follow doctor's directions rather than question them in order to obtain a full understanding.

The reproductive health model

The second stage of evolution, the reproductive health stage, has produced a broader, more comprehensive vision of reproductive welfare. This is based not simply on control of unwanted fertility, but also on preservation of fertility, through, for example, the reduction of reproductive tract infections and unsafe abortion, and the ability, for instance, to space births of children so as to maximize maternal and infant survival and wellbeing. This model reflects an overarching definition of reproductive health found in the Cairo Programme, which explains that reproductive health is:

'a state of complete physical, mental and social wellbeing, and is not merely the absence of disease or infirmity, in all matters relating to the reproductive system and to its functions and processes. Reproductive health therefore implies that people are able to have a satisfying and safe sex life and that they have the capability to reproduce and the freedom to decide if, when and how often to do so. Implicit in this last condition are the rights of men and women to be informed and to have access to safe, effective, affordable and acceptable methods of family planning of their choice, as well as other methods of their choice for regulation of fertility which are not against the law, and the right of access to appropriate healthcare services that will enable women to go safely through pregnancy and childbirth and provide couples with the best chance of having a healthy infant.' (para. 7.2)

The Cairo Programme and the Beijing Platform identify components of the right to the highest attainable standard of reproductive health from a woman's perspective. Both stress the importance of affordable, accessible and acceptable services throughout the life cycle (Cairo paras. 7.5 and 7.23, Beijing paras. 92 and 106(e)), and 'acceptable' services include gender-sensitive standards for delivery of quality services (Cairo para 7.23, Beijing paras. 95, 103, 106(c) and (g)).

For the first time, a UN Population Conference recognizes that maternal deaths arise from unsafe abortion, with global estimates as high as 200 000 each year[21]. The Cairo Programme calls on governments to address unsafe abortion as a leading cause of maternal mortality and a 'major public health concern' (para. 8.25). The call for safe abortion was underscored by the Beijing Platform (paras. 97, 106(j) and (k)). Through the Beijing Platform, governments recognize women's liberty interest by agreeing, for instance, to consider 'reviewing laws containing punitive measures against women who have undergone illegal abortions' (para. 106(k)). Courts at the national level have addressed abortion by finding restrictive criminal abortion provisions unconstitutional for violating women's rights to liberty and security[22].

At the international level, the Human Rights Committee, the committee that monitors the implementation of the International Covenant on Civil and Political Rights, found that in Peru, the abortion law subjected women to inhuman treatment, incompatible with women's equality rights, their rights to life and not to be subjected to degrading treatment, on the basis of evidence provided to them by a non-governmental organization of high rates of maternal mortality[23]. The Committee's Concluding Observation provided an important opportunity to conclude that government neglect to address the causes of high rates of maternal mortality is internationally wrongful. Most states commit themselves to promote and protect the human rights of women through national constitutions and membership of regional and international human rights conventions.

Crude measures of the failure of reproductive health remain national, regional and community rates of maternal mortality. These rates are indicators of violations of international human rights, such as the right to equal access to health care, often associated with state responsibility for failure to provide or to facilitate programs of reproductive health protection. The Women's Convention requires member countries 'to eliminate discrimination against women in the field of health care in order to ensure . . . access to health care services, including those related to family planning' (Article 12(1)).

The women's empowerment or social justice model

The third and most recent stage of evolution is the women's empowerment or social justice stage. This is founded on a transcending concept of social justice and respect for women's dignity in areas by no means limited to reproductive health, whose aim is comprehensive women's empowerment. The empowerment of women includes reproductive self-determination, but as a subtext or essential contributory factor in empowerment rather than as an end in itself. Women's ability to control their reproduction is regarded as only a precondition to women taking charge of their own lives, and lack of such control is regarded as denying women control of other aspects of their lives. The Beijing Platform makes explicit that:

> '[t]he human rights of women include their right to have control over and decide freely and responsibly on matters related to their sexuality, including sexual and reproductive health, free of coercion, discrimination and violence. Equal relationships between women and men in matters of sexual relations and reproduction, including full respect for the integrity of the person, require mutual respect, consent and shared responsibility for sexual behaviour and its consequences.' (para. 96)

The model recognizes the need for women to control the risk of sexually transmitted diseases, because men cannot be relied upon to protect partners against infection. Development of the female condom moves in this direction, although problems of cost, distribution and education in use have to be addressed internationally[24].

The women's empowerment model accepts the challenge laid down in the Women's Convention:

> '[t]o modify the social and cultural patterns of conduct of men and women, with a view to achieving the elimination of prejudices and customary and all other practices which are based on the idea of the inferiority or the superiority of either of the sexes or on stereotyped roles for men and women' (Article 5(a)).

Regarding family life, the model accepts the related challenge to demonstrate 'the common responsibility of men and women in the upbringing and development of their children' (Article 5(b)).

The way forward: a call for an alliance

A strong alliance between the health and legal professions is needed at the national and international level to develop the ethical and legal norms necessary for the implementation of the three models.

Ethical guidance

The Cairo and Beijing documents recommend that the health professions develop, disseminate and implement ethical codes to ensure practitioners' conformity with human rights, ethical and professional standards (Cairo para. 7.17, Beijing para. 106(g)). Promising signs are the development of ethical guidance by medical associations such as the International Federation of Gynecology and Obstetrics[25] and the Commonwealth Medical Association[26].

Guidance for reproductive health laws

The FIGO/WHO Task Force is developing guidance for the health and legal professions to formulate reproductive health laws at the national level. Countries are moving to formulate reproductive health laws that give force to the human rights that serve reproductive health and self-determination (for example, the Reproductive Rights Law of the Russian Federation, 1996). Since the Cairo Conference, Argentina has considered enacting a reproductive health law (Reproductive Health Bill, 1995), and Guyana and South Africa have enacted components of one (Guyana Medical Termination of Pregnancy Act, 1995; South African Choice of the Termination of Pregnancy Law, 1997). State policies that protect and promote reproductive health within a wider program of women's health have been enacted in Colombia[27] and Brazil[28].

Guidance for women's empowerment

The Cairo and Beijing texts also indicate a variety of mechanisms to identify standards for observance of rights to determine whether states are in compliance or violation. The Beijing Platform recommends legal literacy and legal service programs (paras. 232 and 233) and the creation of independent ombudspersons, rights advocates or defenders, with power to investigate alleged violations of reproductive rights, issue periodic reports, advise governmental and other agencies and make recommendations for reforms (para. 232(e)).

Profamilia, the Colombian non-governmental reproductive health association, has over the years developed aspects of the family planning and reproductive health models and is now working to include aspects of the women's empowerment model through programs such as legal services for women and gender training workshops[29]. Profamilia's Legal Services for Women now delivers legal services in six reproductive health centers in those areas of discrimination and oppression that concern reproductive health and family matters, such as divorce and domestic violence. The service provides information, education and counseling to women about their rights, and legal services to implement rights and to seek remedies through litigation for women whose rights have been violated. Through a series of publications[30] and videos[31], the service attempts to expand awareness about women's rights.

Profamilia holds periodic workshops to explain and discuss gender issues and analysis with its doctors and other health personnel. The workshops also explain how the new Colombian health policy proposes to reduce women's existing disadvantages to improve the quality of life of women and respond to women's health concerns in a comprehensive fashion[32]. They show how epidemiological and statistical data, fertility surveys and quality-of-care studies can be used to hold governments and institutions accountable to improve women's health care. Moreover, the workshops show how data can be interpreted and analyzed from a gender perspective. For example, this perspective requires that women's points of view are taken into consideration with the traditional indicators of effectiveness used in family planning, such as acceptance and continuation rates. A gender analysis identifies problems from women's perspectives in areas of access, informed choice and user satisfaction.

References

1. Fathalla, M. F. (1994). Women's health: an overview. *Int. J. Gynecol. Obstet.*, **46**, 105–18
2. Cook, R. J. and Fathalla, M. F. (1996). Advancing reproductive rights beyond Cairo and Beijing. *Int. Family Planning Perspect.*, **22**, 115–21
3. United Nations (1994). *Report of the International Conference on Population and Development*, United Nations, New York, NY, A/Conf.171/13
4. United Nations (1995). *Report of the Fourth World Conference on Women*, United Nations, New York, NY, A/Conf. 177/20
5. Cook, R. J. and Plata, M. I. (1994). Women's reproductive self-determination: evolutionary models. *Development*, **3**, 29–34
6. General Assembly Resolution 217 A (III), United Nations Document A/810 (1948)
7. 18 December 1979, 34 United Nations General Assembly Official Records Supplement, (No 21) at 193, United Nations Document A/Res/34/180
8. General Assembly Resolution 2200 (XXI), 21 United Nations General Assembly Official Record Supplement (No 16) at 52, United Nations Document A/6316, 1966
9. General Assembly Resolution 2200 (XXI), 21 United Nations General Assembly Official Record Supplement (No 16) at 49, United Nations Document A/6316, 1966
10. 213 United Nations Treaty Series 221 (1959)
11. Organization of American States Treaty Series at 1 (1969)
12. Organization of African Unity Document CAB/LEG/67/3/Rev.5 (1981)
13. United Nations, International Human Rights Instruments (1996). *Compilation of General Comments and General Recommendations Adopted by Human Rights Treaty Bodies*, HRI/Gen/1/Rev.2, 29 March
14. Commonwealth Medical Association (1996). *A Woman's Right to Health, Including Sexual and Reproductive Health*. (London: Commonwealth Medical Association); United Nations Population Fund (1996). *Roundtable of Human Rights Treaty Bodies on Human Rights Approaches to*

Women's Health, with a Focus on Reproductive and Sexual Health and Rights, (New York: United Nations Population Fund), 8–11 December

15. See symposium edition on reproductive rights of *American University Law Review*, 44, 4, 1995 and citations to the literature in Cook, R. J. and Oosterveld, V. L. (1995). A select bibliography of women's human rights. *Am. Univ. Law Rev.*, **44**, 1429–71, updated periodically on the internet at http://www.law.utoronto.ca/pubs/h_rghts.htm

16. Catley-Carlson, M. (1994). The challenges of population: reflections on the eve of Cairo. *New World*, 1–3

17. Cook, R. J. and Maine, D. (1987). Spousal veto over family planning services. *Am. J. Public Health*, **77**, 339–44

18. Dixon-Mueller, R. and Germain, A. (1992). Stalking the unmet need for family planning. *Studies Family Planning*, **23**, 330–41

19. Kjeldsen, Busk Madsen and Pedersen v. Denmark, 1 Eur. H. R. Rep. 711 (1976) [Danish Sex Educations case]

20. Open Door and Dublin Well Woman v. Ireland, 14 Eur. H. R. Rep. 131 (1992)

21. World Bank (1993). *World Development Report 1993 – Investing in Health.* (New York: Oxford University Press)

22. R. v. Morgentaler (1988) 44 D.L.R. (4th) 385 (Sup. Ct. Canada)

23. United Nations, International Covenant on Civil and Political Rights (1996). *Third Periodical Report of State Parties: Peru.* CCPR/C/83/Add. 1 21 March 1995; United Nations, *Concluding Observations on the Report of Peru of the Human Rights Committee*

24. Elias, C. and Heise, L. (1993). The development of microbicides: a new method of HIV prevention for women. *Population Council Working Papers*, **6**

25. The FIGO Committee for the Study of Ethical Aspects of Human Reproduction (1994). *Recommendations on Ethical Issues in Obstetrics and Gynecology.* (London: International Federation of Gynecology and Obstetrics)

26. Commonwealth Medical Association (1994). *Medical Ethics and Human Rights: Guiding Principles.* (London: Commonwealth Medical Association)

27. Colombian Ministry of Health (1992). *Salud para la Mujer, Mujer para la Salud* (Health for Women, Women for Health). (Bogota: Ministry of Public Health)

28. Pitanguy, J. (1995). From Mexico to Beijing: a new paradigm. *Health Hum. Rights*, **1**, 454–60

29. Plata, M. I. (1994). Reproductive rights as human rights: the Colombian case. In Cook, R. J. (ed.) *Human Rights of Women: National and International Perspectives*, pp.515–31. (Philadelphia: University of Pennsylvania Press)

30. Profamilia Servicios Legales Para Mujeres (Profamilia Legal Services for Women) (1993). *Amparo a Mis Derechos Fundamentales. La Acción de Tutela* (Safeguard My Fundamental Rights: the Right to Petition), and *La Violencia y los Derechos Humanos de la Mujer* (Violence and the Human Rights of Women). (Bogota: Profamilia)

31. *Erase Una Vez* (Once Upon a Time), 1988; and *Cada Dia, Cada Instante* (Every Day, Every Instant), 1989 (Bogota, Colombia: Profamilia)

32. Calderón, M. C. (1993). *Talleres de Género en 12 Clínicas de Profamilia. Informe de Actividades* (Gender Workshops in 12 Profamilia Clinics: Summary Report). (Bogota: Profamilia)

Violence against women: reproductive consequences

20

B. Schei

Introduction

The United Nations declaration (1992) defines violence against women as:

'Any act of gender-based violence that is likely to result in physical, sexual or psychological harm or suffering to women, including threats of such acts, coercion or arbitrary deprivation of liberty, whether occurring in public or private life.'

Violence affects women all over the world. At all stages in life women might become subject to violence: women can be betrayed by their closest relatives, as young girls sexually abused by their fathers; in adolescence they can be raped by boyfriends and subjected to sexual harassment in schools and workplace; in adulthood marital violence and rape occur; as old women they can be abused by their children and other relatives.

In addition to these types of interpersonal violence, cultural practices harmful to women, such as genital mutilation, have been included as violent acts against women. Man-made disasters, such as wars, unequally affect women. Systematic rape of women and girls as part of ethnic cleansing has recently received international attention, as in the war in former Yugoslavia. Women are also subjected to violence related to trafficking in women, forced prostitution and other types of exploitation of the female gender.

The international community has increasingly acknowledged the problem of violence against women. The Fourth World Conference on Women held in Beijing in 1995 adopted the Beijing Platform of Action that specified the need to take steps to eliminate violence against women[1]. The World Health Organization

(WHO) has declared violence as a public health priority. At the World Health Assembly (WHA) in 1996, a resolution (WHA 49.25) was adopted. For the first time ever it was declared that violence has become a leading international public health problem. Special concern was expressed regarding the increase in violence against women and children.

To examine the reproductive effects of all types of violence is beyond the scope of the present paper. Instead, the focus will be on the violence women are subjected to at home by their intimate partner.

'It is still true that for a woman to be brutally or systematically assaulted, she must usually enter our most sacred institution, the family. It is within marriage that a woman is most likely to be slapped and shoved about, severely assaulted, killed, or raped'[2].

Wife-beating: looking back to understand its presence

A husband's right to beat his wife is deeply embedded in the European culture and also in the legal system of Europe. Before the late 19th century, physical punishment of wives was accepted as adequate behavior under certain conditions:

'The term "rule of the thumb" purportedly derived from the ancient right of the husband to chastise his wife with a stick no thicker than his thumb'[2].

According to Dobash and Dobash, pioneers in the study of violence against women, the first step offering women an opportunity to escape severe violence in England was given in the law of 1853. In 'The Act for Better Prevention and Punishment of Aggravated Assaults upon Women and Children' women were given some of the same protection already extended to animals who were cruelly treated[2]. By the turn of the century, England had even formed a Select Committee on violence in marriage[3]. A public silence fell upon the topic for nearly 100 years until the women's movements brought it back on to the public agenda: in 1971 the first shelter in Europe was established to give protection to battered women[4]. This heralded a new period in Western societies making this part of private life again a public affair. Violence against wives became a matter of public concern and scientific inquiry.

Defining abuse by intimate partner

The term spouse abuse most often refers to violence against wives. Gayford defined a battered woman as 'a woman who has suffered more than one visible injury caused by spousal violence'[3]. A commonly applied definition is that of the American sociologist, Murray Straus. He defined a battered woman as 'a woman who had suffered at least one episode of violent act from her spouse, more severe than slapping'[5].

Additional criteria have been based on recognition of the behavioral dynamics. Walker described three phases in the cycle of violence: the tension-building phase, the explosion of acute battering incidents and the calm, loving phase. She defines the battering relationship 'as a relationship in which these cycles of violence take place'[6]. These cycles, in which the woman experiences her husband's unpredictable transformation from a loving partner to a violent monster and then to a repentant sinner, are important for keeping her trapped in the relationship. Others have described the dynamics of an abusive relationship as a type of mind-control[7].

How common is wife-beating?

One of the first and often cited population-based studies is that of Straus[5]. In a national survey in the USA he found that 3.8% of women had experienced physical abuse by their spouse within the previous year. A Norwegian study gave a similar estimate of 3.6%[8]. Typical estimates of women ever physically abused in a relationship are 10–13% in Western countries. If a broader definition is applied to include all types of violence by the intimate partner, the estimates are 17–38%[7,9]. Limited studies carried out in Africa, Latin America and Asia report even higher rates of physical abuse of up to 60% and more[10]. The legal status of a woman in society is related to the magnitude of the problem. A woman with limited options might not be able to leave her husband even if he is beating her. This is illustrated in a recent study from India. Of the 1842 participating women, 40% gave a positive answer to ever having been beaten by their husbands. Only 5% expressed the view that a woman should leave her husband if she is beaten excessively[11].

Health consequences

Physical injuries

Violence against wives is an important cause of death among women. Statistics from England and the USA show that between 30 and 40% of murdered women are killed by their male partner[12]. A large proportion of wife murderers have been identified as batterers before the killing of their wives. The non-fatal injuries include cerebral hemorrhages, fractures, open wounds, bruises and burns. There is no typical pattern of injuries. Spousal violence is considered one of the most important causes of injuries among women, more important than, for instance, car accidents[13]. Even so, medical journals rarely include this information. In a study from the USA, the proportion of injuries among women recognized as caused by abuse was estimated to be 5.6% when medical journals were used as sources of information. When a standard procedure was introduced including direct questions related to spousal abuse, the estimated proportion of injuries caused by spouse-inflicted violence rose to 30%[12].

Somatic and mental health

To live with a husband who beats her has an impact on the woman's health far beyond the physical injuries. A follow-up study of battered women demonstrated a risk of a variety of health problems registered as admissions to hospital. One of these was attempted suicide. Another important observation was that battered women were often admitted without any definite diagnosis being established[14]. Battered women in a nationally representative sample (USA) reported poor communication with physicians. Only 10% of the battered women had ever discussed the abuse with their doctor[15]. This might lead to misunderstanding and lack of appropriate measures, and might partly explain the overlooking of battered women by the healthcare system.

Mental health problems are a major feature of the poor health of battered women. The feeling of helplessness and constant fear for one's own and children's lives are emotions evoked by the violence, and symptoms of depression[16] and anxiety are prevalent[17]. In addition to these general reactions, battered women report specific symptoms related to the trauma of abuse: nightmares, flashbacks and avoidance such as memory loss or affective numbing; and autonomic arousal such as sleep disturbances, difficulties concentrating, hypervigilance and heightened startle response. These symptoms might reflect a post-traumatic stress disorder (PTSD). Recent studies show that battered women exhibit significantly higher rates of PTSD than other maritally distressed women[18]. Severe mental disorders, such as psychoses, are also considered to be an effect of living with an abusive spouse[19].

Reproductive consequences

Violence against wives: also sexual

Without having any say as to when and how, and under what kind of circumstances she will have sex with her husband, a woman has few reproductive choices. This right of the husband to sexual access to his wife has traditionally been part of the marriage license. Not only has marriage legalized hitting in the past, but it has also been a license to rape. Still in some countries, rape in a legal sense refers to events taking place outside marriage[20]. A woman might experience different types of sexual coercion in a battering relationship. She might be raped as part of a violent attack. She might also submit to sexual activity as an attempt to stop the beating.

Genital infections

The lack of control of her sexual life will expose a woman to unwanted risk of sexually transmitted diseases. Abusers are likely to engage in sex outside marriage, and the woman might have to submit to intercourse even if she knows she runs the risk of disease transmission. Vaginitis, colpitis and pelvic inflammatory diseases can be consequences of abuse[21]. This again might lead to chronic conditions and infertility. Another aspect of the relationship between infections and abuse is that the woman might refrain from following the prescribed treatment after diagnosis of an infection. Abusers often share the common feature of being exceedingly jealous. Discovering that she has an infection might provoke the husband's violence. As an example of this, in a study of perinatal human immunodeficiency virus (HIV) transmission in Kenya, the professionals discovered that enrollment was not always harmless for the women involved. Women who were screened as positive were often blamed for bringing acquired immunodeficiency syndrome (AIDS) to the family, and violence against them was common when the results were conveyed. Learning this, a change in practice in the clinic was established. Women were informed that they had the right not to be told the results[22]. This was an attempt to protect a woman from being beaten if she lived with an abuser.

Women sexually abused in childhood are at risk of being revictimized. During adolescence and adulthood they are also more likely to engage in risk behavior such as promiscuity. A larger proportion of battered women have also been victimized as children compared with a non-battered population. This adds to the total elevated risk of genital infections among women living with abusers.

Unwanted pregnancy

The power and control exhibited by the abuser will also affect a woman's opportunity to decide when, and under what kind of circumstance, she wants to become pregnant. In family planning, the advice on condom use might have an unwanted effect when given to an abused woman. A woman from Uganda was cited in a paper by Heise[23] 'If you advise your husband to use a condom, he may beat you and send you away. Where will you go then?'

The husband can also refuse her access to health-care. Being in control of the economy, the woman might have great difficulty in buying contraceptives. She might also be too afraid to use pills in fear of being discovered taking them. He might also rape her with the explicit purpose to make her pregnant and then less likely to leave him, as conveyed in some case histories. Or he may stop her having a legal abortion as another way of controlling her. Steward and Cecutti reported that almost 90% of all pregnancies among women abused in pregnancy were unplanned[24].

Violence in pregnancy

A woman might hope that her husband will stop beating her when she is pregnant: 30–40% of battered women report that they were not beaten when pregnant[25].

However, 20% of women hit during pregnancy reported an increase in abuse[26]. Men who continue to beat their wives during pregnancy are also considered to be generally more violent both towards their wives and others[27]. Studies of prevalence of violence against pregnant women were recently reviewed[28]. Thirteen studies were found, and all except one from Australia were carried out in North America. The reported rates of violence against pregnant women were between 0.9 and 20.1%. The lowest rate was reported by women attending a private clinic and responding to a self-administered questionnaire. The authors concluded that despite the limitations of the studies they described, there was reason to believe that violence may be a more common problem for pregnant women than pre-eclampsia, gestational diabetes and placenta previa, conditions for which pregnant women are routinely screened and evaluated.

When a pregnant woman is subjected to violence it is certainly a threat to her own health, but the fetus is also at risk. There are case histories describing 'the battered fetus' syndrome as a cause of perinatal death[29]. Injuries caused by interpersonal violence in pregnancy are also demonstrated to be associated with non-fatal adverse pregnancy outcome[30]. Several studies have demonstrated that physical abuse is associated with a range of adverse perinatal outcomes, such as premature birth and low birth weight[31]. The proposed mechanisms whereby abuse might cause adverse outcomes include stress-related factors and genital infections, in addition to the effect of direct physical injuries. Another major influence of abuse on a pregnant woman is on lifestyle. A woman's ability to protect herself and her unborn baby is limited by the abuser. Abused women reported insufficient intake of food, alcohol and drug abuse, and cigarette smoking, which might also influence the health of the unborn child. Psychological problems and suicidal ideation are prevalent among pregnant women who are abused[24].

How to face violence as obstetrician–gynecologists?

General considerations

Violence is a dark side to women's lives which is hard to face. There are still large gaps in the education and training of health-care providers[32]. Helplessness and reluctance to face the problem might be the result. It is important to bear in mind, however, that overlooking abuse might lead to poor quality of diagnosis and evaluation in the physician's daily work. In order to increase knowledge and skills in this area, all physicians training in obstetrics and gynecology should be offered postgraduate training. All patients should be given general information with detailed descriptions of legal rights, shelters and services for battered women in the region. The problems of violence cannot be fully dealt with within the medical setting. In many parts of the world shelters for battered women and networks against violence have been established. Collaboration should be established between reproductive health services and services outside the hospital/clinic. There is also a great need to develop models for best practice within the health-care system. Obstetrician–gynecologists might refrain from facing the problem because of a lack of referral systems and resources in the community to address violence. But it is important to remember that most battered women express a wish that someone asks them about abuse. For an abused woman to encounter a caring obstetrician–gynecologist with knowledge of abuse might be the first step in changing her situation. The following is a summary of some key features to be taken into account in everyday practice.

Gynecological encounters

(1) Consultation should always allow for women to disclose by careful active listening in a safe environment.

(2) Abused women are over-represented among several diagnostic groups, and women with these disorders (e.g. chronic pelvic pain, pelvic inflammatory disease and sexually transmitted diseases) must be carefully examined with reference to abuse history.

(3) Comorbidity, such as psychological problems, PTSD, suicide attempts, injuries and 'unexplained' somatic symptoms should raise the suspicion of abuse.

(4) Abused women might have problems in following certain kinds of treatment, such as antibiotics, as they might be beaten, suspected of extramarital sex.

(5) Abused women might face difficulties in informing their husband of positive testing for, e.g. HIV.

(6) Memories of severe trauma might be triggered by the gynecological examination.

(7) Abused women might be even more severely beaten if the husband knows she has reported the abuse.

(8) Contraceptive advice should take into account the woman's ability to control her sex life.

Antenatal care

(1) The pregnant woman should have an opportunity to communicate without the presence of her spouse.

(2) Abuse in high-risk women (e.g. comorbidity, certain pregnancy complications and disorders in pregnancy) should be assessed.

(3) Likelihood of abuse should be assessed when advice and medical treatment implicitly involve a co-operative partner.

(4) If the woman is abused in pregnancy, the danger should be assessed and individual safety plans made.

(5) In severe cases, legal action should be considered.

Concluding remarks

Obstetrician–gynecologists are among key professionals in the effort to end violence against women. By recognizing abuse as a problem, we can effect change to an individual woman's life through our daily work. By acknowledging that violence is also our professional responsibility, we can improve education and training in this area. By being the abused woman's advocates in society we can urge the authorities to improve the total service for abused women. By saying 'No' to violence we can contribute to the long-term goal of ending all violence against women.

References

1. United Nations (1995). *Report of the Fourth Conference on Women*, A/conf 177/20. (New York: United Nations)
2. Dobash, R. E. and Dobash, R. (1980). *Violence Against Wives*. (London: Open Books)
3. Gayford, J. J. (1975). Wife battering: a preliminary survey of 100 cases. *Br. Med. J.*, 1, 194–7
4. Pizzey, E. (1974). *Scream Quietly or the Neighbours Will Hear You.* (London: Penguin)
5. Straus, M. A. (1977/78). Wife beating: how common and why? *Victimology*, 2, 433–58
6. Walker, L. E. (1979). *The Battered Woman.* (London: Harper and Row).
7. Boulette, T. R. and Andersen, S. M. (1985). 'Mind control' and the battering of women. *Commun. Ment. Health J.*, 21, 109–18
8. Schei, B. and Bakketeig, L. S. (1989). Gynaecological impact of sexual and physical abuse by spouse. A study of a random sample of Norwegian women. *Br. J. Obstet. Gynaecol.*, 96, 1379–83
9. Mullen, P. E., Romans-Clarkson, S. E., Walton, V. A. and Herbison, P. G. (1988). Impact of sexual and physical abuse on women's mental health. *Lancet*, 1, 841–5
10. United Nations (1995). The world's women 1995. *Trends and Statistics*, Social Statistics and Indicators Series K, No. 12. (New York: United Nations)
11. Jejeebhoy, S. and Cook, R. J. (1997). State accountability for wife-beating: the Indian challenge. *Lancet*, 349, sI10–sI12.
12. Sassetti, M. R. (1993). Domestic violence. *Primary Care*, 20, 289–305
13. McLeer, S. V. and Anwar, R. (1989). A study of battered women presenting in an emergency department. *Am. J. Publ. Health*, 79, 65–6
14. Bergman, B. and Brismar, B. (1991). A 5 years follow up study of 117 battered women. *Am. J. Publ. Health*, 81, 1486–9
15. Plichtera, S. B., Duncan, M. M. and Plichta, L. (1996). Spouse abuse, patients–physician communication and patient satisfaction. *Am. J. Prevent. Med.*, 12, 297–303
16. Walker, L. E. (1977/78). Battered women and learned helplessness. *Victimology*, 2, 525–34
17. Jaffe, P., Wolfe, D. A., Wilson, S. and Zak, L. (1986). Emotional and physical health problems of battered women. *Can. J. Psychiatry*, 31, 625–9
18. Astin, M. C., Ogland-Hand, S. M. and Foy, D. W. (1995). Posttraumatic stress disorder and childhood abuse in battered women: comparison with maritally distressed women. *J. Consult. Clin. Psychol.*, 63, 308–12
19. Jacobsen, A. and Richardson, B. (1987). Assault experience of 100 psychiatric inpatients. Evidence of the need for routine inquiry. *Am. J. Psychiatry*, 144, 908–13
20. Russel, D. E. H. (1982). *Rape in Marriage.* (New York: Macmillan Publishing Co.)
21. Schei, B. (1991). Physically abusive spouse – a risk factor of pelvic inflammatory diseases? *Scand. J. Primary Health Care*, 9, 41–5
22. Temmerman, M., Ndiya-Achola, J., Ambasni, J. and Piot, P. (1995). The right not to know HIV-test results. *Lancet*, 345, 969–70
23. Heise, L. L. (1993). Reproductive freedom and violence against women: where are the intersections? *J. Law Med. Ethics*, 21, 206–16
24. Steward, D. and Cecutti, A.(1993). Physical abuse in pregnancy. *Can. Med. Assoc.*, 149, 1257–69
25. Schei, B. (1990). *Trapped in Painful Love. Physical and Sexual Abuse by Spouse – a Risk Factor of Gynaecological Disorders and Adverse Perinatal Outcomes*, Series A: dissertation No. 63. (Trondheim: Tapir)
26. Hillard, P. J. (1985). Physical abuse in pregnancy. *Obstet. Gynecol.*, 66, 185–90
27. Fagen, J. A., Douglas, K. S. and Hansen, K. V. (1983). Violent men or violent husbands. Background factors and situational correlates. In Finkelhor, D., Gelles, R. J., Hotaling, G. H. and Straus, M. A. (eds.) *The Dark Sides of Families*, pp. 49–69. (London: Sage Publications)
28. Gazmararian, J. A., Lazorick, S., Spitz, A. M., Balard, T. J., Saltzman, L. E. and Marks, J. S. (1996). Prevalence of violence against pregnant women. *J. Am. Med. Assoc.*, 275, 1915–20
29. Morey, M. A., Begleiter, D. J. and Harris, D. J. (1981). Profile of the battered fetus. *Lancet*, 2, 1295–6
30. Goodwin, T. M. and Breen, M. T. (1990). Pregnancy outcome and fetomaternal hemorrhage after noncatastrophic trauma. *Am. J. Obstet. Gynecol.*, 162, 665–71
31. Newberger, E. N., Barkan, S. E., Lieberman, E. S., McCormick, M. C., Yllo, K., Gary, L. T. and Schechter, S. (1992). Abuse of pregnant women and adverse outcome. Current knowledge and implication for practice. *J. Am. Med. Assoc.*, 267, 1212–13
32. Chambliss, L. R., Bay, C. R. and Jones, R. F. III (1995). *Am. J. Obstet. Gynecol.*, 172, 1035–8

Violence against women in sub-Saharan Africa: building a response

21

C. Watts

Violence against women in sub-Saharan Africa

Violence against women in its various forms is endemic in all communities and countries around the world. It is a phenomenon which cuts across class, race, age, religious and national boundaries.

In sub-Saharan Africa, violence against women takes many forms. Some types of violence are common world-wide, and include physical assault, sexual harassment, rape and domestic violence. Others, linked to traditional or customary practices, are limited to specific communities or geographical regions. As well as female genital mutilation, these include child marriage and the inheritance of the wife of a deceased man by his brother[1].

The few studies that have been conducted in sub-Saharan Africa indicate that it is common for women to experience multiple forms of violence, primarily by their partners, but also by other family members. Research in Malawi, Uganda and South Africa also shows that for many girls, their first sexual experience was forced (Table 1). Generally, cross-cultural studies find that a large percentage of rapes are perpetrated against girls aged 15 years and under, and that in many cases, the girl or woman will know the perpetrator[2].

Violence against women

In sub-Saharan Africa there are non-governmental organizations (NGOs) in Zimbabwe, South Africa, Namibia, Cameroon, Tanzania, Uganda and Kenya addressing violence against women. For example, in Zimbabwe the Musasa Project provides shelter, counseling and legal services to women experiencing abuse, and conducts advocacy, educational and training activities to challenge the acceptability of violence against women, and to strengthen the services

Table 1 Evidence of extent of violence against women in sub-Saharan Africa

In a representative sample of 966 women aged 18 and over in one province in Zimbabwe, 32% reported experiencing some form of physical abuse; 37% reported experiencing sexual abuse, with 18% reporting that someone had either attempted or succeeded in forcing them to have sex against their will; in most cases, the perpetrator was the woman's husband or partner.

In a detailed family-planning survey of 733 women in Kissi District of Kenya, 42% reported being beaten regularly by their husbands.

In a representative sample of women aged 20–44 and their partners in two districts in Uganda, 40.5% of women report being beaten or physically harmed by a partner; 40.8% of men admit to beating.

In a Ugandan sample of 400 students randomly selected from 40 primary schools (average age 13.9), 49% of sexually active girls said they had been forced to have intercourse; 22% had received gifts or rewards for sex.

In rural Malawi, 55% of 120 adolescent girls interviewed reported that they are often forced to have sex; 66% report having accepted money or gifts for sex.

provided to women experiencing abuse. The present author has been working with this NGO for the past 2 years, and will make reference to some of their experiences and insights in this paper.

Commonly, violence against women is framed as a legal or human-rights issue. As such, it is often seen as being peripheral to women's health concerns. However, violence against women has a number of important health consequences[2] (Figure 1).

Abuse and gynecological problems

There is a strong link between a history of abuse and gynecological problems, including chronic pelvic pain, vaginal discharge, sexually transmitted diseases (STDs) including human immunodeficiency virus (HIV) infection and pelvic inflammatory disease (PID)[2,3]. There are also connections between abuse and unwanted

pregnancy and STDs/HIV. For example, violence can cause pregnancy and STDs directly, may inhibit contraceptive use and consented condom use and may promote early sex and sexual risk-taking behavior. The links are both direct and indirect. A pattern of emotional and behavioral damage puts women at greater risk of early pregnancies and STDs in later life. A young girl who has been sexually abused may be very confused about her sexuality, and may not be able to distinguish between love and someone who is trying to abuse or use her. There is also a tendency for young girls who have been abused to have intercourse at an earlier age and to use alcohol and drugs more than those who have not been abused[2].

Teenage pregnancies

The figures shown in Table 2 suggest that for many girls, their first sexual experience is

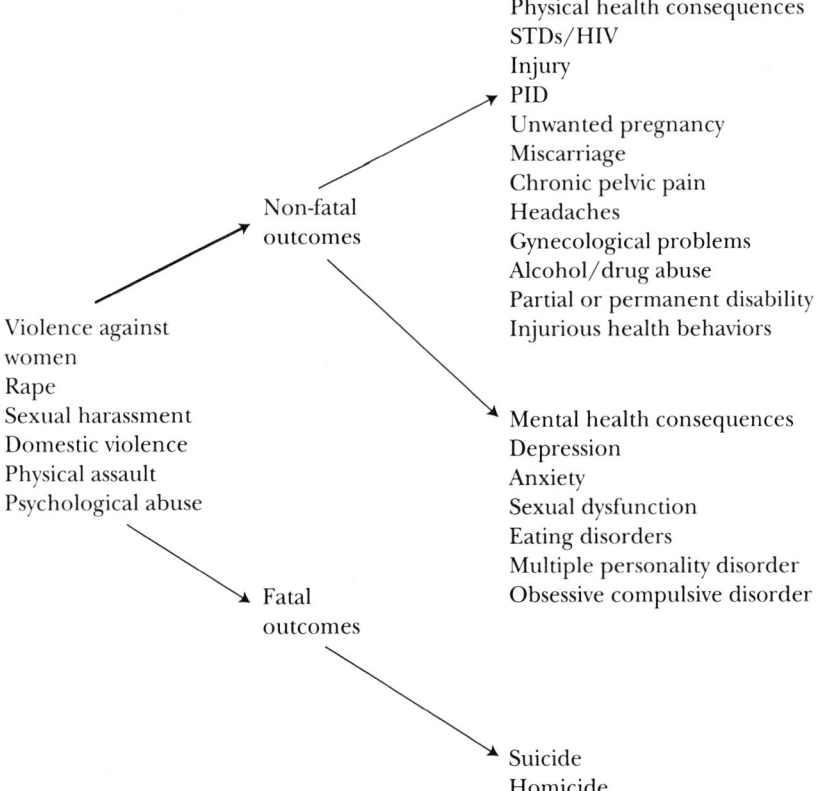

Figure 1 Health consequences of violence against women

forced. It may well be that many teenage pregnancies are as a result of violent and abusive relationships. The findings from a survey of teenage girls attending an antenatal clinic in Cape Town illustrates the degree to which this may occur, with the majority reporting that they had been beaten (a median of 10 times) and forced to have sex by their boyfriends[4]. The girls also feared rejection, scorn, punishment or violence if they did not have sex.

Violence during pregnancy

Several studies in industrialized countries have documented some women's increased vulnerability to violence during pregnancy. Overall, between 9 and 20% of women world-wide experience abuse during pregnancy[2]. Research suggests that such women have a much higher risk of having a premature birth and low birthweight infants, miscarriage and other pregnancy complications. They are also likely to have interference with their prenatal care. In sub-Saharan Africa the extent and health consequences of violence during pregnancy have not been widely acknowledged or explored. However, research from a community survey in Zimbabwe indicates that physical and psychological abuse are common.

The survey found that almost one in five (23%) women who had ever been pregnant reported experiencing some form of physical or psychological abuse during their pregnancy (Figure 2)[5]. One in 15 reported being kicked, bitten, slapped, hit or had objects thrown at them while they were pregnant, and 4% reported being pushed, kicked or hit in the stomach. In the majority of cases, the perpetrator was the woman's partner.

It is likely that some women are more vulnerable to abuse during pregnancy than others. In Zimbabwe it was found that younger women reported a significantly higher level of lifetime experiences of violence during pregnancy than older women, despite having had less time to possibly be abused. This suggests that the different forms of abuse investigated may be more common currently than in the past.

In Zimbabwe, Musasa finds that in some cases violence may be ongoing prior to the pregnancy, but increases in intensity during the pregnancy. For example, one of their clients

Table 2 Extent of violence experienced by teenage mothers in Cape Town[4]

Among teenage girls attending antenatal clinic in Cape Town (mean age 16.3):
   30% reported that their first intercourse was forced
   71% report having had sex against their will
   11% said they had been raped
   60% said that they had been beaten by their partner (median of 10 times)
   less than a quarter had terminated relationships because of abuse

When asked what they thought consequences of refusing sex would be:
   75% said they would be beaten
   38% feared being laughed at
   6% felt they would lose their friends

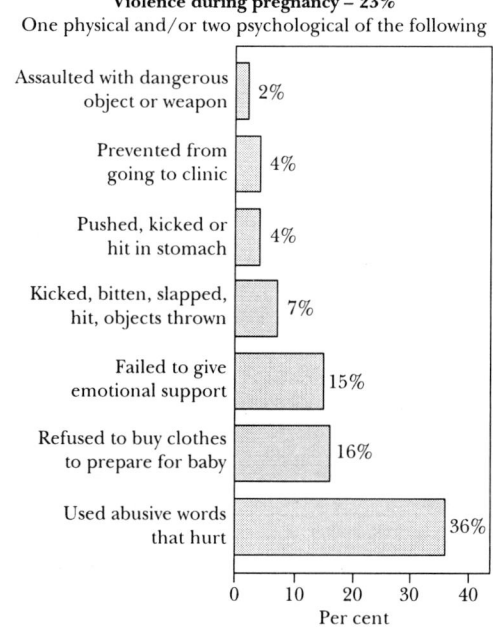

Violence during pregnancy – 23%
One physical and/or two psychological of the following

- Assaulted with dangerous object or weapon 2%
- Prevented from going to clinic 4%
- Pushed, kicked or hit in stomach 4%
- Kicked, bitten, slapped, hit, objects thrown 7%
- Failed to give emotional support 15%
- Refused to buy clothes to prepare for baby 16%
- Used abusive words that hurt 36%

Per cent

Figure 2 Extent that a community sample of women over 18 reported experiencing different forms of violence during one or more pregnancies. Overall prevalence of 23% gives extent that women reported experiencing either one physical and/or two psychological forms of abuse

lives in the rural areas while her husband lives in town. Commonly, when she goes to visit him, he beats her. On one occasion she was severely beaten when she was 7 months pregnant, and subsequently miscarried. Although she wanted to wait before having another child, 3 months later she is pregnant again, as her husband wants another child[1].

Violence may also start during pregnancy. This may occur particularly among young unmarried couples, due to tensions over who is the father of the child.

Strengthening the health sector response

The above examples highlight some of the ways in which violence against women impacts on women's reproductive health in sub-Saharan Africa. At Musasa, clients commonly have experienced abuse for an average of 10 years before turning to outside sources of help. As the following quote illustrates, at this point, often their relationship has reached a crisis situation, and they are seeking counseling and legal advice about the options for themselves and their children:

'Imagine, since 1976 my husband has been beating me. Even when I was highly pregnant my husband used to beat me and I would faint . . . soon after giving birth he resumed beating me'.

Client at Musasa, 1995

Before coming to Musasa, many clients have used clinics or been in hospital several times. In some cases, they have gone to obtain treatment for injuries sustained during violent incidents, or to get medication to relieve pain, to bring down their blood pressure or for depression. In other cases, they have come into contact with health services for unrelated reasons, such as to obtain family planning, for antenatal care or to get treatment for a sick child.

Because abused women use health services for a number of reasons, health workers, including those providing reproductive health services, could potentially identify, support and refer cases of violence at an early stage, when the possibilities for successful intervention are much greater. This is particularly important as violence in relationships commonly escalates in severity over time.

In 1995, Musasa Project held discussions with nurses and doctors to identify how the health-sector response could be strengthened. Clients at Musasa were also interviewed about their experiences when using health services. Quotes from some of the people consulted are used below to discuss possible forms of intervention, focusing on the role of obstetricians and gynecologists, and related reproductive health workers.

Sensitivity training for staff

Fundamentally, before health workers can start to discuss violence with their clients, they should be encouraged to look at themselves, and confront any biases, misconceptions and fears that they may have about the issue. A woman who has been assaulted or raped has already experienced terrible things. They can be revictimized through judgmental or indifferent behavior. Within any intervention, sensitivity training is an important first step to help ensure that doctors contribute to their clients' safety and well-being.

Asking about violence

Some health workers said that, whenever necessary, they did try to discuss violence with their clients. However, many said that they did not have enough time to ask such questions. Several also stated that, out of fear of stigmatization or further violence, many women would not discuss abuse, even if they were asked. This is illustrated by the following quote:

'There is a woman in the wards who claimed that she caught fire from a paraffin stove. The husband came to the matron to confess that he actually poured paraffin on her, and set her alight after a domestic dispute'.

Hospital matron

When clients at Musasa were asked whether they had talked with health workers about their experiences of violence, a number reported that they had not been asked. Others stated that they did not discuss their problem because they did not think that the health workers would be sensitive to their plight. For example, when asked about why she did not discuss the violence that she was experiencing, one client responded:

'They [the nurses] seemed to be enjoying themselves and I concluded that they were making a mockery out of me'.

Client at Musasa

Confidentiality and privacy

A key factor influencing whether a woman will discuss a sensitive topic such as violence is whether or not she feels that confidentiality will be maintained. Health workers described how when a woman is admitted to hospital, it provides hospital staff with the opportunity to discuss violence and provide counseling. However, the following quote illustrates how, unless care is taken, it may be difficult to maintain confidentiality:

'I went to the hospital. My husband beat me when I got pregnant. Of course I got the required treatment. What hurt me was that there was no confidentiality by the doctors and nurses treating me. Everyone in the ward got to know that I had been beaten by my husband'.

Client at Musasa

In addition, any discussion about violence needs to take place in private, in a setting where a woman can feel safe and relaxed. This may require that at least at the hospital level, space and time is set aside for such discussions.

Revision of protocols for the management of rape cases

Obstetricians and gynecologists play an important role in documenting that rape has occurred, providing services to meet the survivor's specific health needs, and starting the healing process. Many hospitals have protocols for the management of rape cases, which discuss the services that need to be provided to women who have been raped. In many cases, these protocols were developed many years ago, and it may be necessary to review their relevance and adequacy.

Women who have been raped have a number of immediate reproductive health needs. Protocols need to stress the importance of providing screening for STDs, emergency contraception and access to abortion, and clearly outline the procedures for obtaining these different services.

It is also important that such protocols highlight the importance of ensuring that all cases are taken seriously, and handled with sensitivity. For example, one doctor in Zimbabwe said that examinations to assess whether the hymen is still intact were commonly performed, even though they were often unnecessary and distressing. Obstetricians and gynecologists need to be at the forefront, highlighting the ambiguity of such evidence in many instances. The importance of ensuring that the process of collecting evidence does not degrade or further distress a woman needs to be stressed also.

Protocols commonly highlight that rape survivors need to be counseled. However, nurses have often not received adequate training in this area. However, with the onset of acquired immunodeficiency syndrome (AIDS) in the region, nurses are increasingly receiving training in counseling. A lack of rape-related counseling skills could possibly be remedied through the provision of additional training in ongoing counseling courses.

Improved documentation and collection of evidence

Even where an assault has not been reported to the police, it is important that accurate and detailed medical records are kept – including details of the perpetrator of the assault. For, even if at the time of the consultation a woman does not want to go to the police, at a later point she may well want to press charges. Then, she may need medical evidence about the history and severity of the abuse. As the quote below illustrates, without detailed medical records the possibilities to gain compensation may be limited:

'In some cases women do not want violence written on their health cards. For example, we had a client who was beaten whilst she was pregnant, aborted and now is infertile. She does not have any records documenting this, and so cannot seek compensation from her husband'.

Key informant, Zimbabwe

If, out of a fear of further violence, the woman does not want details written on her medical card, it may be necessary to register these details on the hospital records.

Reducing delays

Commonly, only government doctors are authorized to document rape or assault. Since there is often a shortage of government doctors, a survivor may have to wait a few days to see a doctor. By this time, most of the evidence may be lost.

Although abortion following rape is legal in many countries, in many cases women are not aware of the availability of this option. For women seeking to terminate a pregnancy following rape there may be numerous bureaucratic hurdles to negotiate: any delay or opposition by the police, the judiciary or medical practitioners can seriously jeopardize whether a woman can obtain the abortion in time. In Zimbabwe, Musasa has had cases where women could not get abortions because the process of obtaining the necessary signatures took too long:

'Obtaining an abortion requires documentation from the police, a magistrate and an affidavit from a doctor. This can be very bureaucratic, and lead to delay. For example, we had one client who couldn't get an abortion as it took too long for her to obtain the signature'.

Key informant, Zimbabwe

Ideally, there should be sufficient numbers of qualified people in each urban center or growth point to ensure that abused women can be promptly attended to. The situation could be improved if the range of people permitted to document abuse and give evidence in court was increased. People who could potentially be authorized to complete affidavits include doctors working outside the public sector (such as private doctors, or doctors working in mission hospitals), and senior nursing staff who could be trained to handle and document cases of sexual and physical assault.

Strengthening systems of referral

Women who have experienced violence may come into contact with a range of different agencies including the police, social welfare and health workers. It is important that at the community level, these agencies work together. If not, a client may travel back and forth between agencies and then just give up. The experience of one client at Musasa in Zimbabwe clearly illustrates the problem:

'I went to the matron. I was then advised to come to Musasa Project. They sent me to social welfare. At social welfare I kept on being referred from one person to another the whole day. I went back the next day and was told to go back to the police station'.

Client at Musasa, Zimbabwe

Methods to streamline systems of referral need to be identified. For example, key focal point persons could be identified within each agency. These people could then meet regularly to review cases, discuss difficulties and generally get to know each other. Then clients could at least be referred between specific people within each agency who are concerned about the issue.

Conclusion

Violence against women is a substantial problem. Currently the issue is primarily being addressed by women's organizations. While they have made substantial gains, often the

155

organizations are small, and on their own can only ever hope to have a limited impact.

Collaborative action by different agencies coming into contact with cases of abuse is needed if substantial change is to be achieved. Reproductive health workers are regularly coming into contact with cases of abuse, and so could play an important role in identifying, supporting and referring cases of violence. Reproductive health services are likely to have regular, and far earlier contact with survivors of violence than other agencies, such as the police. This could provide important opportunities for early identification, when the possibilities for successful intervention are far greater.

However, in sub-Saharan Africa, many of these agencies are over-burdened and have limited financial resources, and feel that if they developed activities to respond, it would further add to their load. However, it is important to recognize that it is costly to the woman, the health sector and society as a whole if only the presenting problem is addressed. With support and training, reproductive health workers could help to identify cases of abuse, and link women with available sources of support. Although it may not always be possible to stop violence, even small actions are important. As the following quote illustrates, even providing a woman with an opportunity to talk can be an important intervention:

'She [the health worker] does not have time to sit down and counsel, or advise the victims because they are so busy. So maybe this person [the abused woman] will continue to suffer because nobody actually took the time to sit down and talk to them'.

Discussion with nurses, Zimbabwe

There are many possible forms and levels of intervention. In resource-constrained settings such as sub-Saharan Africa, priority activities which can be feasibly addressed need to be identified. Collaborative, exploratory research is needed to document the likely consequences of inaction, identify priority areas for intervention and to develop feasible, sustainable and appropriate strategies for action.

Acknowledgements

The research in Zimbabwe was conducted in collaboration with the Musasa Project. I would like to thank Mavis Ndlovu and Eunice Njovana, in particular, for their support. The study was supported by the Health and Development Policy Project USA, and Comic Relief through Womankind Worldwide. This paper draws upon a paper published in *Reproductive Health Matters*, and a presentation given at a Workshop held in Harare to explore strategies for action[6].

References

1. Njovana, E. and Watts, C. H. (1996). Gender violence in Zimbabwe: a need for collaborative action. *Reprod. Health Matt.*, **7**, 45–53
2. Heise, L. (1994). *Violence Against Women: the Hidden Health Burden*, World Bank Discussion Papers 225. (Washington, DC: The World Bank)
3. Heise, L., Raikes, A., Watts, C. H. and Zwi, A. B. (1994). Violence against women: a neglected public health issue in less developed countries. *Soc. Sci. Med.*, **39**(9), 1165–79
4. Jewkes, R., *et al.* (1997). He forced me to love him: putting violence on the adolescent sexual health agenda. Unpublished document
5. Watts, C., Ndlovu, M., Njovana, E. and Keogh, E. (1997). Violence against women in Zimbabwe: survey results. Unpublished report, Musasa Project
6. Snowsill, F., Watts, C., Ndlovu, M. and Nyamunzi, V. (eds.) (1997). Violence against women in Zimbabwe: identifying strategies for action. Unpublished workshop report, Musasa Project

Violence against women: a physician's concern? 22

A. F. P. L. d'Oliveira and L. B. Schraiber

Violence and health

For the past 3 years, we have been working on the relationship between violence against women and health services in a Medical School in São Paulo, Brazil. This project aims at training health professionals and investigating the growth of violence-related health problems in health-care services and the medical attitude towards it. The Integrated Project for Professional Training and the Development of Technologies to Assist Women Victims of Violence began in October 1994. It is a partnership between the Preventive Health Department of the School of Medicine of the University of São Paulo and the non-governmental organization (NGO) Coletivo Feminista Sexualidade e Saúde, and it is sponsored by the FORD Foundation. The goal of the Project is to contribute to the organization of basic services and to the development of fully integrated health-care for women. With this paper we wish to draw attention to the Project and contribute to making 'violence against women' an actual health-services problem.

São Paulo is a very large city in Brazil, with over 13 million inhabitants. Violence is a huge problem, as it is in all metropolitan areas in Brazil. Mortality rates due to external factors grew by 40.7% from 1980 to 1989 in Brazil[1]. Urban violence is expressed mainly by homicide rates relating to young males in the outskirts of town. The victims are younger by the day, and the violence against children on the streets of the large cities is known world-wide, including the murder of groups of children who live on the streets.

There is also, in São Paulo, an active movement to fight and prevent violence against women. In 1985, the first Women's Police Station in Brazil was opened in São Paulo. Today there are 10 of these Police Stations in the city and over 100 in the state. The rates of domestic violence are supposedly high, but since domestic violence results rather in morbidity than in mortality, these data are not available on a population basis for Brazil. There are, nevertheless, some figures which are indicative of the situation.

Notwithstanding male mortality by homicide being extremely high, the authors of these two types of crime seem to be different: they are men, in the majority in both cases, but in the group where the victims are women, they are men who are seemingly very close to the victims, generally a relative or the victim's spouse. A survey in the city of Diadema showed that external factors were the first cause of death among women in their prime (25.2%). Of these deaths, 13% were homicides which were committed, in 60% of the cases, by their partners[2].

In Brazil, as disclosed by IBGE (Brazilian Institute of Geography and Statistics), the statistical data for 1988 show that, while relatives were responsible for 31.9% of the aggressions against women, they represented only 10.6% of the crimes against men. As for the place of occurrence, while 18% of the cases of violence to men happened at home, these figures rose to 48% when the victim was a woman[3].

These data are not isolated findings. It is consensus, however, that violence against women is quite common. Representative national surveys in the United States consistently indicate that approximately 20% of adult women have been physically abused at least once by a male intimate[4]. Research from all over the world presents even higher rates, with some countries presenting 40% of women reporting physical violence from their partners, or even higher rates[5].

A great deal of research has been carried out, and now we have a large amount of evidence that links both domestic and non-domestic violence to many usual health problems, in addition to the injuries themselves. Violence against women has been associated with depression, anxiety, suicide and other psychological disorders, drug and alcohol abuse, sexual dysfunction, functional gastrointestinal disorders, headaches, chronic pain and multiple somatic symptoms[5,6]. In the area of reproductive health, violence against women is associated with inflammatory pelvic disease, chronic pelvic pain, high risk for acquired immunodeficiency syndrome (AIDS) and sexually transmitted disease (STD), unwanted pregnancy and abortion[5]. Women are at higher risk when they are pregnant, and between 17%[7] and 25%[4] of all women attending antenatal care are abused during pregnancy.

Violence against women is associated with increased use of health-care[4-6]. Medical professionals, however, find it difficult to detect the problem, and so it is tremendously underestimated[4-6,8].

This information raises some very concrete issues for all who are concerned with the organization of public health-care services, training professionals in the area and planning and managing a basic health unit. For those who specifically act in primary care, social violence is closely related to the professionals, for they face a demand with countless problems which are immediately social at this level of interaction.

Violence is not a pathology. It is an important social problem that leads to a large number of pathologies. Health services know everything about pathologies, but social issues are troublesome, especially for medical work. This is because modern medicine is based on theories that work and are extremely effective through the very reduction of social and historical man to the individual biological body, the basis of diagnostic reasoning[9,10]. This is how health-care works and it has been shown to be effective in connection with countless pathologies. That is why, in the specific case of violence, the immediate injury is treated, but the 'root' of the problem remains intact and shall go on causing physical, psychological and social damage.

Violence is a social problem, but it is reflected as a demand on health-service centers. We must find ways to recognize and handle the matter also from this angle, somehow incorporating the social issues in health-care and re-directing individual cases to the proper authorities. Omission in this field has brought about successively recurring pathologies and therapeutic failures.

Interdisciplinary work, where the physician acknowledges the other members of the team and is acknowledged by them, is essential. It is necessary because different methods of capturing and working on the demands that arise out of violent situations, from the medical examination to educational groups, from nursing to psychotherapeutic activities, are required. Various forums for dialoging, reception and solution of the problem, through a combination of several professionals working together, are also needed.

The response of institutions to violence seems to be fundamental for its perpetuation. We believe that domestic and social violence is socially built, not an individual problem restricted to the victim or the aggressor. Domestic violence isolates the woman, and rape makes her ashamed and prevents her from looking for help and denouncing her aggressor. Institutional response is fundamental to avoid reinforcing and perpetuating the *status quo* through omission, but at the same time one has to respect the woman in question and to be very careful not to annul her subjectivity and her choices of what kind of help she would want and what she intends to do her with her life. Preserving the range of possible options for women, or even amplifying it, is fundamental in order to prevent the usual scope of the institutions from perpetuating violence.

Training and research in Brazilian health services

The Project we have been working on is divided into two parts: training program and research program, and aims at improving the institutional response to violence against women. The training program has already trained 121 people. Our students came mostly from health services – nurses, psychologists, social workers and physicians. We have also trained activists who work with social movements and in women care. The program provides basic understanding in violence, covering the legal, police and health areas, including reproductive health, mental health and health service organizations from the management perspective. It also comprises panels on violence and the media, institutional violence, and race and violence. The program has been extremely successful. Students said that it would change the way in which they work, because now they could see, gather and treat or refer violence-related problems, despite the difficulties in finding adequate references for the different issues arising all over town. We hope that our training program is contributing to a greater perception of the subject in the health services in town.

The research program is divided into several investigations. We shall briefly report here on two of them, the first already completed and the second in the process of completion. The research team multidisciplinary, comprising psychologists, nurses and medical students enrolled in the fourth year with a scholarship for scientific initiation granted by the CNPq (National Research Council).

The first investigation is related to the making and publishing of a *Guide of the Services Available to Women Exposed to Violence*. This guide was developed as a reference material to facilitate the integration of social services of different natures, so that health services would easily recognize situations of violence, thus increasing the possibility of proper intervention. First, the

universally encompassing services especially directed to the care of women subject to violence in the city of São Paulo were surveyed. Through the answers to a standardized questionnaire especially designed for this purpose, 36 services were visited and evaluated for the assistance given. The schedule contained an identification of the services relating to their nature of assistance and relating to the logic of their organization, comprising its physical area, type of attendance expected, activities to be held, human and material resources, management, supervision and work appraisal. Five modalities of service were recognized: police assistance, judicial assistance, health assistance, specialized psychosocial assistance and basic guidance. Eight hundred booklets were distributed to public and private health services, NGOs and Women's Police Stations. After a year, we shall evaluate the effective use of this material.

It was observed that, at present, the police modality is the gateway to this 'assistance network'. This fact gives rise to a lot of problems, because women's demands greatly surpass the possibilities of assistance that the police can offer, and the police are often embarrassed by the large number of women who are not willing to register or who want to withdraw the complaints against their partners. Incorporating social workers in Police Stations was a hard task, due to the aggressive and punishing character of the police in Brazil, often extremely violent in itself. It seems that health services could be an important alternative gateway, being more receptive and intervening in a less direct way. The whole effort put into making and distributing the guide, and into the training program, is directed towards diversifying the gateways and options of assistance presented to women subject to violence, integrating the different possibilities of assistance and making better use of each of them. We seek a wider range of options for handling the cases and directing them to the different professionals working in the health services.

The second investigation is related to the search in primary health-care settings for violent situations, how they emerge, their modalities, their acknowledgement or not and what kind of intervention occurred. For this purpose, we performed an exploratory study in order to understand not only *how many times* but mainly *how* violence presents itself in the actions of PAISM (Integral Attention to Women's Health Program)* in primary care services.

The partial results of this ongoing research are presented here. The investigation is intended to study: (1) the form in which domestic and sexual violence is presented by female health-service users, and perceived as a health issue; (2) the spontaneous emergence (without active search) of reports on violent situations from assistance activities and records in a basic health unit; and (3) the ways in which these issues are treated in terms of communicability, reception and dialog by the professionals. The research uses three complementary data collection techniques: observation of the PAISM assistance activities, records and interviews of the 'life history' type with key informants at the women's homes.

We shall present here the results related to the first of the data collection techniques being used in this study. We gave preference to educational/assistance group activities, that are also a PAISM priority, as a forum for the discussion of issues connected with gender relationships. They are: family planning activities, receiving Papanicolaou results and education in women's health.

All activities were observed and taped, and the gestures, expressions, emphasis and other factors of importance observed by the researcher were reported in writing. Tapes were transcribed and annexed to the observation report, resulting in a final report in conjunction with observations from the researcher. Between March and August 1995, 16 groups were observed, comprising a total of 115 women. The majority of the groups (11) were conducted by assistant nurses, and the five groups dealing with

women's health had a physician and a psychologist (both women) as co-ordinators. The ages of the women observed ranged from 14 to 53 years, distributed mainly within the 14–30 band (69.1%). As for their marital status, 72.9% lived with their partners. The great majority of them had only 4 years of formal schooling, worked as domestic servants, cleaning women or housewives and lived in slums.

The first great difficulty in analyzing the material was defining violence, because when we adopted the gender-relationship reference for this analysis, we observed that gender and violence issues are often converging and treated as having the same conceptual definition. We have included here, however, only those reports that included deliberately inflicted physical or sexual damage (or perceived as such by the subject).

Results

Since there was no screening or active search, we were surprised by spontaneous reports arising in seven of the groups studied. The data collected were grouped by themes related to reproductive health (body, STD/AIDS, reproduction, sexuality) and analyzed from two different standpoints: relationships between women and men, and the relationship between women and the health services.

From the first standpoint, the situations of violence observed were mainly related to non-consensual sexual intercourse reports (three groups). There was also a report of domestic violence that did not emerge in connection with sexuality but rather with vague symptoms of dizziness and discomfort (one group). As to the relationship with the health services, situations of violence were raised in connection with hospital services, especially during childbirth (three groups).

As for sexuality, in almost every group there were accounts of hardships which were related

*PAISM is a 13-year-old federal health program, its main feature being that it was planned and implemented with the participation of women's movements. It was established having epidemiological references and with emphasis on primary care and educational activities.

to men. Among the most discussed issues were the trouble the women had convincing their men to use condoms, to treat their STDs and to assume responsibilities related to fatherhood. Another recurring theme was related to the fact that men are adamant in deciding themselves when and where to have sexual intercourse.

In one of the groups in which violence was found, an attempted rape which had taken place in childhood was reported. The account was roused by a discussion on the causes of lack of sexual pleasure among women. Two other women in the same group reported physical and sexual abuse from their husbands, maybe stimulated by this account. It is interesting to note that when something was reported to the group other similar reports arose, which suggests that the problem was underestimated but emerged when a suitable forum was provided for dialog and reception.

In another group, a woman began by complaining about the trouble she had trying to make her husband treat a STD, told about the interference of the health service and ended by reporting a sexual violence episode:

Conceição: '. . . The doctor said that my husband and I had to take the medicine, but my husband wouldn't take it. He'd say: "You're the one who's sick . . ."'

Conceição: 'I took him there to see the doctor, at the hospital, the doctor talked to him, but he kept on saying that I was the one who was sick . . .'

Conceição: (Another time) 'The lady doctor had to write a letter to my husband. The doctor said I had to put a cream there, that I couldn't have intercourse and he wouldn't believe me. So the doctor had to write him a letter.'

Health Service (HS): 'And if he wants to have intercourse and you don't, then what happens?'

Conceição: 'We quarrel . . .' (laughter).

Later, while the group is discussing the reasons for these attitudes that men show, someone says that it is because they are stronger and the following dialog takes place:

Conceição: '. . . When he beats you, beat him too, my mother used to say.'

HS: 'Your mother said that?'

Conceição: 'Yes . . . there was no dialog.'

HS: 'And he is stronger . . .'

Conceição: 'Yeah, of course.'

HS: 'And you never lodged a complaint?'

Conceição: 'No . . . It wasn't so that he would beat me . . . The two of us, right? Not of him beating me, right? But we used to stick together too. There was this one night when he spent the whole night trying and I didn't want to, I closed my legs like this and he kept on trying . . . my legs were all bruised by the morning . . . When he wants he won't let go.'

This woman has been suffering from a recurring gleet for 9 years and she is also being treated for infertility. The difficulty arising from this situation of violence for the intervention of the health center in connection with the STD becomes evident here, and sterility is probably a consequence of this difficulty. It is important, then, to acknowledge and approach the subject of violence in order to obtain success.

However, what surprised us most were reports regarding the health services. They were negative in their great majority. Complaints in connection with health services were mainly directed to mistreatment in childbirth assistance. In one of the family-planning groups, the subject arose, then the discussion was interrupted by the co-ordinator, and emerged again at the end as a topic for a lengthy discussion when the co-ordinator left the group by itself, to proceed with the necessary forwarding and prescriptions. Most women had a story to tell the others:

Maria: 'Me too. I don't want to [give birth] not even if I'm paid for it' (quite affirmative).

HS: 'Why, was it that traumatic?'

Maria: 'Many hours of pain . . . the more the pain . . . I had never felt so much pain in my life . . . At the hospital . . . they made it hurt down below, it wasn't up above, it was down below, the nurses: "Shut up, you enjoyed the f..., didn't you?" It can't be like this, right? I think that the person must be more . . .'

HS: 'What did you do when she said "You enjoyed the f..."?'

Maria: 'Ha, there you are lying there, you're submitted to it, right, we just keep still because they . . . It's no use in screaming. You're full of pain all over, what is there to answer? It is hurting already. They treat you like if it was nothing. I think that if they said a caring word, a loving word, but no . . . it would lessen. It is not our fault . . .'

In most cases, complaints of mistreatment referred to female nurses or physicians. It is curious that they should have been women. In this case, the discriminative institutional logic seemed to be stronger than gender alliances. The co-ordinator suggested reaction and confrontation as possibilities in these situations. When she left and the subject returned, another woman reported an episode in which she stressed her attempt to reverse, at least in part, an unfavorable situation by taking an active position and arguing heatedly:

Clara: 'Then the second one, the girl, she was born there. The doctor, he came to me and said: "You aren't going to . . . we are not going to take you in, I'm leaving right now." He even said to me: "You have an hour and a half at most to go to another hospital to have your baby born, otherwise your daughter is going to be born on the street."'

HS: 'How awful!'

Clara: '"Your child is going to be born on the street." Then it was enough, I got as hot as hell, started screaming at him. Anything, no hospital accepts transferral from other hospital.'

Maria: 'That's absurd!'

Clara: 'Then the doctor got tired of sending us away to another hospital. We stayed there and suffered as hell. And when I got there, kid, time was almost up and they still made me have that serum.'

Maria: 'Ouch! It's too much!'

Clara: 'It looked like it was going to kill me.'

In these institution–user relationships, there seems to be no real possibility of negotiation and dialog. In a city like São Paulo, only a small percentage of the population has access to private health services and a place in a hospital secured when the time for delivery comes. The rest go from hospital to hospital looking for a vacancy. Compelled to get assistance, women find in public hospitals a brutality that they think is best to endure quietly instead of screaming, resisting and fighting back, risking retaliation. As a patient wondered: 'And if I start complaining and he makes a bigger cut, on purpose, so as to get it infected?' However much truth is in this statement, the possibility of this woman cogitating this image is persuasive enough to demonstrate the status of the health institution–user relationship. This injustice felt by women includes criticisms of hospital routines that are widely non-recommended in the medical literature but are largely used in Brazil, such as routine episiotomy and quick delivery induction. It is interesting to recognize this dissatisfaction displayed by women because, although its basis is completely different from that of a scientific study, it can be combined with a variety of technical information for the use of the professionals concerned. Concrete experience is always very persuasive:

Vanda: 'The last one was born in the hospital . . . God have mercy on me! I think that if I had to give birth to another child the last place I'd go to would be a hospital.'

HS: 'What happened?'

Vanda: 'Ha, they cut then they came with that needle to apply' (she laughs). 'She comes with this anesthetic to apply and I says: "What?! You are not going to apply no injection there! I didn't tell you to cut me! I had children already, there was no need!" "Ha, then you'll be wide open and that's the way it's going to be." And I says: "I don't care! It's my [body], isn't it?" And I left' (laughs).

Vanda: 'So they put me in bed the way I was, all open up, they hadn't put one single stitch. Then the hemorrhage began. The doctor she came and she wanted to inject the anesthetic and I says: "No!" "So it shall be in cold blood!" and I says: "Okay" and they sewed me in cold blood but I didn't let them inject the anesthetic in me.'

Neusa: 'Anesthesia is better, it doesn't hurt, right?'

Dolores: 'Only the first little prick.'

162

E: ' You had yours in the hospital? How was it?'

It is not clear if this woman really knew that anesthesia would reduce the suture pain. But what calls our attention is the absurd lack of dialog with, and reception to, this woman who experienced irrational and inhuman hospital procedures for the first time, even though there was a possibility of a technical solution in this case and it could easily have been done.

We believe that these small excerpts taken from a vast amount of material are sufficient for the discussion we intend to bring about. In addition to detecting situations of violence, which is fundamental for successful action in reproductive health, health services must also acknowledge their own violence, especially in underdeveloped countries. Lack of access, or access to services lacking quality, may have serious consequences and represent real violence.

From the health-services standpoint, it is important to understand that even when solution of an individual case by an isolated professional is impossible, there is always the possibility of the team being able to solve the case. There is need for information, acknowledgement of sociopolitical rights, education, support and treatment of pathologies. A formal complaint against bad professionals is also a way of guaranteeing the prestige of the rest of them, who are actively engaged in making things better for the population from the health point of view. We do not intend to reinforce defensive medicine, where each action is preceded by calculation of possible judicial disputes, but we cannot defend the underdeveloped authoritarian services where users have no rights either.

To make all this possible, it is necessary that we endeavor to give heed to the problem, being receptive to it as health professionals. That is why we must improve the dialog, searching for the problem when it is not evident and being really interested in the life histories, which are sometimes extremely painful, of our patients. Only a service open to real communication with the users will be able to hear (and provoke a response from) a problem of such importance for health work that is still greatly under-reported, in order to increase the assistance response of the service directed towards its prevention and solution.

References

1. Souza, E. R. and Minayo, M. C. S. (1995). O impacto da violência social na saúde pública do Brasil: década de 80. In Minayo, M. C. S. (ed.) *Os Muitos Brasis. Saúde e População na Década de 80*, pp. 87–106. (Rio de Janeiro: Hucitec-Abrasco)
2. Vianna, L. A. C. (1990). Características da mortalidade das mulheres (10 anos e mais) residentes em Diadema/São Paulo. Doctorate thesis, Faculdade de Saúde Pública, University of São Paulo
3. Brazilian Institute of Geography and Statistics Foundation (1990). *Participação Político-Social – Justiça e Vitimização*, Vol.1. (Rio de Janerio: FIBGE)
4. Stark, E. and Flitcraft, A. (1991). Spouse abuse. In Rosemberg, M. L. and Fenley, M. A. (eds.) *Violence in America – a Public Health Approach*, pp.123–57. (New York: Oxford University Press)
5. Heise, L. (1994). Gender-based abuse: the global epidemic. In *Cadernos de Saúde Pública*, **10**(suppl. 1), 135–45
6. McCauley, J., Kern, D. E., Kolodner, K., Dill, L., Schroeder, A. F., Dechant, H. K., Ryden, J., Bass, E. B. and Derogatis, L. R. (1995). The 'battering syndrome': prevalence and clinical characteristics of domestic violence in primary care internal medicine practices. *Ann. Intern. Med.*, **123**(10), 737–48
7. McFarlane, J., Parker, B., Soeken, K. and Bullok, L. (1992). Assessing for abuse during pregnancy. J. Am. Med. Assoc., **23**(267), 3176–8
8. Stark, E., Flitcraft, A. and Frazier, W. (1983). Medicine and patriarchal violence: the social construction of a 'private' event. In Fee, E. (ed.) *Women and Health: the Politic of Sex in Medicine*, pp. 177–209. (New York: BayWood Publishing Co.)
9. Canguilhem, G. (1992). *O Normal e o Patológico*, 2nd edn. (Rio de Janeiro: Forense Universitária)
10. Foucault, M. (1980). *O Nascimento da Clínica*, 2nd edn. (Rio de Janeiro: Fornese Universitária)

Violence against women: WHO's response

C. Garcia-Moreno

Following nearly two decades of women's activism and work on violence against women, this issue has finally been recognized in the international arena as a major concern for women's human rights. It is only more recently that there has been a growing awareness of the impact of violence on women's mental, physical and reproductive health and of the contributions that public health can make to addressing violence. With this in mind, the World Health Organization (WHO) has begun an initiative to help define the role of the health sector in prevention efforts and in the management of the health consequences of violence against women.

At the previous FIGO Congress in Montreal, the WHO/FIGO Task Force organized a Pre-Congress Workshop on the elimination of female genital mutilation and the FIGO General Assembly adopted a resolution on this topic. At the 1997 Congress, the WHO/FIGO Workshop was on 'The Elimination of Violence Against Women: in Search of Solutions'. Presenters from several parts of the world talked about their experiences in helping to address this problem, and particularly about the role that obstetrician/gynecologists and other health-care providers can play in this.

For WHO, this was an important event, as underlying the work on violence against women is the building of partnerships. The WHO is working to raise awareness of this issue among health providers and professional associations and to build partnerships for action. Worldwide, obstetrican/gynecologists are uniquely well placed to assist women suffering from abuse and to reduce the long-term disability and damage caused by such violence. However, practitioners should not feel that they have to rectify everything by themselves. First are needed partnerships between health providers (doctors, midwives, nurses and primary health-care workers). Second, we need to recognize that violence against women is a complex and multifactorial problem and that the health sector alone will not resolve it. So, obstetrician/gynecologists also need to build partnerships with other sectors: the legal and judicial systems, the social and other community services and, finally, with the women's organizations working on this issue. In many countries, such organizations have been at the forefront of providing support and other services for women. We must learn from their years of experience. Health practitioners do not need to fix everything, but can listen, provide support and help find solutions, working with other colleagues in the health and in other sectors.

There is one particular interphase of sectors which is particularly relevant to medical practitioners. In many cases, the judiciary service cannot act without medical evidence, yet doctors are usually not trained to collect this evidence. In some countries, they can act as gatekeepers to the legal system rather than as facilitators.

Qualitative research undertaken in 16 Latin American countries by WHO Regional Office for the Americas/Pan American Sanitary Bureau found endless stories of women who tried and tried to gain access into the legal system, but gave up, because of the many barriers they faced. One of these barriers was the reluctance of doctors to submit reports. Other studies have shown that this evidence may be taken in an insensitive manner that blames women and, at worst, revictimizes them. On this issue, the resolution recently adopted by the FIGO General Assembly recommends that obstetricians and gynecologists assist in the legal prosecution of cases of sexual abuse and rape by careful and sensitive documentation of the evidence.

Violence against women is present in all societies, often accepted as part of the order of things. Because much of it is hidden inside the home, it is extremely difficult to document and even harder to prevent.

One of the tasks of WHO is to increase the available knowledge about the magnitude of the problem and its health consequences among health providers, policy makers and program planners.

Existing data are still scattered and anecdotal, and mostly from developed countries. Furthermore, there is no universally accepted definition of violence. All societies have forms of violence that are socially prescribed and others that are tolerated or at times encouraged by social customs and norms. Whether socially condoned or not, these acts as well as their effects on women's health need to be recorded. Yet we know that there is huge underreporting and that recording is often incomplete and inconsistent.

This is important because reporting standards influence work on many levels. Individual women are more likely to receive appropriate care and services if health-care providers accurately identify them and record information in a systematic manner. At community and national levels, data support changes to health-care, legal and social-services systems. At international level, adequate data are needed to strengthen advocacy. This is not just about measuring things, but about naming them and making them visible.

In the same research from Latin America above-mentioned, many of the women interviewed had never told the health sector of their situation when they went to seek treatment. They reported going for broken bones, sexually transmitted diseases, insomnia, depression and anxiety, but they were never directly asked about violence and they never volunteered the infor-

mation. Those health workers who did suspect what was going on, in some cases, would prescribe tranquilizers without delving further into the situation; a few others did, in fact, encourage the women to seek help and gave guidance on where to find it. In several countries, women reported being referred to the psychiatrist or psychologist, which contributed to their fears of being abnormal or crazy.

Most women come into contact with the health service at least once in their lifetime, either when they seek contraception or pregnancy care, or give birth. Thus, if they are experiencing abuse, this is an opportunity for identification and care or referral. Moreover, some data seem to suggest that pregnancy is a particularly vulnerable time for abuse, although further research into this is needed.

WHO's response to violence against women

The World Health Organization seeks to strengthen the capacity of the health sector at all levels to identify and respond appropriately to women who have been abused, mentally, physically and sexually.

First, WHO *will develop standards for the identification, adequate care and referral of women suffering from abuse* for different levels of the health service. Few health-care professionals are presently able to identify violence, even when injuries or symptoms are highly suggestive. Studies show that, with proper training and protocols, health-care providers can significantly improve their sensitivity to this problem.

Second, WHO is initiating a *multi-country study on the prevalence, health consequences and risk and protective factors for violence against women in families.* A major challenge is to design valid and reliable methodologies to generate data that are persuasive to policy makers and that serve as the basis for interventions. While the ultimate goal of the study is to generate new knowledge, WHO also seeks to strengthen local research capacity, to develop and test new instruments for measuring violence and its consequences, across cultures, and to promote research that meets the needs of women and that values the experience of women's groups working on the issue.

Third, WHO has set up a *database* to collect information from around the globe on prevalence and health consequences (of domestic violence, rape and sexual assault). This includes hard-to-access unpublished data. More than 700 items have been compiled, to date, from all regions. This will allow WHO in future to monitor trends in the same way as for maternal mortality, unsafe abortion and other such issues.

Fourth, WHO is producing *tools to help health providers, policy makers and others* fully *recognize the extent of violence* against women *and its implications* for health policies and programs. One of these is this an information package on *Violence Against Women*.

Fifth, WHO is supporting the *systematic evaluation and documentation of existing interventions in the health sector* and the development and testing of new ones. For example, with proper training and protocols, health-care workers detect significantly more cases of battering and domestic violence. These kinds of protocols need to be evaluated and, if reliable, disseminated. In general, we need to look at how effective interventions are, and how appropriate and sustainable they are in resource-poor settings. We must beware of taking interventions that have worked in certain settings, particularly in the North, and transposing them to the South. We need to see what works in a particular setting. For example, what a health provider can do where facilities for referral exist is different to what he or she can do in places where no support services for

women exist, and what can be done in an accident and emergency department is different to what is appropriate for a rural health center.

Obstetricians and gynecologists have a unique opportunity as they interact with women who are already victims of violence and with those who may be at risk of violence. We need to make use of this opportunity, but with caution: one of the issues that was underlined in the 1997 Pre-Congress Workshop is that, at times, the health sector, including obstetrician/gynecologists, may further, unwittingly, victimize women. We need to be aware of this and to ensure that, with all good intentions, any interventions do not further victimize women or put them at risk, that we do not turn women into the problem, or 'a case', depersonifying them and moving the focus away from the real problem, which is violence by men. Rather, health providers need to create a supportive environment and communicate with all patients in a way that makes them feel confident that they can bring their problems to us. We need to listen and remember that the only experts on violence against women are women themselves, those who survive it.

In the 1997 WHO/FIGO Pre-Congress Workshop, it was agreed that an appropriate response is long overdue, that there is something which can and should be done. As the FIGO resolution recommends: health-care providers should educate themselves more with regard to this problem and increase their skills in order to best respond to the needs of the women they care for.

Efficacy of emergency contraception 24

C. Ellertson

Introduction

Efficacy is one of the most important characteristics of any medication. Without an idea of how well a method is likely to work, women and their health-care providers cannot balance trade-offs with side-effects, compare the regimen to other options, or prepare themselves adequately for contingencies. Moreover, without estimates of efficacy, drug regulatory agencies are unlikely to approve a new drug, or a new indication for an existing drug. For this reason, it is important to calculate the best possible efficacy estimates of emergency contraceptives.

The simplest measure of how well an emergency contraceptive works is the failure rate. In this measure, the number of observed pregnancies is divided by the number of women treated. The quotient tells health-care providers roughly what proportion of their patients, who present for treatment at a mixture of cycle days, will likely become pregnant despite treatment with emergency contraception.

One analytical problem with using the failure rate as the sole measure of how well a method works is that the failure rate depends heavily on the mixture of days in the cycle that women in a study have had unprotected intercourse and have sought treatment. Women who present for treatment are not evenly distributed throughout their cycles. Indeed, they may be most likely to present following unprotected intercourse that occurred at times such as during mid-cycle intercourse, when the probability of pregnancy is highest. For this reason, it is difficult to compare failure rates strictly across different studies and methods when little information is available about the cycle days on which women had unprotected intercourse.

A more rigorous metric is method efficacy, or the proportionate reduction in pregnancy. In the case of emergency contraception, however, efficacy is difficult to measure. Measures of contraceptive efficacy compare the pregnancy rate among women who use the method to an expected pregnancy rate among similar (sometimes hypothetical) women who did not use the method. Not all women who take emergency contraception would have become pregnant if the therapy were not available to them.

A major determinant of a fecund woman's chances of becoming pregnant following an act of unprotected intercourse is the cycle day on which the intercourse occurred[1]. Without sophisticated technology, however, few women can accurately pinpoint the exact day on which ovulation occurs in a given month and report it to researchers conducting clinical trials of the various methods. For this reason, the number of expected pregnancies that researchers calculate would have occurred without emergency contraception is subject to error. Without an accurate yardstick against which to compare the observed number of pregnancies, the estimates of efficacy that are derived from a clinical trial will also be inaccurate.

Estimates of the number of expected pregnancies in most published research are calculated from the Dixon estimates[2], shown in Table 1. To calculate the expected number of pregnancies, researchers multiply the number of women apparently having had unprotected intercourse on each cycle day by the probability of conception on that day. They can then sum these results to calculate the number of pregnancies that might have been expected in the absence of treatment with emergency

Table 1 Probability of conception in absence of contraception, by cycle day of coitus. Adapted from reference 2

Coital day	Risk of conception
−8	0.001
−7	0.007
−6	0.025
−5	0.055
−4	0.104
−3	0.146
−2	0.169
−1	0.173
0	0.141
1	0.091
2	0.049
3	0.019
4	0.005
5	0.001

contraception. This expected number can be compared with the observed number in order to derive an estimate of efficacy. Estimates based on the Dixon table, however, should be regarded as lower bounds. The figures are based in part on probabilities derived from artificial insemination using frozen sperm, and in part on data from couples who may have been selected for lower then average fecundity[3,4].

Efficacy of main regimens available in clinical practice

Three methods of emergency contraception are widely available in at least some countries. These are: the Yuzpe regimen of combined estrogen and progestin, the levonorgestrel-only regimen, and the postcoital copper intrauterine device (IUD) insertion. Efficacy information on these regimens has been published in some detail elsewhere[3,5,6], but will also be reviewed here.

Yuzpe regimen

The Yuzpe regimen is the best-studied method of oral postcoital contraception[7-16]. This regimen consists of 200 µg of ethinylestradiol and 1.0 mg of levonorgestrel. Women begin treatment within 72 h after unprotected intercourse and take half the treatment (100 µg

ethinylestradiol and 0.5 mg levonorgestrel) immediately. They take the other half (100 µg ethinylestradiol and 0.5 mg levonorgestrel) 12 h later.

Based on the 10 available studies that contain information on cycle day of intercourse[7-16], it is possible to calculate a proportionate reduction in the likelihood of pregnancy associated with the use of the Yuzpe regimen. By comparing observed to expected pregnancies, investigators have demonstrated that the Yuzpe regimen reduces the chances of pregnancy by about 75%[3,4,6]. The failure rate is about 2%, and ranges from about 1 to 3%[17].

Levonorgestrel

The levonorgestrel emergency contraceptive regimen consists of 0.75 mg levonorgestrel taken twice at 12 h apart and started within 48 h of unprotected intercourse. Although progestins were among the first drugs used in postcoital contraception, few published studies have analyzed the emergency levonorgestrel regimen in a way that controls for cycle day of unprotected intercourse.

The best and most recent of the levonorgestrel emergency contraceptive trials was conducted in Hong Kong[14] and indicates a failure rate of 2.4% and a proportionate reduction in pregnancy of 60%. The study randomized women reporting for treatment within 48 h of unprotected intercourse to either a Yuzpe or a levonorgestrel arm. During the trial, 410 women used the levonorgestrel method. Investigators did not detect a statistically significant difference between the levonorgestrel and Yuzpe method. This study is being replicated in a multinational trial sponsored by the World Health Organization (WHO)[18].

Copper intrauterine device

The copper IUD offers the highest efficacy of any known emergency contraceptive. A meta-analysis of 19 studies of postcoital IUDs[6] reveals that the copper IUD inserted postcoitally has a failure rate of approximately 0.1%. While IUDs are typically far more expensive than the hormonal methods, the IUD can provide up to 10 years of contraceptive protection if the woman chooses to leave the device in place following emergency insertion.

New developments in efficacy research

As noted earlier, estimates of the number of expected pregnancies calculated from the Dixon table are not unbiased. For this reason, the number of pregnancies that a researcher might expect to see among women in a trial in the absence of emergency contraception would be too low, and the estimated efficacy of an emergency contraceptive assessed against this metric would be too low.

A recent study[1] of conception probabilities by cycle day of intercourse promises to shed new light on efficacy research in emergency contraception. In this study, 221 couples in the United States were recruited at the time they stopped using their regular methods of contraception in order to conceive. Couples were followed until they conceived, or for up to 6 months. Daily urine samples and coital logs were used to assess the risk of pregnancy on each day of the cycle. Conception rates were estimated as 8, 17, 8, 36, 34 and 36% on cycle days −5, −4, −3, −2, −1 and 0 respectively, where 0 indicates the day of ovulation. Interestingly, the study found no conceptions occurring after the day of ovulation. The study also found that approximately 25% of the pregnancies that could be chemically detected were lost before they could be clinically confirmed. For this reason, the study included many pregnancies that would have been missed in other studies relying on clinical confirmation only. Finally, the study also measured ovulation in a way that differs slightly from other published research. The implication of these points is that the efficacy of the emergency contraceptives discussed above is incorrect and may be too high. Further analysis, however, will be available in a few months' time along with revised estimates of the cycle day of conception suitable to replace those based on the Dixon method.

Conclusions

Several methods of emergency contraception are sufficiently effective to justify their widespread use in clinical practice. The copper IUD is the most efficacious method, followed by the Yuzpe and levonorgestrel-only regimens.

Further research is currently under way to gather additional information about the efficacy of the Yuzpe regimen and the levonorgestrel-only regimens. Additional research will refine understanding of the manner in which efficacy is measured.

It should be noted, however, that because of the special circumstances of emergency contraception and lack of other options, even efficacy rates that are as low as 50% (or lower) might be acceptable to women. Women, in consultation with their health-care providers, should be allowed to make that determination for themselves.

Acknowledgements

I am grateful to Paul Van Look and James Trussell for valuable comments on an earlier draft, and to the Alan Guttmacher Institute for allowing me to draw upon material from a manuscript published in *International Family Planning Perspectives*[5].

References

1. Wilcox, A. J., Weinberg, C. R. and Baird, D. D. (1995). Timing of sexual intercourse in relation to ovulation: effects on the probability of conception, survival of the pregnancy, and sex of the baby. *N. Engl. J. Med.*, **333**, 1517–21

2. Dixon, G. W., Schlesselman, J. J., Ory, H. W. and Blye, R. P. (1980). Ethinyl estradiol and conjugated estrogens as postcoital contraceptives. *J. Am. Med. Assoc.*, **244**, 1336–9

3. Trussell, J., Ellertson, C. and Stewart, F. (1996). The effectiveness of the Yuzpe regimen of emergency contraception. *Fam. Plann. Perspect.*, **28**, 59–64, 87

4. Trussell, J. and Stewart, F. (1992). The effectiveness of postcoital hormonal contraception. *Fam. Plann. Perspect.*, **24**, 262–4

5. Ellertson, C. (1996). History and efficacy of emergency contraception: beyond Coca-Cola. *Int. Fam. Plann. Perspect.*, **22**, 52–6

6. Trussell, J. and Ellertson, C. (1995). Efficacy of the copper IUD and of the Yuzpe regimen of post-coital contraception. *Fertil. Control Rev.*, **4**, 8–11

7. Yuzpe, A. A. and Lancee, W. J. (1977). Ethinyl-lestradiol and dI-norgestrel as a postcoital contraceptive. *Fertil. Steril.*, **28**, 932–6

8. Yuzpe, A. A., Percival-Smith, R. and Rademaker, A. W. (1982). A multicenter clinical investigation employing ethinyl estradiol combined with dI-norgestrel as a postcoital contraceptive agent. *Fertil. Steril.*, **37**, 508–13

9. Glasier, A., Thong, K. J., Dewar, M., Mackie, M. and Baird, D. T. (1992). Mifepristone (RU486) compared with high-dose estrogen and progestogen for emergency postcoital contraception. *N. Engl. J. Med.*, **327**, 1041–4

10. Bagshaw, S. N., Edwards, D. and Tucker, A. K. (1988). Ethinyl oestradiol and d-norgestrel is an effective emergency post-coital contraceptive: a report of its use in 1 200 patients in a family planning clinic. *Aust. NZ J. Obstet. Gynaecol.*, **28** 137–40

11. Van Santen, M. R. and Haspels, A. A. (1985). Interception II: postcoital low-dose estrogens and norgestrel combination in 633 women. *Contraception*, **31**, 275–93

12. Percival-Smith, R. K. L. and Abercrombie, B. (1987). Postcoital contraception with dl-norgestrel/ethinyl estradiol combination: six years experience in a student medical clinic. *Contraception*, **36**, 287–93

13. Zuliani, G., Colombo, U. F. and Molla, R. (1990). Hormonal postcoital contraception with an ethinylestradiol–norgestrel combination and two danazol regimens. *Eur. J. Obstet. Gynecol. Reprod. Biol.*, **37**, 253–60

14. Ho, P. C. and Kwan, M. S. W. (1993). A prospective randomized comparison of levonorgestrel with the Yuzpe regimen in post-coital contraception. *Hum. Reprod.*, **8**, 389–92

15. Webb, A. M. C., Russell, J. and Elstein, M. (1992). Comparison of Yuzpe regimen, danazol, and mifepristone (RU486) in oral postcoital contraception. *Br. Med. J.*, **305**, 927–31

16. Tully, B. (1983). Post coital contraception – a study. *Br. J. Fam. Plann.*, **8**, 119–24

17. Van Look, P. F. A. and von Hertzen, H. (1993). Emergency contraception. *Br. Med. Bull.*, **49** 158–70

18. von Hertzen, H. and Van Look, P. F. A. (1996). Research on new methods of emergency contraception. *Int. Fam. Plann. Perspect.*, **22**, 62–8

Emergency contraception: the users and the services   25

A. Glasier

Introduction

Emergency contraception is for use by women who are at risk of pregnancy usually as a result of either unprotected intercourse or the failure of a barrier method, e.g. burst condom. While condom failures are not always recognized, in a recent study of condom breakage and slippage[1], between 4 and 7% of couples in the USA experienced a recognized condom failure over a study period of up to 3 months. In all such cases, emergency contraception might prevent pregnancy.

It is not usually appropriate to prescribe emergency contraception for missed oral contraceptive pills since effective rules involving secondary use of a barrier method make physiological sense and are easy to follow.

The users

In the UK, women seeking emergency method contraception are often young and nulliparous[2]. The characteristics of users in other countries have not been described.

Knowledge among providers and potential users

Emergency contraception is not universally available. In countries where a marketed product has existed for some considerable time, such as the UK and The Netherlands, most doctors and nurses (the usual providers) and probably the majority of potential users know of the existence of emergency contraception. Even in these countries, knowledge of the practical details (among both providers and users) is often surprisingly poor. A survey[3] of mainly 14- and 15-year-old schoolchildren undertaken in Scotland in 1996 demonstrated that, while over 90% of the teenagers had heard of emergency contraception, less than one-half of them knew the correct time limits. In a random sample of 2000 women aged between 18 and 47 years and living in the north of Scotland[4], only 39% of women knew the correct timing for emergency contraception use. Among professionals, a small survey of general practitioners (family doctors) in London (A. Graham, unpublished data) revealed gaps in their knowledge and prejudices about how often it was safe to use the combined estrogen–progestogen regimen (Yuzpe, Tetragynon®) of emergency contraception. In countries where no marketed products exist (such as the USA) or where licensing of emergency contraception has only recently been discussed (such as South Africa), ignorance abounds among both the public and professionals. In such countries, service providers are often reluctant[5] to provide emergency contraception because they confuse the method with abortion. As all marketed hormonal emergency contraceptives must be taken within 72 h of intercourse, they cannot possibly induce abortion since implantation will not have taken place within this period of time and pregnancy is not therefore established. A survey of university students[6] undertaken in the USA showed that potential users may also confuse emergency contraception with abortion. Interestingly, in this survey, 32% of students had 'ethical concerns' about emergency contraception.

Myths and misunderstandings about the safety of emergency contraception are also common. Fifty-seven per cent of US university students[6] were concerned about the health risks of emergency contraceptive pills. Scottish teenagers not uncommonly believe that repeated use can cause infertility. In their as yet unpublished survey of general practitioners, Graham and colleagues reported that 4% of doctors thought of the Yuzpe regimen as a 'harmful drug' while a further 10% appeared to have reservations about safety aspects. These concerns about safety together with a not uncommon tendency to moralizing about emergency contraceptive use leads to frequent refusals to prescribe hormonal emergency contraception more than once, certainly in the same cycle and quite often in the same year. Misconceptions among providers only add to those of potential users, so that it is not only lack of knowledge of the method among the general public which limits the use of emergency contraception.

It is interesting to note that almost one-half of the women surveyed in the north of Scotland[4] thought that emergency contraception should not be made available over the counter. The most common reason for disapproval was the fear that emergency contraception would become too easy to use or would be used inappropriately. Almost 20% of respondents felt that the move would encourage casual or unsafe sex. Moralizing on the issue is not only limited to providers!

Provision of services

In the UK, as in many other countries, emergency contraception must be prescribed by a doctor. For this reason it is only widely and reliably available from general practitioners and community family planning clinics. Recently, attempts have been made to improve provision, and many genitourinary medicine clinics now provide emergency contraception. It is still not available from all hospital accident and emergency departments, but in many hospitals arrangements for provision through gynecological wards are in place. In reality, hormonal emergency contraception is not available 24 h per day in most places, but then it does not need to be because potential users have 72 h to act. In the USA a National Emergency Contraception Hotline was set up in February 1996 which gives toll-free information about emergency contraception and where it can be obtained locally.

The recently established Consortium for Emergency Contraception, which is committed to making emergency contraception a standard part of reproductive health-care world-wide, has produced a resource packet for health-care providers and program managers which gives advice about possible service delivery systems. For widespread use of emergency contraception to be possible, supplies must be available from a source which is accessible in terms of geography and time of day and in a manner which is regarded by potential users as approachable. Precise service arrangements will depend on whether or not emergency contraception has to be prescribed by doctors and on the manner in which contraceptive services are usually provided.

There has recently been widespread discussion about making hormonal emergency contraception available over the counter. The marketed product equivalent to the Yuzpe regimen (PC4) has been licensed in the UK since 1984 and prescribed to well over 4 million women. Recognizing its potential role in preventing unwanted pregnancy, the Royal College of Obstetricians and Gynaecologists, Royal College of General Practitioners and Royal Pharmaceutical Society all approved the over-the-counter availability in 1995, but the manufacturers are reluctant to seek the appropriate change in the product license. This is perhaps not surprising in view of an increasing tendency of the public in the UK to sue pharmaceutical companies. In New Zealand too, despite requests from the government[7], PC4 has not been made available over the counter. Very recently, the decision of the South African government not only to license PC4 but to license it off prescription may well delay the introduction of the drug.

Conclusion

In summary, anyone who has had unprotected intercourse or an accident with a barrier method, and yet who wishes to avoid pregnancy, is eligible to use emergency contraception. Widespread use is limited by lack of knowledge and misinformation among both potential users and providers. Widespread use is only possible if methods of emergency contraception are available and genuinely accessible from an approachable source of provision.

References

1. Steiner, M., Piedrahita, C., Joanis, C., Glover, L. and Spruyt, A. (1994). Condom breakage and slippage rates among study participants in eight countries. *Int. Fam. Plann. Perspect.*, **20**, 55–8
2. Glasier, A., Thong, K. J., Dewar, M., Mackie, M. and Baird, D. T. (1992). Randomised trial of mifepristone (RU486) and high dose estrogen–progestogen as an emergency contraceptive. *N. Engl. J. Med.*, **327**, 1041–4
3. Graham, A., Green, L. and Glasier, A. (1996). Teenagers' knowledge of emergency contraception: questionnaire survey in south east Scotland. *Br. Med. J.*, **312**, 1567–9
4. Smith, B. H., Gurney, E. M., Aboulela, L. and Templeton, A. (1996). Emergency contraception: a survey of women's knowledge and attitudes. *Br. J. Obstet. Gynaecol.*, **103**, 1109–16
5. Ramsay, S. (1995). What is the problem with emergency contraception? *Lancet*, **345**, 1169
6. Harper, C. C. and Ellertson, C. E. (1995). The emergency contraceptive pill: a survey of knowledge and attitudes among students at Princeton University. *Am. J. Obstet. Gynecol.*, **173**, 1438–45
7. Williams, C. (1996). New Zealand doctors resist emergency contraception. *Br. Med. J.*, **312**, 463

Emergency contraception: a brighter future? 26

P. F. A. Van Look

Introduction

For centuries women have adopted measures, or used devices or preparations, in their attempts to prevent pregnancy after intercourse has taken place. Violent physical exercise to try dislodging the ejaculated semen from the genital tract; potions, seeds or herbs taken orally or placed in the vagina; and postcoital douching are all known to have been used, some of them as long ago as 1500 BC[1].

The origin of today's hormonal methods of emergency contraception can be traced back to the mid-1920s when it was demonstrated for the first time that ovarian extracts with estrogenic activity had an antifertility effect in several species of lower mammals. This finding led to the veterinary use of estrogen for pregnancy prevention, but it was only in the 1960s that the first human trials of postcoitally administered high-dose estrogen were undertaken[2,3]. The combined estrogen–progestogen regimen, often referred to as the Yuzpe regimen after its inventor, the Canadian gynecologist Albert Yuzpe, was introduced in the early 1970s[4,5] and has now largely replaced the high-dose estrogen approach, while postcoital insertion of an intrauterine device (IUD) for emergency contraception was first reported in 1976[6].

There is no doubt that greater use of emergency contraception could prevent a substantial proportion of the tens of millions of unplanned pregnancies which occur every year. Meta-analysis of trials conducted on the effectiveness of the Yuzpe regimen indicates that this method prevents, on average, about three-quarters of the unplanned pregnancies that would occur if no treatment is given[7]. In the case of postcoital insertion of an IUD, effectiveness is even greater, in the order of 99% or more[8].

In spite of its proven efficacy and the fact that it employs contraceptive technologies that have been available for more than 30 years, emergency contraception has remained very much in the shadows of reproductive health-care, its use in most countries restricted to rape victims and university health centers. This paper reviews some of the major barriers that exist in countries around the world to full utilization of this important method of contraception. Subsequently, some encouraging developments that have taken place during the past 2 years will be discussed, giving hope that emergency contraception may be poised to emerge from the relative obscurity it has suffered over the past 30 years. In the preparation of this review, use has been made of several of the present author's recent reviews on the topic of emergency contraception to which the reader is referred for additional detail[9–11].

World-wide barriers to use of emergency contraception

In virtually every country, major barriers still exist to widespread use of emergency contraception. Reasons underlying this unfortunate state of affairs can be grouped into four main categories.

Product-related reasons

All methods currently available for emergency use have limitations. That they can only be administered within a few days after intercourse (3 days for hormonal methods; 5 days for post-coital IUD insertion) restricts their usefulness and disqualifies for treatment women who cannot meet these deadlines. Moreover, the methods, and the hormonal regimens in particular, may cause unpleasant side-effects such as nausea, vomiting, headaches, dizziness and breast tenderness. These side-effects can limit compliance and, in the case of vomiting, may affect the methods' efficacy.

Emergency methods are generally not as effective as other contraceptive methods. As stated above, even when the Yuzpe regimen is administered within the recommended 72 h, it fails to prevent one-quarter of the pregnancies that would be expected without the therapy[7]. Also, although insertion of an IUD after unprotected intercourse is more effective[8] and can be initiated later than the hormonal regimens, its usefulness is limited because of the risk of infection, especially in victims of sexual assault or following intercourse with a new partner. Insertion of an IUD is also not usually recommended for nulliparous women, and such women constitute a sizable proportion of those requesting emergency contraception[12].

In addition to the drawbacks of the existing methods, their variety is very limited; a woman seeking emergency contraception has few choices at her disposal. Thus, there is a clear need for new and improved methods, particularly methods that can be easily administered

and would be appropriate for over-the-counter provision.

A second product-related reason that is affecting the wider use of emergency contraception is the absence, in most countries of the world, of a dedicated preparation specifically marketed for emergency-contraceptive use. Until September 1996 only one pharmaceutical company (Schering AG) had a proprietary preparation of the estrogen–progestogen combination (Yuzpe regimen) for emergency-contraceptive use and this product was registered in very few countries (UK, New Zealand, Germany, Switzerland, Norway, Finland, Sweden and South Africa). This preparation is relatively expensive and only four tablets are supplied. For these reasons, many doctors in these countries are making up their own supplies using packets of an appropriate oral contraceptive-pill preparation that contains the same hormones, i.e. ethinylestradiol and levonorgestrel (or *dl*-norgestrel) (Table 1). This is considerably cheaper and extra pills can be given should vomiting occur. In September 1996, the Hungarian pharmaceutical company, Gedeon Richter, acquired a license to market its Yuzpe-type preparation in Hungary. According to company sources applications for registration in other countries are planned.

In countries where a dedicated Yuzpe-type product is not available, use of tablets from an appropriate oral contraceptive-pill preparation is the only available option and this approach is

Table 1 Examples of formulations and dose required for Yuzpe regimen of emergency contraception

Formulation	Common brand name	Tablets per dose	Doses required	Timing of administration
EE 50 μg + LNG 250 μg	Duoluton, Eugynon 250, Monovar, Neogynon, Noral, Ovidon, Ovran, Stediril-d	2	2	First dose within 72 h of unprotected sex. Second dose 12 h later
EE 50 μg + NG 500 μg	Eugynon, Eugynon-50, Ovral, Primovlar, Stediril	2	2	
EE 30 μg + LNG 150 μg	Levlen, Microgynon, Nordette, Ovranet, Rigevidon	4	2	First dose within 72 h of unprotected sex. Second dose 12 h later
EE 30 μg + NG 300 μg	Lo-Femenal, Lo-Ovral	4	2	

EE, ethinylestradiol; LNG, levonorgestrel; NG, *dl*-norgestrel (or norgestrel) which contains half the amount of active ingredient as levonorgestrel

certainly followed in several countries. However, since the practice involves the use of oral contraceptive pills for a non-approved indication, practitioners are reluctant to employ pills for this purpose, thus hampering wider availability and use.

Client-related reasons

Knowledge of emergency contraception among women takes a long time to disseminate, even in countries where a dedicated product is on the market. For example, in the UK, where the Schering product has been registered since 1984, a survey of a general practice-based population 10 years later, in 1994, showed that 21% of 878 women aged 16–50 years had not heard of emergency contraception and only 14% knew the correct time limit for using it[13]. The main reason underlying this ignorance is, of course, the failure of family planning services and providers and of the education system to give information about emergency contraceptives to potential users, particularly those at risk of unprotected intercourse and unplanned pregnancy such as adolescents, women not using contraception, users of a barrier method and those requesting pregnancy termination.

The impact of well-designed and intensive information, education and communication campaigns cannot be underestimated. For instance, in the UK, significant efforts have been made in the past 2 years to make emergency contraception better known in an attempt to lower the rates of unplanned pregnancy and abortion among teenagers. These efforts appear to have paid off as illustrated by recent findings from Scotland[14,15]. Using a confidential questionnaire survey of fourth-year pupils, aged 14–16 years, in 20 secondary schools in and around Edinburgh, it was found that 93% of the pupils had heard of emergency contraception[14]. A total of 194 girls (33%) and 168 boys (28%) had experienced sexual intercourse, and nearly one-third (31%) of these 194 girls had used emergency contraception. Asked where they had learnt about emergency contraception, pupils gave school (437 pupils; 39%) and magazines

Table 2 Sources of knowledge about emergency contraception[14]

Source	Percentage of pupils* ($n = 1121$)
School	39.0
Magazines	37.9
Friend	22.6
Family member	17.6
Leaflet or poster	16.6
General practitioner, family-planning clinics, etc.	9.2
TV and radio	4.6
Cannot recall	21.6

*Since more than one source could be recorded, percentages add up to more than 100%

(425 pupils; 38%) as the most common sources (Table 2). Similarly, in a postal survey of a stratified random sample of 2000 Grampian women aged 18–47 years, 94% of respondents were aware of emergency contraception although far fewer (39%) knew the correct timing for its use[15]. These figures were generally higher among younger, single women. The popular media represented the most common source of information, whereas general practitioners and family-planning clinics were cited rarely.

Failure to use emergency contraception is not always a matter of ignorance, however. In a recent study, also from the UK, among 167 teenagers (aged 13–19 years) requesting pregnancy termination ($n = 95$; 57%) or having their first antenatal visit ($n = 72$; 43%), 135 girls (81%) had heard of emergency contraception but 119 did not obtain it. In just over two-thirds of these 119 teenagers, the girl was aware that she was at risk of pregnancy but 'took a chance' rather than obtain emergency contraception[16]. Clearly, counseling about the risk of unplanned pregnancy following unprotected intercourse must be given greater emphasis in sex education, family-planning counseling, etc.

Provider-related reasons

The role that service providers and other types of health-care personnel play in ensuring availability and use of emergency contraception cannot be underestimated, but few data have been reported in the literature on knowledge, attitudes and practices (KAP) of these professional groups in respect of this method of contraception. A recently published KAP study[17] from New South Wales, Australia, among rural and urban general practitioners (GPs) indicated that 5% of the rural GPs and 22% of the urban GPs did not know about emergency contraception. Among those who knew, 58% of urban GPs and 52% of rural GPs used the Yuzpe regimen. Two per cent said they did not know what to prescribe and the remainder prescribed a variety of regimens including triphasic pills, but did not state which strength tablet of the triphasic regimen was used, and administration ranged from one to six doses per day over a period ranging from 2 to 72 h. Less than one-third of GPs included information about emergency contraception in routine contraceptive counseling. In addition, the survey results suggested that some doctors never provided information or prescribed emergency contraception, probably because of moral or religious objections.

Service-related reasons

Data from a survey conducted by the International Planned Parenthood Federation among its affiliate members indicate that several family-planning programs do not provide emergency contraception because of the mistaken belief that its mode of action is an abortifacient one[18]. Where such misconception does not exist and emergency contraception is available, a number of service-related factors frequently hamper accessibility and wider use.

Hormonal emergency contraception must be started within 72 h of intercourse and, in the few countries where a dedicated product is licensed, it can only be prescribed by a doctor. The greatest need for emergency contraception is often at weekends, when clinics and doctors' offices are closed, and on Monday mornings, when they are at their busiest. Many people, particularly the young, often find it difficult to obtain emergency contraception from their

family doctor and not all hospital accident and emergency departments will supply it. For people living at a distance from a doctor or clinic where emergency contraception can be obtained, accessibility is an even greater problem. For these reasons, and in view of the potential of emergency contraception for reducing unwanted pregnancies, the possibility of making it available over the counter from pharmacists has been discussed in the UK, New Zealand and Norway. Another approach, taken in China, is to give barrier-method users emergency contraceptive pills prophylactically, for back-up use in case of mishap with the barrier method.

Overcoming the obstacles

During the past couple of years a number of significant events have taken place that bode well for a wider acceptance and use of emergency contraception. In this context, three developments in particular need to be mentioned: (1) the discovery of new hormonal methods of emergency contraception that are more effective and/or have less side-effects than the Yuzpe regimen; (2) increasing evidence suggesting that the Yuzpe regimen, and probably the levonorgestrel regimen also, act primarily through inhibition of ovulation rather than prevention of implantation; and (3) rising international interest in emergency contraception.

New hormonal methods

Progestogen-only pills A variety of progestogen-containing pills, the so-called 'visiting pills' or 'vacation pills', are being used in China as a method of contraception by couples who are living apart for most of the year and can have intercourse only intermittently, during brief visiting spells and vacation periods[19]. The efficacy of various progestogens given alone for post-coital contraception was also examined during the 1970s in several studies conducted mostly in South America[20]. Most of these trials examined the potential of progestogens for regular post-coital use, an application for which they were found unsuitable primarily because of the high incidence of cycle disturbances. If used infrequently, such as is the case in emergency contraception where treatment is generally limited to one occasion, such cycle disturbances are less of an issue and, in fact, tablets of 750 μg of levonorgestrel for 'occasional' contraceptive use are marketed in several countries under the trade name of Postinor®. The recommended regimen of this preparation is to take one tablet as soon as possible after intercourse. In the case of more than two successive acts of intercourse, a second tablet must be taken 8 h later. For any given cycle, the manufacturers (Gedeon Richter) recommend that the total dose should not exceed four tablets.

The effectiveness of these levonorgestrel tablets (one tablet followed 12 h later by a second tablet) for emergency contraception has recently been tested against the Yuzpe regimen in a randomized trial; both treatment regimens were initiated within 48 h after unprotected intercourse in this study. The results showed that the levonorgestrel regimen was as effective as the Yuzpe regimen but that it was associated with significantly less nausea and vomiting (Table 3)[12]. To further study this approach in comparison with the Yuzpe regimen, a large multinational trial has been organized by our Programme in which the time limit for treatment has been extended to 72 h. Results from this study are expected to be published in early 1998.

Antiprogestogens Antiprogestogens, such as mifepristone (RU 486), which neutralize the effects of progesterone by binding to its receptors, are capable of blocking ovulation and retarding endometrial development, depending on whether they are administered before or after ovulation[21]. In view of these actions, it seemed probable that mifepristone would be effective as an emergency contraceptive, and this assumption was confirmed to be correct in two randomized clinical trials supported by our Programme and conducted in the UK[22,23]. In the two studies combined there were no method-related pregnancies among the 597 women treated with mifepristone while nine pregnancies occurred in the group of 589 women who received the Yuzpe regimen. In addition, the women in the mifepristone group reported less nausea and vomiting as well as fewer other side-effects than the women treated with the Yuzpe regimen. However, women given mifepristone were more likely to have a delayed onset of menstruation (42% vs. 13% in the Yuzpe group), presumably because the inhibitory effect of the antiprogestogen, when given in the preovulatory phase, on follicular development and ovulation causes lengthening of the cycle.

The dose of mifepristone used in these two studies was a single dose of 600 mg which is also the dose recommended when the antiprogestogen is used together with prostaglandin for inducing abortion[21]. Data from a recently completed multinational trial co-ordinated by our Programme indicate, however, that a low, 10-mg dose of mifepristone is as effective as 600 mg, although neither of these two doses was 100% efficacious as was the case in the earlier two, single-center studies (Table 4). Research is currently under way in which low doses of the antiprogestogen with the Yuzpe regimen and levonorgestrel are being compared in

Table 3 Incidence of side-effects after emergency contraception (%)[12]

	Levonorgestrel	*Yuzpe regimen*
Nausea	16.1*	46.5*
Vomiting	2.7*	22.4*
Fatigue	23.9*	36.8*
Breast tenderness	15.9	20.8

*Significant between-group differences, $p < 0.001$

Table 4 Efficacy of three doses of mifepristone in emergency contraception

Dose (mg)	Women (n)	Observed pregnancies (n)	Pregnancy rate (%)	Expected pregnancies* (n)	Efficacy (%)
10	565	7	1.24	42	83
50	561	7	1.25	39	82
600	559	7	1.25	41	83
Total	1685	21	1.25	122	83

*Calculated using conception probabilities of reference 24

randomized trials to evaluate the advantages and disadvantages of these various approaches to hormonal emergency contraception.

New insights into mechanisms of action

Although the mode of action of hormonal methods of emergency contraception has not been fully elucidated, the view is gradually gaining ground that suppression of ovulation rather than prevention of implantation is the primary mode of action. For example, a recent study[25] has shown that the Yuzpe regimen given before ovulation disrupts normal follicular development and maturation resulting in anovulation or delayed ovulation with deficient luteal function. In contrast, when administered on the second day after the luteinizing hormone (LH) peak, i.e. at the time when ovulation has occurred and fertilization may have taken place, the treatment had no effect on ovarian hormone secretion and only a modest effect on the morphometrical characteristics of the endometrium. These observations suggest that failure may be more likely if ovulation and fertilization have already taken place at the time of treatment and, thus, that prevention of implantation may not be a primary mode of action of the Yuzpe regimen.

Similarly, in the case of levonorgestrel, an early study in which women received 1.6 mg of levonorgestrel on day 10 of their cycle showed that the treatment seemed to suppress the mid-cycle LH peak, but did not appear to influence the formation and function of the corpus luteum, since the urinary excretion of pregnanediol (the main metabolite of progesterone) was normal[26].

Another study, which examined the effects of a daily dose of 0.75 mg of levonorgestrel administered for 4 days before ovulation, around the time of ovulation or after ovulation, indicated that the impact of levonorgestrel depends on the time of administration[27]. When levonorgestrel was given during the early follicular phase, the total cycle length was significantly prolonged as a result of the increased duration of the follicular phase. Post-treatment biopsies taken on cycle days 20–22 still showed proliferative endometrium in accordance with the delay in ovulation.

When levonorgestrel was administered around the time of ovulation, however, the effects were variable: ovulation was blocked in some women, while in others follicular activity was followed by deficient luteal function, and still other women ovulated normally. On the other hand, administering levonorgestrel during the luteal phase did not affect cycle length or cause any significant endometrial changes.

If further research confirms that the Yuzpe and levonorgestrel regimens act primarily, if not exclusively, through inhibition of ovulation, the findings should have a positive impact on acceptability of this method of contraception among those who, for religious or other reasons, do not wish to use any contraceptive method that acts after fertilization has occurred.

As for mifepristone, administration of a single dose on the second day after the urinary LH peak, i.e. shortly after ovulation, has been shown to have a profound inhibitory effect on the secretory transformation of the endometrium[28] and on fertility in both rhesus monkeys[29] and women[30]. Thus, compared with the Yuzpe and levonorgestrel regimens, prevention of implantation may play a more prominent role in the mode of action of mifepristone and this could explain the superior efficacy of the antiprogestogen.

Rising international interest

Within the past 2 years, many health and family-planning organizations have undertaken efforts to bring emergency contraception into the mainstream of reproductive health-care.

First, in October 1994, the International Medical Advisory Panel (IMAP) of the International Planned Parenthood Federation issued substantially liberalized guidelines[31] designed to make emergency contraceptive pills more easily accessible through 'the most practical delivery systems' and to remove virtually all contraindications for their use. The nearly complete lifting of contraindications was prompted by the World Health Organization (WHO) review of medical eligibility criteria for contraceptive use[32] which concluded that there are no absolute medical contraindications to the use of the Yuzpe regimen with the exception of pregnancy. In this last situation emergency contraceptive pills should not be used, not because they are thought to be harmful to either the mother or the early pregnancy but because they are no longer effective[32].

Second, in April 1995, experts from around the world meeting in Bellagio, Italy, produced a 'Consensus statement on emergency contraception', calling on family-planning providers to educate themselves about the regimens and to ensure that women everywhere 'have access to these safe and effective ways to prevent unwanted pregnancy'[33]. The participants recommended, among other things, that emergency contraceptives be added to essential drugs lists, a recommendation acted upon in December 1995 by the WHO Expert Committee on the Use of Essential Drugs.

Third, in June 1995, an Inter-agency Symposium on Reproductive Health in Refugee Situations was organized by the United Nations High Commissioner for Refugees (UNHCR) and the United Nations Population Fund (UNFPA), in collaboration with the United Nations Children's Fund (UNICEF) and WHO, and with the participation of some 50 governmental and non-governmental institutions. The Symposium led to the development of *An Interagency Field Manual on Reproductive Health in Refugee Situations* and the formulation of a 'minimum initial service package' which includes emergency contraception[34]. As a result of this initiative, emergency contraception now forms part of the core reproductive health activities recommended for implementation in the initial phase of a newly identified refugee or emergency situation.

Fourth, to test new strategies for expanding knowledge and appropriate use of emergency contraceptive pills and to work with industry to make dedicated products widely available at reasonable cost, seven major organizations

established, in late 1995, the Consortium for Emergency Contraception. The member organizations of the Consortium are the Concept Foundation, the International Planned Parenthood Federation, the Pacific Institute for Women's Health, Pathfinder International, the Population Council, the Program for Appropriate Technology in Health and our Programme at WHO. The Consortium's goal is to identify, through model introductions and operations research, the specific 'best practices' needed to broaden access to hormonal emergency contraceptives while ensuring their safe and appropriate use.

Fifth, national campaigns have been launched in, *inter alia*, the UK, Sweden, the USA and other countries to educate women and providers about emergency contraception. In the USA, an Emergency Contraception Hotline was launched on Valentine's Day 1996. The toll-free Hotline provides callers with information about methods of emergency contraception and offers a list of health-care providers in each caller's area who can prescribe emergency contraception. Information about emergency contraception and the more than 2000 practitioners across the USA who are providing it can also be found on the World Wide Web (http://opr.princeton.edu/ec/).

Sixth, large multicenter clinical trials of the standard Yuzpe regimen, the antiprogestogen mifepristone, and the new levonorgestrel-only approach under the sponsorship of our Programme are expected to put additional impetus behind efforts to broaden access to information and services.

Seventh, in June 1996, an Advisory Committee of the US Food and Drug Administration (FDA), on an unusual initiative, declared the Yuzpe method safe and effective and urged its wider availability. This action should facilitate approval of a Yuzpe-type preparation in the USA. In early 1997, a newly established company announced its intention to apply to the FDA for registration of such a product.

Finally, in October 1996, the American College of Obstetricians and Gynecologists (ACOG) issued *Practice Patterns* on 'Emergency contraception'. A revised version was published in December 1996[35]. Because ACOG issues *Practice Patterns* so infrequently, these guidelines are highly influential and serve to mainstream new and innovative medical practices. The ACOG *Practice Patterns* on emergency contraceptive pills provides further encouragement for health-care professionals in the USA to prescribe emergency contraception.

Conclusion

Given the chance, women will wish to prevent an unplanned pregnancy rather than having to face the difficult decision whether or not to seek recourse to abortion if such a pregnancy occurs. The primary goal of any family-planning program, therefore, must be the prevention of unintended pregnancies through the provision of services that are easily accessible, affordable and acceptable to the women and men they are intended to serve. As stated very clearly in the 'Programme of Action' adopted at the International Conference on Population and Development (ICPD) held in Cairo in 1994, 'Governments should take appropriate steps to help women avoid abortion, which in no case should be promoted as a method of family planning'.

Unplanned pregnancies do occur – and will continue to occur – however, irrespective of the quality of the services, the prevalence of contraceptive use and the degree of motivation of contraceptive users to avoid such pregnancies. In some instances these pregnancies are entirely unexpected, such as when a woman conceives with an intrauterine device *in situ* or following sterilization. Many unintended pregnancies in contraceptive users, however, are due to a failure of the contraceptive method in use that was recognized at the time when it occurred. Typical examples of such situations include the breakage or slippage of a condom, or displacement of a diaphragm, during intercourse; or failed coitus interruptus with ejaculation in the vagina or on the external genitalia. In these instances, as well as in all situations in which sexual intercourse took place without using any method of family planning, emergency contraception offers a last-chance, secondary method of contraception to avoid unplanned pregnancy.

Given that current methods of emergency contraception rely on technology that has been available for some 30 years, family-planning programs and practitioners not yet offering this effective means of preventing unplanned pregnancy should seriously consider doing so.

Acknowledgements

I am grateful to the Alan Guttmacher Institute and Irvington Publishers, Inc. for permission to reproduce copyrighted material from other review papers written by me and published or about to be published by them. The views expressed in this paper are mine and do not necessarily reflect those of the UNDP/UNFPA/WHO/World Bank Special Programme of Research, Development and Research Training in Human Reproduction or of its cosponsoring agencies.

References

1. Van Look, P. F. A. and von Hertzen, H. (1993). Emergency contraception. *Br. Med. Bull.*, **49**, 158–70
2. Morris, J. M. and van Wagenen, G. (1966). Compounds interfering with ovum implantation and development. III. The role of estrogens. *Am. J. Obstet. Gynecol.*, **96**, 804–15
3. Morris, J. M. and van Wagenen, G. (1967). Post coital oral contraception. In Hankinson, R. K. B., Kleinman, R. L., Eckstein, P. and Romero, H. (eds.) *Proceedings of the Eighth International Conference of the International Planned Parenthood Federation*, pp. 256–9. (London: International Planned Parenthood Federation)

4. Yuzpe, A. A. and Lancee, W. J. (1977). Ethinyl-estradiol and *dl*-norgestrel as a potential contraceptive. *Fertil. Steril.*, **28**, 932–6
5. Yuzpe, A. A., Smith, R. P. and Rademaker, A. W. (1982). A multicenter clinical investigation employing ethinylestradiol combined with *dl*-norgestrel as a postcoital contraceptive agent. *Fertil. Steril.*, **37**, 508–13
6. Lippes, J., Malik, T. and Tatum, H. J. (1976). The post-coital copper-T. *Adv. Planned Parenth.*, **11**, 24–9
7. Trussell, J., Ellertson, C. and Stewart, F. (1996). The effectiveness of the Yuzpe regimen of emergency contraception. *Fam. Plann. Perspect.*, **28**, 58–64, 87
8. Trussell, J. and Ellertson, C. (1995). Efficacy of emergency contraception. *Fertil. Control Rev.*, **4**(2), 8–11
9. von Hertzen, H. and Van Look, P. F. A. (1996). Research on new methods of emergency contraception. *Int. Fam. Plann. Perspect.*, **22**, 62–8
10. Van Look, P. F. A. and Stewart, F. H. (1998). Emergency contraception. In Hatcher, R. A., Trussell, J., Stewart, F., Stewart, G. K., Kowal, D., Guest, F. and Cates, W. Jr (eds.) *Contraceptive Technology*, 17th rev. edn. (New York: Irvington Publishers)
11. Van Look, P. F. A. (1997). Emergency contraception: the Cinderella of family planning. In: Rodriguez, O. *et al.* (eds.) *Clinical Infertility and Contraception*. (Carnforth, UK: Parthenon Publishing)
12. Ho, P. C. and Kwan, M. S. W. (1993). A prospective randomized comparison of levonorgestrel with the Yuzpe regimen in post-coital contraception. *Hum. Reprod.*, **8**, 389–92
13. George, J., Turner, J., Cooke, E., Hennessey, E., Savage, W., Julian, P. and Cochrane, R. (1994). Women's knowledge of emergency contraception. *Br. J. Gen. Pract.*, **44**, 451–4
14. Graham, A., Green, L. and Glasier, A. F. (1996). Teenagers' knowledge of emergency contraception: questionnaire survey in south east Scotland. *Br. Med. J.*, **312**, 1567–9
15. Smith, B. H., Gurney, E. M., Aboulela, L. and Templeton, A. (1996). Emergency contraception: a survey of women's knowledge and attitudes. *Br. J. Obstet. Gynaecol.*, **103**, 1109–16
16. Pearson, V. A. H., Owen, M. R., Phillips, D. R., Pereira Gray, D. J. and Marshall, M. N. (1995). Pregnant teenagers' knowledge and use of emergency contraception. *Br. Med. J.*, **310**, 1644
17. Weisberg, E., Fraser, I. S., Carrick, S. E. and Wilde, F. M. (1995). Emergency contraception. General practitioner knowledge, attitudes and practices in New South Wales. *Med. J. Aust.*, **162**, 136–8
18. Senanayake, P. (1996). Emergency contraception: the International Planned Parenthood Federation's experience. *Int. Fam. Plann. Perspect.*, **22**, 69–70
19. Lei, H. P. and Hu, Z. -Y. (1981). The mechanisms of action of vacation pills. In Chang, C. F. and Griffin, D. (eds.) *Recent Advances in Fertility Regulation*, pp. 70–82. (Geneva: Atar SA)
20. Rinehart, W. (1976). Postcoital contraception – an appraisal. *Population Reports*, Series J, No. 9. (Baltimore: Johns Hopkins University, Population Information Program)
21. Van Look, P. F. A. and von Hertzen, H. (1995). Clinical uses of antiprogestogens. *Hum. Reprod. Update*, **1**, 19–34
22. Glasier, A., Thong, K. J., Dewar, M., Mackie, M. and Baird, D. T. (1992). Mifepristone (RU 486) compared with high-dose estrogen and progestogen for emergency postcoital contraception. *N. Engl. J. Med.*, **324**, 1041–4
23. Webb, A. M. C., Russell, J. and Elstein, M. (1992). Comparison of Yuzpe regimen, danazol and mifepristone (RU 486) in oral postcoital contraception. *Br. Med. J.*, **305**, 927–31
24. Dixon, G. W., Schlesselman, J. J., Ory, H. W. and Blye, R. P. (1980). Ethinylestradiol and conjugated estrogens as postcoital contraceptives. *J. Am. Med. Assoc.*, **244**, 1336–9
25. Swahn, M. -L., Westlund, P., Johannisson, E. and Bygdeman, M. (1996). Effect of post-coital contraceptive methods on the endometrium and the menstrual cycle. *Acta Obstet. Gynecol. Scand.*, **75**, 738–44
26. Kesserü, E., Garmendia, F., Westphal, N. and Parada, J. (1974). The hormonal and peripheral effects of *d*-norgestrel in postcoital contraception. *Contraception*, **10**, 411–24
27. Landgren, B. -M., Johannisson, E., Aedo, A. -R., Kumar, A. and Shi, Y. -E. (1989). The effect of levonorgestrel administered in large doses at different stages of the cycle on ovarian function and endometrial morphology. *Contraception*, **39**, 275–89
28. Swahn, M. L., Bygdeman, M., Cekan, S., Xing, S., Masironi, B. and Johannisson, E. (1990). The effect of RU 486 administered during the early luteal phase on bleeding pattern, hormonal parameters and endometrium. *Hum. Reprod.*, **5**, 402–8
29. Ghosh, D., De, P. and Sengupta, J. (1994). Luteal phase contraception with mifepristone (RU 486) in the rhesus monkey. *Indian J. Physiol. Pharmacol.*, **38**, 17–22
30. Gemzell-Danielsson, K., Swahn, M. L., Svalander, P. and Bygdeman, M. (1993). Early luteal phase treatment with mifepristone (RU 486) for fertility regulation. *Hum. Reprod.*, **8**, 870–3

31. International Planned Parenthood Federation (1994). *Statement on Emergency Contraception.* (London: International Planned Parenthood Federation)

32. World Health Organization (1996). *Improving Access to Quality Care in Family Planning. Medical Eligibility Criteria for Contraceptive Use,* Doc. WHO/FRH/FPP/96.9. (Geneva: World Health Organization)

33. Anonymous (1995). Consensus statement on emergency contraception. *Contraception,* **52,** 211–13

34. United Nations High Commissioner for Refugees (1995). *Reproductive Health in Refugee Situations. An Inter-agency Field Manual.* (Geneva: United Nations High Commissioner for Refugees)

35. American College of Obstetricians and Gynecologists (1996). Emergency oral contraception. *ACOG Practice Patterns.* (Washington, DC: American College of Obstetricians and Gynecologists)

Induced abortion: a global perspective on a controversial issue* 27

P. F. A. Van Look

Introduction

Even before more reliable information started to become available in the 1970s about the number of induced abortions, including those performed under unsafe conditions, the public health aspects of induced abortion were already a matter of concern to many nations. As early as 1967, the World Health Assembly of the World Health Organization (WHO) passed a Resolution (WHA 20.41) which stated that '. . . abortions . . . constitute a serious public health problem in many countries . . .' and requested '. . . the Director-General: (a) to continue to develop the activities of the World Health Organization in the field of health aspects of human reproduction; . . .'[1].

The International Conference on Population, held in Mexico City in 1984, urged governments '. . . to take appropriate steps to help women avoid abortion, which in no case should be promoted as a method of family planning and – whenever possible – to provide for the humane treatment and counselling of women who have had recourse to abortion'[2]. The recent International Conference on Population and Development, held in Cairo in 1994, also approved a Programme of Action that states: 'In no case should abortion be promoted as a method of family planning. All Governments and relevant intergovernmental and non-governmental organizations are urged to strengthen their commitment to women's health, to deal with the health impact of unsafe abortion as a major public health concern and to reduce the recourse to abortion through expanded and improved family planning services. Prevention of unwanted pregnancies must always be given the highest priority and every attempt should be made to eliminate the need for abortion . . .'[3]. The Fourth World Conference on Women, which took place in Beijing in 1995, echoed these sentiments in its Plan for Action[4].

From the standpoint of public policy, few would disagree that reducing the number of unintended pregnancies and abortions worldwide is a desirable goal. However, opinions differ as to the most effective means of achieving that goal. As is evident from the declarations quoted above, international gatherings of a primarily political nature emphasize prevention through a wider provision of family-planning services rather than decriminalization or 'liberalization' of existing restrictive legislation. This emphasis on prevention rather than on legislative change reflects the divergent views – and the consequent need for political compromise – on a subject that religious and moral beliefs keep at the center of an intense public controversy about the status of the fetus and a woman's right to make choices about pregnancy and motherhood[5].

This paper reviews the world-wide occurrence of induced abortion and some of the factors that can influence trends in the number of abortions carried out. The causes and consequences of induced abortion will be discussed.

---

*The views expressed in this paper are those of the author and do not necessarily represent the opinions or stated policies of the World Health Organization or of its Member States

Special consideration will be given to unsafe abortion which, in the words of a recent WHO report, is '. . . one of the great neglected health problems of health care in developing countries and . . . a serious concern to women during their reproductive lives'[6].

Global estimates of induced abortions

Annual number

The number of pregnancies aborted each year throughout the world is unknown. Even in countries where legal restrictions are minimal and induced abortion is widely accepted, statistics are not always reliable due to under-reporting. Not all procedures performed by physicians are reported, and those provided by traditional, non-medical practitioners do not appear in the official statistics. For example, in India, official statistics put the number of induced abortions at about 600 000, but most experts, including Indian Government officials, agree that the figure is more likely to be in the region of 1.5 million. Estimating the number of clandestine abortions is even more difficult; various approaches have been proposed over the years, but complete accuracy will probably remain elusive[7]. Indirect methods that have been – and are being – used include surveys of the numbers of women admitted to hospital with conditions that can be attributed to clandestine abortion, such as pelvic infection or reproductive tract injury; information on death certificates; and surveys of samples of women[8,9].

Henshaw[10] has estimated that the number of legal abortions performed world-wide in 1987 was approximately 28 million, but may have ranged from 26 to 31 million. The number of clandestine abortions during that year was estimated at 15 million (range 10–22 million), giving an estimated world-wide total of between 36 and 53 million. Demographers calculate that from one-third to one-half of all women undergo at least one induced abortion during their lifetime.

Rates and ratios

The occurrence of abortion is usually measured by rates or ratios. Both approaches yield different but complementary information and both are needed for an understanding of induced abortion from a demographic perspective[11].

Abortion rates can be expressed in several ways[12]. The crude abortion rate is the number of abortions per year per 1000 total population at mid-year; it corresponds to other crude rates in vital statistics, such as the crude birth rate. A more refined, and more preferable, measurement is the general abortion rate per 1000 women of reproductive age (usually defined as 15–44 years). Abortion rates are also frequently calculated for successive ages, usually at 5-year intervals. Cumulation of these age-specific rates over the entire reproductive period gives the total abortion rate per 1000 women during their lifetime in the same way as the total fertility rate is calculated. The total abortion rate thus represents the number of abortions that would be experienced by 1000 women during their reproductive lifetimes, assuming the present age-specific abortion rates (from which the total abortion rate is calculated) remain unchanged.

Abortion ratios may be computed per 100 (or 1000) live births or deliveries or per 100 (or 1000) known pregnancies. The abortion ratio per 1000 deliveries is most often used in studies of legal abortions, especially if such abortions are relatively infrequent. Age-specific abortion ratios per 100 (or 1000) pregnancies are usually computed in terms of age at conception, but age-specific abortion ratios per 100 (or 1000) live births are often based on when the pregnancy ends. The latter calculation may introduce a substantial error for the youngest age group and smaller errors for all other age groups if a significant proportion of conceptions among women of the youngest age group occurs towards the end of the age period. For example, women who conceive between 19 years and 3 months and 19 years and 9 months of age will most likely appear in the 'under-20' age group if the pregnancy ends in abortion, while most of them will be in the '20–24' age group if they continue the pregnancy and give birth. The displacement of births into the next higher age group produces an inflation of the abortion ratio for the youngest age group. Conversely, the abortion ratios for all higher age groups are reduced, especially that for the highest age group.

Examples of abortion rate, abortion ratio and, where known, total abortion rate are shown for selected countries in Table 1. Differences between countries are the result of a complex interaction between several factors that include, *inter alia*, desired family size, the status of women in society, the use of contraception and the provision and availability of family-planning services.

Among countries thought to have complete and reliable statistics, The Netherlands has the lowest reported abortion rate in the world, which contradicts the claim made by groups opposed to abortion that a non-restrictive abortion law inevitably results in a large number of abortions and a reliance on abortion as a method of family planning. The high rates and ratios in Central and Eastern European countries reflect a desire for smaller families in societies that had then – and often continue to have now – limited access to modern contraceptives. In the former USSR, the official data for 1987 indicated a rate of 112 per 1000 women aged 15–44 years, but estimates derived from survey data suggested that the rate may have been as high as 181 per 1000. Abortion rates in most of the other developed countries range from 10 to 20 per 1000 women of reproductive age, but the USA rate is somewhat higher at 28 per 1000. In Great Britain, the rate for Scotland is only about two-thirds that of England and Wales and, like the rate for The Netherlands, is below the range found in most developed countries.

Table 1 Number of abortions, abortion rate per 1000 women aged 15–44, abortion ratio per 100 known pregnancies and total abortion rate for selected countries. From reference 10

Country (year)	Number of abortions	Rate	Ratio	Total rate
Complete statistics				
Australia (1988)	63 200	16.6	20.4	484
Bulgaria (1987)	119 900	64.7	50.7	u
Canada (1987)	63 600	10.2	14.7	299
China (1987)	10 394 500	38.8	31.4	u
Czechoslovakia (1987)	156 600	46.7	42.2	1400
Denmark (1987)	20 800	18.3	27.0	548
England and Wales (1987)*	156 200	14.2	18.6	413
Finland (1987)	13 000	11.7	18.0	356
Hungary (1987)	84 500	38.2	40.2	1137
Netherlands (1986)	18 300	5.3	9.0	155
New Zealand (1987)	8 800	11.4	13.6	323
Norway (1987)	15 400	16.8	22.2	493
Scotland (1987)[†]	10 100	9.0	13.2	255
Singapore (1987)	21 200	30.1	32.7	840
Sweden (1987)	34 700	19.8	24.9	600
USA (1985)	1 588 600	28.0	29.7	797
Incomplete statistics				
France (1987)	161 000	13.3	17.3	406
India (1987)	588 400	3.0	2.2	u
Ireland (1987)[‡]	3 700	4.8	5.9	139
Italy (1987)	191 500	15.3	25.7	460
Japan (1987)	497 800	18.6	27.0	564
Soviet Union (1987)	6 818 000	111.9	54.9	u

*Residents only; [†]including abortions obtained in England; [‡]based on Irish residents who obtained abortions in England; u, unknown

Trends

Owing to incomplete statistics and uncertainty about the number of clandestine abortions, it is not known whether the world-wide total number of induced abortions is decreasing or increasing. In fact, even within a given country, changes in annual abortion statistics may be difficult to interpret. For example, in countries where reporting is less than optimal and both the numerator and denominator used in calculating a rate or ratio are subject to substantial errors, a change in the extent of underreporting can have a large effect. Likewise, increases or decreases in abortion rates and ratios can be caused by simple shifts in the age-structure of a population rather than by profound changes in women's attitudes to – and requests for – abortion. Transient rises in the reported number of abortions have been observed in some countries following the accident at the Chernobyl nuclear plant[13] and in the wake of 'pill scares'. For instance, the recent reports of increased risk of venous thromboembolism in users of combined oral contraceptive pills containing so-called third-generation progestogens (gestodene and desogestrel)[14–17], and the recommendation of the UK Medicines Control Agency that pills containing these progestogens should preferably be avoided, are thought to have been responsible for a transient increase in the number of abortions in Britain[18].

Effect of abortion on fertility rate

In the demographic transition from high to low fertility, induced abortion is an unavoidable factor, although its importance as a proximate determinant of the fertility rate varies depending on the stage of the demographic transition process. Generally, as couples become motivated to limit the size of their family, the abortion rate frequently rises, initially because the provision of contraceptives is often still low and couples are poorly informed about their use. At this point in the demographic transition, the lowering effect of abortion on the fertility rate is highest. Subsequently, when contraceptive use becomes sufficiently widespread and smaller families are achieved, the resort to abortion (legal or clandestine) diminishes, but many developing countries have not yet reached this point[10].

Reasons for induced abortions

According to WHO estimates, some 100 million acts of sexual intercourse take place each day, resulting in approximately 910 000 conceptions[6]. About 50% of these conceptions are unplanned and some 25% of them are definitely unwanted. About one-half of the unwanted pregnancies (i.e. between 100 000 and 150 000 every day or 36–53 million in a year) are terminated by induced abortion. Most of the unplanned pregnancies occur in women who were not using any method of contraception at the time of conception.

Over the past three decades, there has been an impressive rise in the use of contraceptives all over the world. In 1990, in the developing part of the world, up to 57% of all married women of reproductive age or their husbands were using a method of contraception. This represents an increase of 6% over the prevalence in 1983 and of nearly 50% compared with the early 1960s.

These figures do not tell the whole story, however. For example, in the least developed countries, which have some 540 million people, the total fertility rate in 1992 was still 6.1 births per woman, which corresponds to an estimated prevalence of contraceptive use of only 14%. In developing countries, it is estimated that there are over 100 million women who are married or in a union who are not practicing family planning even though they say that they do not want to become pregnant[19]. To this figure should be added the women with unmet need who are not sampled in traditional surveys but are at high risk of unplanned pregnancy, namely adolescent girls and unmarried women. Clearly, fulfilling these large unmet needs is bound to have favorable repercussion on the numbers of unplanned pregnancies and induced abortions.

The magnitude of the shortfall between contraceptive need and use has been shown, for instance, in a series of recent investigations conducted under the auspices of our Programme. In a study carried out in Nepal, unplanned pregnancy accounted for 95% of induced abortions; most of the women having abortion were not using contraception. Similarly, in a study in the Dominican Republic, scarcely 25% of the women having induced abortions were using a contraceptive method when they unintentionally became pregnant, while in a project carried out in Colombia, 79% of unwanted pregnancy was due to the non-use of contraception. Even in China, where contraception is easily and widely accessible, non-use was found to be a primary reason for unwanted pregnancy and abortion.

The situation in developed countries is generally not much different. For example, in The Netherlands, where there are no barriers to obtaining contraceptives, not even for high-risk groups such as adolescents, about 20% of native Dutch women who request pregnancy termination did not use contraception during the 6 months prior to the abortion[20]. Among a similar group of 769 women in the United Kingdom, 210 (27%) did not use contraception at the time of conception[21]. For women not using contraception and for those who have a contraceptive mishap, such as a torn condom, timely use of emergency contraception can avoid unplanned pregnancy in many cases[22].

Use of a contraceptive method is no absolute guarantee against unplanned pregnancy, however. Many of the current methods of family planning are difficult for some couples to use, and no method is completely effective. The yearly number of pregnancies resulting from contraceptive failure has been estimated at between 8 and 30 million[23]. It is uncertain how many of these unplanned pregnancies are terminated, but they almost certainly contribute substantially to the total number of abortions carried out annually throughout the world.

Risks associated with induced abortion

Owing to its controversial nature, abortion has been intensively studied. Indeed, more is known today about the safety of abortion than any other operation. In countries where legislation is not restrictive, induced abortion is one of the safest operations in contemporary practice. In the USA, for example, the case-fatality rate of legal induced abortion is now 0.6 per 100 000 procedures, making it as safe as an injection of penicillin[24]. Abortions induced under unsafe conditions, on the other hand, are a major cause of maternal morbidity and mortality; of the approximately 580 000 women who die every year due to pregnancy-related causes, some 70 000 deaths are the result of complications of abortions induced in clandestine circumstances[7].

Legal abortions

Morbidity, mortality and the occurrence of complications following legal abortion, with focus on reports with large numbers of patients published since 1980, were recently reviewed by Grimes[25].

Morbidity Where safe, legal abortion is available and easily accessible, complications from the procedure are infrequent. National health statistics have conclusively shown that abortions performed at an early stage of pregnancy are safer than later procedures, and that rates of complications for both first-trimester and second-trimester procedures have diminished in recent decades. The improved safety over time reflects a shift to earlier procedures, more skilled clinicians, improved abortion techniques and greater sophistication in managing complications[26].

Reports published since 1980 from countries where abortion legislation is not restrictive consistently indicate complication rates for first-trimester abortion of less than 10 per 1000 operations (Table 2). A recent large report described the experience of a few highly

Table 2 Complication rates per 1000 procedures in selected large case-series reports. From reference 25

Reference	27	28	29	30
Country	USA	Sweden	Denmark	Canada
No. of patients	170 000	1000	5851	351 879
Gestational age (weeks)	≤ 14	≤ 14	≤ 12	all
Dates	1971–87	1987	1980–85	1975–80
Complication				
infection	4.6	47	24	1.8
cervical laceration	0.1	NR	1	3.5
incomplete abortion	0.28	NR	NR	19.6
uterine perforation	0.09	0.0	4	1.3
hemorrhage	0.07	0.0	42	2.5
twin intra-/extrauterine pregnancy	0.02	NR	NR	NR
Hospitalization	0.71	28	61	NR
Total complications	9.05	56	61	NR

NR, not reported

experienced physicians operating on low-risk patients with established protocols. The overall complication rate among 170 000 first-trimester abortions was nine per 1000 abortions; fewer than one per 1000 required hospitalization[27].

Mortality Where legal abortion is accessible, mortality trends have paralleled those of morbidity. In countries such as Sweden and the USA, deaths from abortion have become rare[26,31]. In these two countries, the risk of death from induced abortion is about one-tenth that of giving birth. For instance, in Sweden, the mortality rate for legal abortions between 1971 and 1980 was 0.7 per 100 000 procedures[31], while the corresponding figure for the USA between 1979 and 1985 was 0.6 per 100 000 procedures[26]. Recent national data from countries in Europe and North America have revealed abortion mortality rates of two or fewer deaths per 100 000 procedures[25].

Illegal (unsafe) abortions

Unsafe abortion has been defined by the WHO as a procedure for terminating an unwanted pregnancy either by persons lacking the necessary skills or in an environment lacking the minimal medical standards, or both[7].

Unsafe abortion may be induced in unhygienic conditions by the woman herself, by a non-medical person or by a health worker. It may be provoked by insertion of a solid object (usually a root, twig or catheter) into the uterus, an improperly performed dilatation and curettage procedure, ingestion of harmful substances or exertion of external force. The mortality and morbidity risks depend on the facilities and skill of the provider, the method used and certain characteristics of the woman herself (for example, her general health, age, parity, presence of genital tract infection, etc.). The risks are also dependent on the availability, utilization and quality of treatment facilities when complications occur[7].

The number of unsafe abortions and the risks associated with them can only be indirectly estimated. A summary of the WHO's most recent global and regional estimates on incidence of, and mortality from, unsafe abortions is given in Table 3. World-wide, some 20 million unsafe abortions take place each year; this represents nearly one in 10 pregnancies, or a ratio of one unsafe abortion to seven births. Almost 90% of unsafe abortions occur in developing countries.

An estimated 70 000 women die each year due to complications of unsafe abortions. Inevitably, this estimate has a large margin of error and the number could be as low as 50 000 or as high as 100 000. The figures in Table 4 indicate that, in 1990, the risk of dying from an unsafe abortion was at least 13 times greater in

Table 3 Global and regional estimates for incidence of, and mortality from, unsafe abortions*. From reference 7

Region	No. of unsafe abortions (1000s)	Unsafe abortions per 1000 women 15–49 years	No. of deaths from unsafe abortion	Mortality from unsafe abortion per 100 000 live births	Percentage of maternal deaths
World total	20 000	15	70 000	49	13
More developed countries[†]	2 340	8	600	4	14
Less developed countries	17 620	17	69 000	55	13
Africa	3 740	26	23 000	83	13
Asia[†]	9 240	12	40 000	47	12
Europe	260	2	100	2	10
Latin America	4 620	41	6 000	48	24
Oceania[†]	20	17	< 100	29	5
USSR (former)	2 080	30	500	10	23

*For North America, where the incidence of unsafe abortion is negligible, no estimate has been made; [†]Australia, Japan and New Zealand have been excluded from the regional estimates, but are included in the total for developed countries; numbers may not add to totals due to rounding

Table 4 Global and regional estimated risk of death from unsafe abortion. From reference 7

Region	No. of unsafe abortions (1000s)	No. of deaths from unsafe abortion	Case-fatality per 1000 unsafe abortions
World total	20 000	70 000	4
More developed countries*	2 340	600	0.3
Less developed countries	17 620	69 000	4
Africa	3 740	23 000	6
Asia*	9 240	40 000	4
Europe	260	100	0.4
Latin America	4 620	6 000	1
Oceania*	20	< 100	2
USSR (former)	2 080	500	0.3

*Australia, Japan and New Zealand have been excluded from the regional estimates, but are included in the total for developed countries; numbers may not add to totals due to rounding

developing countries than in industrialized countries, and as much as 40–50 times greater in some regions of the world.

As is evident from Table 3, there are large differences in incidence of, and mortality from, unsafe abortion between regions. Among developing regions, Asia has the lowest abortion rate at 12 per 1000 women of reproductive age, but the largest absolute number of unsafe abortions because it has the largest population of women in the reproductive age group. In Latin America, the unsafe abortion rate of 41 per 1000 women of reproductive age corresponds to more than one unsafe abortion for every three births, and the abortion mortality ratio of 48 per 100 000 live births represents nearly one-quarter of all maternal deaths in that region. In Africa, the abortion mortality ratio is over 80 per 100 000 live births, and the absolute number of deaths represents one-third of the world-wide total. Although induced abortion is legal in the countries of the former USSR, services are inadequate and their quality is often poor resulting in a high unsafe abortion rate of 30 per 1000 women of reproductive age, the world's second highest after Latin America. Almost 25% of maternal deaths in the region are related to unsafe abortion.

Epilogue

The 70 000 women who die each year from botched abortions are a tragic illustration that neither restrictive abortion laws nor lack of access to professional care prevent women from seeking abortion. Many of the unintended pregnancies can be avoided by increasing access to acceptable and affordable methods of family planning , including emergency contraception. However, neither the methods that are presently available nor the people who use them are perfect, and it would be unrealistic to believe that the recourse to abortion can be totally eliminated. The mere recognition of this fact would go a long way towards finding appropriate solutions for the public-health problems due to unsafe abortion, '. . . one of the great neglected problems of health care in developing countries . . .'.

References

1. World Health Organization (1967). *WHO Official Records*, No. 160, 25
2. United Nations (1984). *Report of the International Conference on Population, 1984*. Mexico City, 6–14 August 1984. Mexico City, 6–14 August 1984. (New York: United Nations)
3. United Nations (1994). *Report of the International Conference on Population, 1994*. Cairo, 5–13 September 1994. (New York: United Nations)
4. United Nations (1995). *Plan for Action. Fourth World Conference on Women*, Beijing, 4–15 September 1995, Document A/Conf. 177/20. (New York: United Nations)
5. Jacobson, J. L. (1990). *The Global Politics of Abortion*. Worldwatch paper 97. (Washington, DC: Worldwatch Institute)
6. Fathalla, M. F. (1992). Reproductive health in the world: two decades of progress and the challenge ahead. In Khanna, J., Van Look, P. F. A. and Griffin, P. D. (eds.) *Reproductive Health: a Key to a Brighter Future*, pp. 3–31. (Geneva: World Health Organization)
7. World Health Organization (Maternal Health and Safe Motherhood Programme) (1993). *Abortion. A Tabulation of Available Data on the Frequency and Mortality of Unsafe Abortion*, 2nd edn. (Geneva: World Health Organization Division of Family Health)
8. Paxman, J. M., Rizo, A., Brown, L. and Benson, J. (1993). The clandestine epidemic: the practice of unsafe abortion in Latin America. *Stud. Fam. Plann.*, **24**, 205–26
9. Barreto, T., Campbell, O. M., Davies, J. L., Fauveau, V., Filippi, V. G., Graham, W. J., Mamdani, M., Rooney, C. I. and Toubia, N. F. (1992). Investigating induced abortion in developing countries: methods and problems. *Stud. Fam. Plann.*, **23**, 159–70
10. Henshaw, S. K. (1990). Induced abortion: a world review, 1990. *Fam. Plann. Perspect.*, **22**, 76–89
11. Van Look, P. F. A. and von Hertzen, H. (1995). Induced abortion: a global perspective. In Baird, D. T., Grimes, D. A. and Van Look, P. F. A. (eds.) *Modern Methods of Inducing Abortion*, pp. 1–24. (Oxford: Blackwell Science)
12. World Health Organization (1970). *Spontaneous and Induced Abortion*. WHO Technical Report Series, No. 461. (Geneva: World Health Organization)
13. Spinelli, A. and Osborn, J. F. (1991). The effects of the Chernobyl explosion on induced abortion in Italy. *Biomed. Pharmacother.*, **45**, 243–7
14. World Health Organization Collaborative Study of Cardiovascular Disease and Steroid Hormone Contraception (1995). Venous thromboembolic disease and combined oral contraceptives: results on international multicentre case–control study. *Lancet*, **146**, 1575–82
15. World Health Organization Collaborative Study of Cardiovascular Disease and Steroid Hormone Contraception (1995). Effect of different progestogens in low oestrogen oral contraceptives on venous thromboembolic disease. *Lancet*, **346**, 1582–8

16. Jick, H., Jick, S. S., Gurewich, V., Myers, M. W. and Vasilakis, C. (1995). Risk of idiopathic cardiovascular death and nonfatal venous thromboembolism in women using oral contraceptives with differing progestagen components. *Lancet*, **346**, 1589–93

17. Bloemenkamp, K. W. M., Rosendaal, F. R., Helmerhorst, F. M., Büller, H. R. and Vandenbroucke, J. P. (1995). Enhancement by factor V Leiden mutation of risk of deep-vein thrombosis associated with oral contraceptives containing a third-generation progestagen. *Lancet*, **346**, 1593–6

18. Dillner, L. (1996). Pill scare linked to rise in abortions. *Br. Med. J.*, **312**, 996

19. Robey, B., Ross, J. and Bhushan, I. (1996). Meeting unmet need: new strategies. *Population Reports*, Series J, No. 43, 1–35. (Baltimore: Johns Hopkins University, Population Information Program)

20. Rademakers, J. (1992). *Abortus in Nederland 1989/1990*. Jaarverslag van de landelijke abortusregistratie. (Utrecht: Stimezo-onderzoek)

21. Bromham, D. R. and Cartmill, R. S. V. (1993). Knowledge and use of secondary contraception among patients requesting termination of pregnancy. *Br. Med. J.*, **306**, 556–7

22. Van Look, P. F. A. and von Hertzen, H. (1993). Emergency contraception. *Br. Med. Bull.*, **49**, 158–70

23. Segal, S. J. and LaGuardia, K. D. (1990). Termination of pregnancy – a global view. *Baill. Clin. Obstet. Gynaecol.*, **4**, 235–47

24. Gold, R. B. (1990). *Abortion and Women's Health. A Turning Point for America.* (New York and Washington, DC: The Alan Guttmacher Institute)

25. Grimes, D. A. (1995). Sequelae of abortion. In Baird, D. T., Grimes, D. A. and Van Look, P. F. A. (eds.) *Modern Methods of Inducing Abortion*, pp. 95–111. (Oxford: Blackwell Science)

26. Council of Scientific Affairs, American Medical Association (1992). Induced termination of pregnancy before and after Roe *v* Wade. *J. Am. Med. Assoc.*, **268**, 3231–9

27. Hakim-Elahi, E., Tovill, H. M. M. and Burnhill, M. S. (1990). Complications of first-trimester abortion: a report of 170 000 cases. *Obstet. Gynecol.*, **76**, 129–35

28. Fried, G., Ostlund, E., Ullberg, C. and Bygdeman, M. (1989). Somatic complications and contraceptive techniques following legal abortion. *Acta Obstet. Gynecol. Scand.*, **68**, 515–21

29. Heisterberg, L. and Kringlebach, M. (1989). Early complications after induced first-trimester abortion. *Acta Obstet. Gynecol. Scand.*, **66**, 201–4

30. Wadhera, S. (1982). Early complication risks of legal abortions, Canada, 1975–1980. *Can. Med. Assoc. J.*, **73**, 396–400

31. Hogberg, U. and Joelsson, I. (1980). Maternal deaths related to abortions in Sweden, 1931–1980. *Gynecol. Obstet. Invest.*, **20**, 169–78

Advances in methods of inducing abortion

28

D. T. Baird and K. Joo Thong

Introduction

Although widespread use of effective contraception can reduce the incidence of unplanned pregnancy, access to safe methods of terminating an unwanted pregnancy ('safe abortion') is one of the prerequisites of reproductive health[1]. It has been estimated that throughout the world approximately 50 million women resort to abortion to terminate an unwanted pregnancy. Although modern methods of inducing abortion are extremely effective and safe, each year 50 000–100 000 women die and countless others suffer infertility and ill health from the complications of unsafe abortion. The most effective way of reducing this unnecessary toll of morbidity and mortality is to provide legal abortion within the services providing reproductive health-care. In the past decade, several advances in methods of inducing abortion have become available which allow women and their providers a choice of safe methods. The most important development has been the availability of compounds which block the action of progesterone by binding to the progesterone receptor[2]. These compounds used in combination with prostaglandin analogs will terminate pregnancy at any gestation, i.e. for induction of abortion or parturition. In addition, they have potential to complement the traditional surgical methods owing to their action on the cervix.

This paper will summarize the advantages and disadvantages of the use of antigestogens and prostaglandins for induction of abortion at three stages of pregnancy: (1) early first trimester (up to 9 weeks' gestation); (2) late first trimester (9–14 weeks'); (3) mid-trimester (12–24 weeks').

Antiprogestogens

In 1980, chemists at Roussel-UCLAF synthesized a derivative of norethisterone (RU 486 or mifepristone) which had the property of binding to the progesterone and glucocorticoid receptors and, hence, blocked the action of the natural ligand[3]. Although several hundred antiprogestogens have been synthesized since then, clinical experience has been confined virtually exclusively to mifepristone which has been shown to be an effective agent for inducing abortion in the first and second trimester of pregnancy. By 24 h of oral administration of mifepristone, there is an increase in spontaneous uterine activity followed within 72 h by vaginal bleeding[4]. The exact mechanism by which mifepristone induces abortion is not entirely clear, but withdrawal of the biological action of progesterone is accompanied by an increase in gap junctions between myometrial cells, an increase in decidual prostaglandins and a decrease in their metabolism, and an influx of neutrophils (especially monocytes) into the decidua[5,6].

Two other groups of compounds have been investigated as medical abortifacients although they have not achieved widespread use. Inhibitors of the enzyme 3β-ol steroid dehydrogenase, such as epostane and trilostane, decrease the synthesis of progesterone and result in changes similar to those induced by antigestogens[7,8]. Antimetabolites, such as methotrexate, inhibit division of the trophoblast and, hence, death of the embryo or fetus[9]. However, neither of these approaches has proved as successful as antigestogens because several days elapse before abortion commences. Moreover, methotrexate in high doses has teratogenic actions in animals and, hence, there is a risk of fetal deformity if the pregnancy continues[10]. In a recent study in which 756 women at gestation of less than 7 weeks received methotrexate 50 mg/m^2 in combination with 500–750 µg misoprostol vaginally, the complete abortion rate was only 88.8%[11]. Vacuum aspiration was necessary in 7.5% of women with ongoing pregnancies and all of the nine fetuses which were examined had congenital abnormalities including missing digits and stunted limbs. For these reasons, these compounds have not gained the same acceptance as antigestogens and will not be considered further.

First-trimester abortion

Initial studies of women in early pregnancy (< 7 weeks' gestation) demonstrated that although bleeding was usually provoked by the administration of mifepristone, complete abortion only occurred in 60–80% of women[12]. However, when a small dose of prostaglandin (sulprostone or gemeprost) was given 36–48 h after the mifepristone, the complete abortion rate could be increased to > 95%[4,13].

Large clinical trials in France and the UK confirmed these initial studies and this combination was licensed for induction of abortion at up to 7 weeks' gestation in France (1988), and up to 9 weeks' gestation in the UK (1991) and Sweden (1992)[14–17]. Subsequent postmarketing experience in these countries has confirmed that this combination is a safe, effective alternative to vacuum aspiration of pregnancy. National data in Scotland demonstrate a slow increase in the number of abortions performed medically[18] (Figure 1). By 1994, 3 years after its introduction, mifepristone was used in 17% of all abortions and in 31% of those of under 10 weeks' gestation. When both methods are freely available as in France and Scotland, over one-half of the women who are suitable choose a medical method[19,20]. In our own hospital, the proportion of abortions performed medically has increased progressively since mifepristone was licensed in 1991 (Figure 2). By 1994, 57% of

abortions under 9 weeks' gestation were performed medically (Figure 3). Those who choose medical abortion tend to be of higher socioeconomic class, and prefer to remain in control of the procedure and wish to avoid instruments in the uterus. In contrast, many women choosing vacuum aspiration wish to be unaware of the abortion and perceive the method as quicker. Thus, each method appeals to different types of women.

A number of issues surrounding the use of mifepristone for induction of first-trimester abortion are still not fully resolved.

Dose of mifepristone

Initial studies of mifepristone employed a range of doses (25–100 mg) at intervals of 12 h over several days. However, it was soon demonstrated that because of the long half-life of mifepristone (~ 20 h), a single large dose, e.g. 600 mg, was as effective as several smaller doses and this more convenient regimen was adopted for licensing[21]. A large World Health Organization (WHO)-sponsored multicenter trial demonstrated that 200 mg was as effective as 600 mg[22], although in a subsequent trial a single dose of 50 mg in combination with 1 mg gemeprost resulted in a lower rate of complete abortion

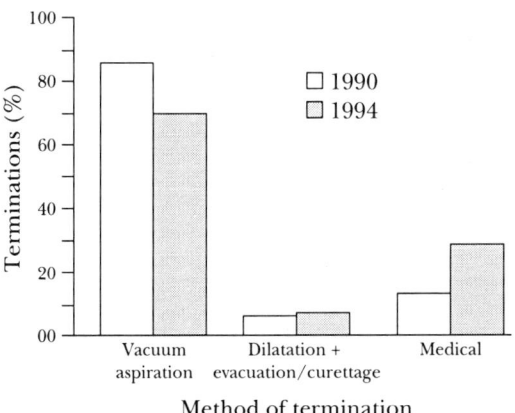

Figure 1 Method of termination of pregnancy in Scotland[18]: total number each year is approximately 11 000

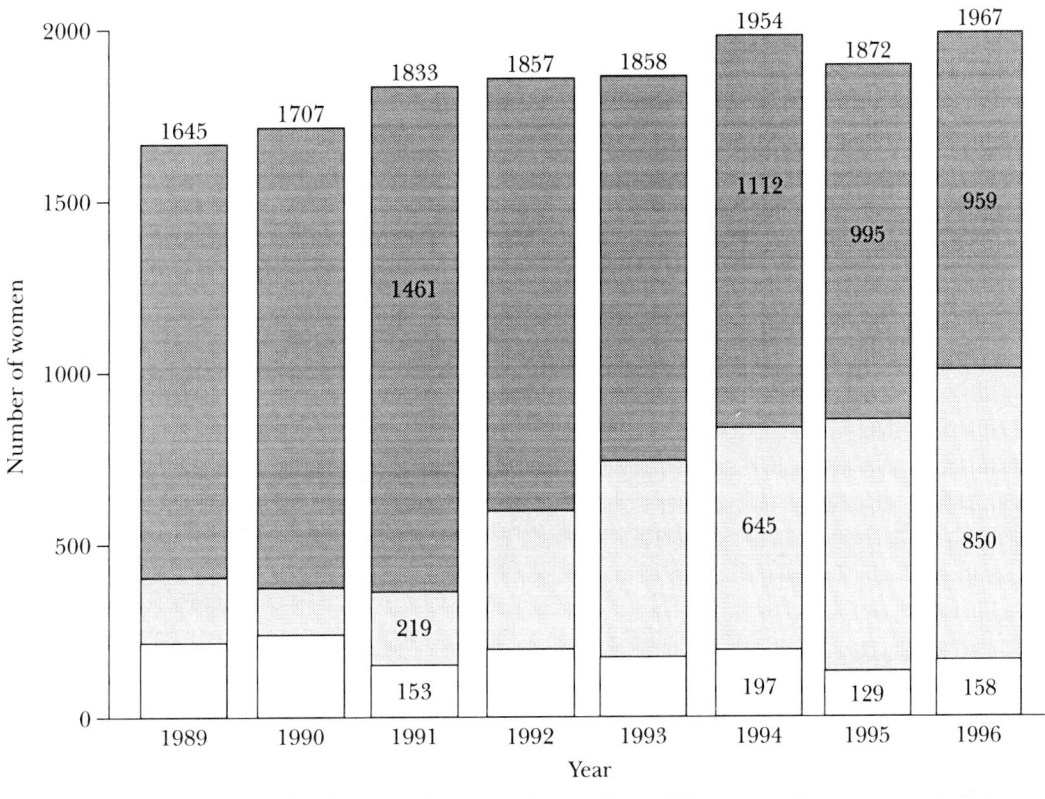

Figure 2 Therapeutic abortions in Royal Infirmary of Edinburgh 1989–96: mifepristone was licensed in July 1991. Adapted from reference 20

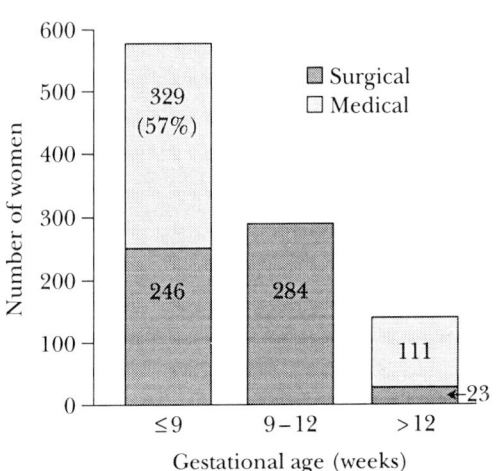

Figure 3 Methods of abortion at different gestational ages in Royal Infirmary of Edinburgh between January and June 1994

(90%)[23]. However, the regimen used in China (25 mg every 12 h for five doses) is reported to be as effective[24]. The minimum dose which induces complete abortion in ~ 95% of women is probably between 100 and 200 mg.

Gestation

The incidence of incomplete abortions and ongoing pregnancies that occur after attempts to induce abortion medically is related to the gestational age. With mifepristone alone, the complete abortion rate ranged from 85% in women within 10 days of a missed menstrual period to approximately 50% at 9 weeks' gestation[7]. The addition of a suitable prostaglandin increases the number of complete abortions at all gestational ages, although the number of failures and the amount of bleeding are greater at more advanced gestation. With a large dose of a potent prostaglandin, e.g. 1 mg gemeprost by vaginal pessary, the incidence of failures and ongoing pregnancies is not significantly greater at gestations of 7–9 weeks as compared to < 7 weeks, although the amount of bleeding and pain is increased[15]. As will be discussed below, the interaction between gestational age and the amount, type and route of administration of prostaglandin is critically important in determining success.

Type of prostaglandin

For over 20 years, prostaglandins in various forms have been used for termination of pregnancy. Initially, natural prostaglandins $PGF_{2\alpha}$ and PGE_2 were infused systemically or injected into the uterus[25]. Longer-acting analogs of the natural prostaglandins, e.g. sulprostone or gemeprost, were developed to be used for cervical ripening prior to vacuum aspiration and for induction of second-trimester abortion. Although abortion can be induced in over 90% of women in the first trimester using repeated administration of these prostaglandins, the side-effects, e.g. vomiting and diarrhea, preclude their routine use in clinical practice[26,27]. However, because antigestogens sensitize the uterus to prostaglandins, the dose required to complete the abortion is very much lower than when used alone and, hence, the side-effects are much reduced.

A range of prostaglandins has been tried in combination with mifepristone for induction of abortion. Sulprostone given by intramuscular injection was used in the initial trials in France, but has been abandoned following a number of cardiovascular catastrophies including a death. Gemeprost in the form of 1-mg vaginal pessaries is licensed for this use in France, the UK and Sweden, and is extremely effective with complete abortion rates of ~ 95% even in pregnancies of up to 9 weeks' gestation. However, the dose of gemeprost is probably excessive and a significant number of women suffer prostaglandin-related side-effects. Randomized trials

Table 1 Medical abortion by gestation using 200 mg mifepristone (oral) and 0.5 mg gemeprost (vaginal pessary). From Baird and Thong, unpublished data

Gestation (weeks)	n	Complete abortion (n)	Incomplete abortion (n)	Ongoing pregnancy (n)
≤ 7	507	493 (97.3%)	11	3
7–9	501	483 (96.4%)	15	3
Total	1008	976 (96.8%)	26	6 (0.6%)

have demonstrated that one-half of a pessary (~ 0.5 mg gemeprost) is as effective as a whole pessary in combination with either 600 or 200 mg of mifepristone[23,28]. Importantly, even in women of gestation > 7 weeks, the incidence of ongoing pregnancies is less than 1%[29] (Table 1). Using one-half of a gemeprost pessary reduces the side-effects and cost, but has the inconvenience that it must be used within a few hours of removal from the vacuum-sealed packet because it is relatively unstable at room temperature. Although gemeprost pessaries are highly effective preparations, the requirement for refrigeration and their high cost limit their widespread use particularly in the developing world.

In a search for a more convenient form of prostaglandin, we originally investigated the uterotonic effect of misoprostol, an orally active stable analog of prostaglandin E_1[30]. Misoprostol is widely used as a therapy for gastric ulcer throughout the world and is stable for long periods at room temperature. We demonstrated that 600 mg of mifepristone in combination with 600 μg of misoprostol orally could induce abortion in pregnancies of up to 56 days[31]. Large clinical trials in France confirmed our original pilot studies that oral misoprostol was a useful alternative to gemeprost or sulprostone, and it received a Product License for use in France for induction of abortion at gestations of < 7 weeks[32]. In our initial studies, we noticed that there were several ongoing pregnancies using oral misoprostol, and a randomized control trial confirmed that at gestations of 7–9 weeks

Table 2 Duration of pregnancy and abortion using 600 mg mifepristone and 600 μg oral misoprostol. Adapted from reference 34

Gestation (days)	n	Complete abortion (n)	Incomplete abortion (n)	Ongoing pregnancy (n)
< 42	123	120 (97.6%)	2	1 (0.8%)
42–49	364	345 (94.8%)	14	5 (1.4%)
50–56	380	355 (93.4%)	19	6 (1.6%)
57–63	235	204 (86.8%)	19	12 (5.1%)
Total	1102	1024 (92.9%)	54	24 (2.2%)

the failure rate was significantly higher than that observed with gemeprost[33]. Of particular concern, the incidence of ongoing pregnancies at this gestation (2–3%) was too high to allow misoprostol to be acceptable for routine clinical use[29]. A large open study conducted by Roussel came to the same conclusion and, as a result, the use of misoprostol is restricted to women of gestation < 7 weeks in France[34] (Table 2).

Although misoprostol is marketed for use orally, several groups have investigated its use placed in the posterior fornix of the vagina. A comparative trial conducted in Aberdeen demonstrated that 800 μg misoprostol vaginally was more effective than a similar dose given orally and was associated with fewer side-effects[35]. However, in the original comparative trial, no analysis was reported with respect to gestation, although a subsequent publication of 360 women using 200 mg mifepristone in combination with 800 μg vaginal misoprostol reported 93% complete abortion (confidence interval 87–97%) in the 105 women at gestations of 7–9 weeks[36]. Comparison of over 1000 abortions performed in women given 200 mg mifepristone showed no overall difference between 0.5 mg gemeprost (Edinburgh) and 800 μg misoprostol (Aberdeen). However, detailed analysis demonstrates that in contrast with those given gemeprost, the ongoing pregnancy rate in women given vaginal misoprostol is significantly higher in women between 7 and 9 weeks' than in those at < 7 weeks' gestation (2.2% vs. 0.34%; $p < 0.004$, Fisher exact test). While it is accepted

that up to 5% of women having medically induced abortion in the first trimester may require vacuum aspiration, there is a risk that the development of the fetus may be compromised if the woman decides to continue with the pregnancy following failure. Although the majority of babies born to women who opt to continue with the pregnancy after failed attempt at medical abortion are normal, fetal abnormalities ranging from mild talipes to absent limbs have been reported to Hoechst-Marion-Roussel.

In summary, misoprostol given by either the oral or vaginal route is a useful, cheaper alternative to gemeprost as the prostaglandin used in combination with mifepristone, but at gestation of 7–9 weeks, the incidence of ongoing pregnancies is too high to be clinically acceptable.

Cervical dilatation

Vacuum aspiration is a well-established, safe technique for termination of pregnancy of up to 14 weeks' gestation, although complications associated with anesthesia, cervical damage and uterine perforation occasionally occur, particularly in young nulliparous women, at advanced gestation and at high parity[37]. These risks can be reduced by 'softening' the cervix with hygroscopic agents, e.g. laminaria, or a range of pharmacological agents which include prostaglandin analogs and antigestogens. In the first trimester, intravaginal gemeprost and misoprostol appear to be equally as effective as oral misoprostol and mifepristone, although the latter approaches have the disadvantage that they require to be given at least 12 h before the vacuum aspiration[38].

Some form of cervical preparation is essential prior to termination of pregnancies at gestations of > 14 weeks in order that the cervix can be safely dilated to a diameter to allow surgical evacuation of the uterus (D & E). There are no published comparisons of the use of prostaglandins and antigestogens for this purpose, although used in combination these drugs are highly effective at inducing abortion medically at this stage.

Mid-trimester abortion

For the past 25 years, the standard method of terminating pregnancy between 14 and 20 weeks' gestation has been D & E[39]. Studies in North America demonstrated that the morbidity and mortality rate was lower using D & E than inducing abortion medically using intra-amniotic hypertonic saline or $PGF_{2\alpha}$. However, a number of large series from Europe have reported successful induction of mid-trimester abortion with either natural prostaglandin E_1 given extra-amniotically or analogs of prostaglandin given by vaginal pessaries[40]. Pretreatment with mifepristone (200–600 mg)[41,42] or epostane[43] prior to administration of the prostaglandin markedly increases the sensitivity of the uterus to prostaglandins. Using this combination, the dose of prostaglandin necessary to induce abortion is reduced markedly with a corresponding reduction in side-effects such as pain, diarrhea and vomiting. Misoprostol can be used either orally or vaginally in place of gemeprost as the prostaglandin in combination with mifepristone for induction of abortion in the mid-trimester of pregnancy[44]. In one randomized study, the mean time from administration of the prostaglandin to abortion was reduced from 15.8 h in the placebo group receiving gemeprost pessaries alone to 6.8 h in the women who were pretreated with 600 mg mifepristone 36 h previously[42]. In subsequent studies, it was demonstrated that equivalent results could be obtained by reducing the dose of mifepristone to 200 mg and that of gemeprost to 1 mg every 6 h[45]. In 365 women (12–24 weeks' gestation) consecutively treated with this regimen in our Center, the median prostaglandin–abortion interval was 8.6 h (range 2–52 h) (Thong and Baird, unpublished data). The cumulative abortion rates were 94 and 99% at 24 and 48 h, respectively. There was a low incidence of side-effects (8% diarrhea) and only one woman suffered local trauma to the cervix. A disadvantage of medically induced abortion is that a minority (~ 10%) require surgical evacuation of the uterus to remove the placenta in whole or in part. However, this surgical procedure is technically less demanding and may have fewer complications than D & E, although uterine rupture has been reported following the use of both gemeprost[46] and misoprostol[47].

Conclusions

In summary, the use of antigestogens in combination with prostaglandin analogs has provided a safe alternative to surgical methods of inducing abortion at all stages of pregnancy. In the very early first trimester (less than 6 weeks' amenorrhea), it is probably more effective than vacuum aspiration and should be the preferred method. From 6 to 9 weeks' gestation, medical and surgical methods are equally effective and safe, and offer women a real choice of method. Studies have demonstrated that women choose different methods for different reasons and that they are more likely to be satisfied with the procedure if they have chosen the method. Thus, by offering women a choice of method, there is an opportunity to make an unpleasant episode less stressful. In the mid-trimester, current evidence suggests that modern medical methods are equally as effective and safe as D & E and demand a lower level of surgical expertise. Thus, at this gestation, the 'best method' may depend not only on the woman's preference but also the facilities and surgical expertise of the medical staff.

References

1. Van Look, P. F. A. and Von Hertzen, H. (1995). Induced abortion: a global perspective. In Baird, D. T., Grimes, D. A. and Van Look, P. F. A. (eds.) *Modern Methods of Inducing Abortion*, pp. 1–24. (Oxford: Blackwell Science)

2. Baird, D. T. (1992). Medical termination of pregnancy. In Edwards, C. R. and Lincoln, D. W. (eds.) *Recent Advances in Clinical Endocrinology and Metabolism*, Vol. 14, pp. 83–94. (Edinburgh and London: Churchill Livingstone)

3. Baulieu, E. E. and Ulmann, A. (1986). Antiprogesterone activity of RU 486 and its contragestive and other applications. *Hum. Reprod.*, **1**, 107–10

4. Bygdeman, M. and Swahn, M.-L. (1985). Progesterone receptor blockage: effect on uterine contractility and early pregnancy. *Contraception*, **32**, 45–51

5. Garfield, R. E. and Baulieu, E. E. (1987). The antiprogesterone steroid RU 486: a short pharmacological and clinical review with emphasis on interruption of pregnancy. *Baill. Clin. Endocrinol. Metab.*, **1**, 207–21

6. Kelly, R. W. (1994). Pregnancy maintenance and parturition: the role of prostaglandin in manipulating the immune and inflammatory response. *Endocr. Rev.*, **15**, 684–706

7. Van Look, P. F. A., and Bygdeman, M. (1989). Antiprogestational steroids: a new dimension in human fertility regulation. *Oxford Rev. Reprod. Biol.*, **11**, 1–60

8. Van der Spuy, Z. M., Jones, D. L., Wright, C. S. W., Piura, B., Paintin, D. B., James, V. H. T. and Jacobs, H. S. (1983). Inhibition of 3-beta-hydroxy steroid dehydrogenase activity in first trimester human pregnancy with trilostane and WIN 32729. *Clin. Endocrinol.*, **19**, 521–32

9. Creinin, M. D. and Darney, P. D. (1993). Methotrexate and misoprostol for early abortion. *Contraception*, **48**, 339–48

10. Darab, D. J., Minkoff, R., Sciote, J. and Sulik, K. K. (1987). Pathogenesis of median facial clefts in mice treated with methotrexate. *Teratology*, **36**, 77–86

11. Wiebe, E. R. (1997). Abortion induced with methotrexate and misoprostol: a comparison of various protocols. *Contraception*, **55**, 159–63

12. Couzinet, B., Le Strat, N., Ulmann, A., Baulieu, E. E. and Schaison, G. (1986). Termination of early pregnancy by the progesterone antagonist RU 486 (mifepristone). *N. Engl. J. Med.*, **315**, 1565–70

13. Cameron, I. T., Michie, A. F. and Baird, D. T. (1986). Therapeutic abortion in early pregnancy with antiprogestogen RU 486 alone or in combination with prostaglandin analogue (gemeprost). *Contraception*, **34**, 459–67

14. UK Multicentre Trial (1990). The efficacy and tolerance of mifepristone and prostaglandin in the first trimester of pregnancy. *Br. J. Obstet. Gynaecol.*, **97**, 480–6

15. UK Multicentre Trial (1997). Final results. The efficacy and tolerance of mifepristone and prostaglandin in termination of pregnancy of less than 63 days gestation. *Contraception*, **55**, 1–5

16. Silvestre, L., Dubois, C., Renault, M., Rezvani, Y., Baulieu, E. E. and Ulmann, A. (1990). Voluntary interruption of pregnancy with mifepristone (RU 486) and a prostaglandin analog. *N. Engl. J. Med.*, **322**, 645–8

17. Ulmann, A., Silvestre, L., Chemama, L., Rezvani, Y., Renault, M., Aguillaume, C. J. and Baulieu, E. E. (1992). Medical termination of early pregnancy with mifepristone (RU 486) followed by a prostaglandin analog. *Acta Obstet. Gynecol. Scand.*, **71**, 278–83

18. Common Services Agency (1994). Abortion statistics. In *Health Briefing 95/23*. (Scotland: Information and Statistics Division, Common Services Agency)

19. Bachelot, A., Cludy, L. and Spira, A. (1992). Conditions for choosing between drug-induced and surgical abortions. *Contraception*, **46**, 435–42

20. Cameron, S. T., Glasier, A. F., Logan, J., Benton, L. and Baird, D. T. (1996). Impact of the introduction of new medical methods on therapeutic abortions at the Royal Infirmary of Edinburgh. *Br. J. Obstet. Gynaecol.*, **103**, 1222–9

21. Rodger, M. W. and Baird, D. T. (1987). Induction of therapeutic abortion in early pregnancy with mifepristone in combination with a prostaglandin pessary. *Lancet*, **2**, 1415–18

22. WHO Task Force on Postovulatory Methods of Fertility Regulation (1993). Termination of pregnancy with reduced doses of mifepristone. *Br. Med. J.*, **307**, 532–6

23. World Health Organization (1995). *Annual Technical Report of WHO Special Programme of Research, Development and Research Training in Human Reproduction*, p. 39. (Geneva: World Health Organization)

24. Sang Guo-wei, Weng Li-ju, Shao Qing-xiang, Du Ming-kun, Wu Xue-zhe, Lu Yu-lan and Cheng Li-nan (1995). Termination of early pregnancy by two regimens of mifepristone with misoprostol and mifepristone with PG 05 – a multicentre randomized clinical trial in China. *Contraception*, **50**, 501–10

25. Bygdeman, M. (1979). In Karim, S. M. N. (ed.) *Practical Applications of Prostaglandins and their Synthesis Inhibitors*, pp. 267–82. (Lancaster: MTP Press)

26. Norman, J. L. E., Thong, K. J., Rodger, M. W. and Baird, D. T. (1992). Medical abortion in women of ≤ 56 days amenorrhoea: a comparison between gemeprost (a PGE$_1$ analogue) alone and mifepristone and gemeprost. *Br. J. Obstet. Gynaecol.*, **99**, 601–6

27. Smith, S. K. and Baird, D. T. (1980). The use of 16-16 dimethyl trans Δ^2 PGE$_1$ methyl ester

(ONO 802) vaginal suppositories for the termination of early pregnancy: a comparative trial. *Br. J. Obstet. Gynaecol.*, **87**, 712–17

28. Rodger, M. W., Logan, A. L. F. and Baird, D. T. (1989). Induction of early abortion with mifepristone (RU 486) and two different doses of prostaglandin pessary (gemeprost). *Contraception*, **39**, 497–502

29. Baird, D. T., Sukchareon, N. and Thong, K. J. (1995). Randomized trial of misoprostol and cervagem in combination with a reduced dose of mifepristone for induction of abortion. *Hum. Reprod.*, **10**, 1521–7

30. Norman, J. E., Thong, K. J. and Baird, D. T. (1991). Increase in uterine contractility and induction of abortion in early pregnancy by misoprostol and mifepristone. *Lancet*, **338**, 1233–6

31. Thong, K. J. and Baird, D. T. (1992). Induction of abortion with mifepristone and misoprostol in early pregnancy. *Br. J. Obstet. Gynaecol.*, **99**, 1004–7

32. Peyron, R., Aubeny, E., Targosz, V., Silvestre, L., Renault, M., Elkik, F., Leclerc, P., Ulmann, A. and Baulieu, E. E. (1993). Early termination of pregnancy with mifepristone (RU 486) and the orally active prostaglandin misoprostol. *N. Engl. J. Med.*, **328**, 1509–13

33. McKinley, C., Thong, K. J. and Baird, D. T. (1993). The effect of dose of mifepristone and gestation on the efficacy of medical abortion with mifepristone and misoprostol. *Hum. Reprod.*, **8**, 1502–5

34. Aubeny, E., Peyron, R., Turpin, C. L., Renault, M., Targosz, V., Silvestre, L., Ulmann, A. and Baulieu, E. E. (1995). Termination of early pregnancy (up to and after 63 days of amenorrhoea) with mifepristone (RU 486) and increasing doses of misoprostol. *Int. J. Fertil.*, **40** (Suppl. 2), 85–91

35. El-Rafaey, H., Rajasekar, D., Abdalla, M., Calder, L. and Templeton, A. A. (1995). Induction of abortion with mifepristone (RU 486) and oral or vaginal misoprostol. *N. Engl. J. Med.*, **332**, 983–7

36. Penney, G. C., McKessock, L., Rispin, R., El-Refaey, H. and Templeton, A. (1995). An effective, low cost regimen for early abortion. *Br. J. Fam. Plann.*, **21**, 5–6

37. Ho, P. C. (1995). Termination of pregnancy between 9 and 14 weeks. In Baird, D. T., Grimes, D. A. and Van Look, P. F. A. (eds.) *Modern Methods of Inducing Abortion*, pp. 54–69. (Oxford: Blackwell Science)

38. Ngai, S. L. W., Yeung, K. C. A., Lao, T. and Ho, P. C. (1996). Oral misoprostol versus mifepristone for cervical dilatation before vacuum aspiration in the first trimester nulliparous pregnancy: a double blind prospective randomised study. *Br. J. Obstet. Gynaecol.*, **103**, 1120–3

39. Grimes, D. A. and Schulz, K. F. (1985). The comparative safety of second trimester abortion methods. In Porter, R. and O'Connor, M. (eds.) *Abortion: Medical Progress and Social Implications*, Ciba Foundation Symposium 115, pp. 83–96. (London: Pitman)

40. Cameron, I. T. and Baird, D. T. (1984). The use of 16,16-dimethyl-trans Δ_2 prostaglandin E$_1$ methyl ester (gemeprost) vaginal pessaries for termination of pregnancy in the early second trimester. A comparison with extra-amniotic prostaglandin E$_2$. *Br. J. Obstet. Gynaecol.*, **91**, 1136–40

41. Urquhart, D. R. and Templeton, A. A. (1990). The use of mifepristone prior to prostaglandin-induced midtrimester abortion. *Hum. Reprod.*, **5**, 883–6

42. Rodger, M. W. and Baird, D. T. (1990). Pretreatment with mifepristone (RU 486) reduces prostaglandin abortion interval in mid trimester therapeutic abortion. *Br. J. Obstet. Gynaecol.*, **97**, 41–5

43. Selinger, M., MacKenzie, I., Gillmer, M. D., Phipps, S. L. and Ferguson, J. (1987). Progesterone inhibition in mid-trimester termination of pregnancy: physiological and clinical effects. *Br. J. Obstet. Gynaecol.*, **94**, 1218–22

44. El-Refaey, H. and Templeton, A. (1995). Induction of abortion in the second trimester by a combination of misoprostol and mifepristone: a randomized comparison between two misoprostol regimens. *Hum. Reprod.*, **10**, 475–8

45. Thong, K. J. and Baird, D. T. (1993). Induction of second trimester abortion with mifepristone and gemeprost. *Br. J. Obstet. Gynaecol.*, **100**, 758–61

46. Norman, J. E. (1995). Uterine rupture during therapeutic abortion in the second trimester using mifepristone and prostaglandin. *Br. J. Obstet. Gynaecol.*, **102**, 332–3

47. Phillips, K., Berry, C. and Mathers, A. M. (1996). Uterine rupture during second trimester termination of pregnancy using mifepristone and a prostaglandin. *Eur. J. Obstet. Gynecol. Reprod. Biol.*, **65**, 175–6

Epidemiological–biological interactions in ovarian cancer

29

R. E. Leake

Introduction

Ovarian cancer remains a major challenge to both cancer researchers and to clinicians. The introduction of platinum-based therapies has significantly improved overall survival, but patients eventually relapse and new therapies are required to treat such patients. In addition to identifying new targets against which to develop these new therapies, it is important to explore whether there is any biological basis for proposing new approaches to reducing the incidence of ovarian cancer. This review examines the biology of the mechanisms by which ovarian cancer is induced and promoted. It also considers the biological fall-out from epidemiological analysis of the disease and then combines the two sets of information to predict possible avenues for future studies on both prevention and treatment.

Epidemiology of ovarian cancer

Preamble

Ovarian cancer is the most frequent cause of death from gynecological malignancy worldwide. Ovarian cancer is the sixth most frequent form of cancer world-wide with an estimated 162 000 incident cases in 1985[1]. Epithelial cystadenocarcinomas constitute the large majority of ovarian malignancies although reliable population-based incidence rates for different histological subtypes of disease are absent. The less frequent germ cell tumors have a younger age distribution. The range of geographical variation for this disease is surprisingly small when compared with the ranges for cancers of other reproductive tissues such as prostate and breast. For example, in northern Europe the estimated incidence rate for 1985 is 12.2/1000 000 per year (based on 8300 cases); in western Europe it is 11.0/100 000 (based on 14 000 cases); in central and eastern Europe it is 10.7/100 000 (8300 cases) and in southern Europe it is 7.8/100 000 (7800 cases).

This relatively small geographical range indicates that diet is not a major factor in incidence of ovarian cancer, and worthwhile approaches to prevention will have to be based on other factors of the disease. It is very clear that there is a genetic component to ovarian cancer risk which is particularly important at younger ages. It has been estimated that women who carry mutations to the *BRCA1* gene (on chromosome 17q) have a 60% lifetime risk of ovarian cancer. A recent series of 30 Canadian families, with either breast or ovarian cancer, identified 12 (40%) with *BRCA1* mutations[2]. Such mutations were found in six of the eight families that contained at least two cases of early-onset breast cancer and two cases of ovarian cancer. This large genetic component of ovarian-cancer risk presents a problem when it comes to the interpretation of epidemiological studies, since many of these studies will have been based on cases who are not homogenous for ovarian-cancer risk. Thus, identification of susceptibles in epidemiological studies, and proper investigation of the interaction of lifestyle factors with susceptibility, will be an important area for future research strategies in understanding ovarian-cancer causation.

Descriptive epidemiology

As can be seen from Table 1, the highest incidence rate of cancer of the ovary is 17.3/100 000 in Ardeche in France, then St Gall in Switzerland (17.0/100 000). High rates are also recorded from four Scandinavian countries: Iceland (16.6/100 000), Denmark (14.9), Sweden (14.6) and Norway (14.6). The other Scandinavian country, Finland, has the 82nd highest rate (9.9). Again, this shows that there is relatively little geographical pattern to the regions with the highest or lowest rates.

Hawaiians and Pacific Polynesian Islanders have higher rates of ovarian cancer than Maoris in whom the incidence is similar to that of non-Maoris in New Zealand. Rates around 15/100 000 are reported in Israel for women born in Europe or America. Most rates in Europe and North America range between 8 and 12/100 000. Rates for US Afro–Americans are about two-thirds of those for Caucasian women in the same community. While women in Asia have a relatively low incidence of ovarian tumors, in the range of 5–7/100 000, Chinese and Japanese who reside in the United States tend to have slightly higher rates, although less than in the white population.

A recent study of migrants from Cyprus, Egypt, Iran, Iraq, Israel, Lebanon, Syria and Turkey to Australia demonstrated lower rates of ovarian cancer in this group than in an Australian-born group[3].

Temporal trends in incidence

There are few long-term series of ovarian-cancer incidence statistics available. In the Nordic countries[4], there have been small increases in incidence rates since the late 1940s. In Denmark, the incidence rate increased from 11.5/100 000 in 1946–50 to 14.9/100 000 in 1983–87. In Finland, the rates have always been lower than in Denmark but they increased from 6.4/100 000 in 1953–55 to 9.9/100 000 in 1983–87. In Norway, the increase was from 10.6/100 000 in 1953–55 to 14.6/100 000 in 1983–87, while in Sweden, the increase was from 12.5/100 000 in 1958–60 to 14.6 in 1983–87. The incidence rates in Norway, Sweden and Denmark for the latter period are very similar and higher than the incidence rate recorded in Finland. The increase in incidence in all countries is small.

Temporal trends in mortality

More data are available to investigate temporal trends in mortality. These data, however, do not necessarily reflect the underlying incidence rate of the disease and are open to influences of variation in the quality of diagnosis and recording on the death certificate, as well as to influences of differences and changes in the outcome of treatment. Nine countries were chosen to give a representative selection of international trends.

In Canada, ovarian-cancer mortality rates remained stable between 1955 and 1973. They declined thereafter, especially when assessed as the truncated rates. Birth-cohort examination

Table 1 Relative incidence of ovarian cancer by geographical site (per 100 000 population)

Registry	n	Incidence
France, Ardeche	155	17.3
Switzerland, St Gall	307	17.0
Iceland	118	16.6
Israel (born Europe or America)	742	15.2
Denmark	3058	14.9
Canada, North-West Territories and Yukon	15	4.7
UK, NE Scotland	300	14.6
Sweden	507	14.6
Norway	2300	14.6
UK, SE Scotland	680	14.0
Czechoslovakia, Bohemia & Morava	5195	13.6
Italy, Latina	38	4.3
USA, Los Angeles (Korean)	10	4.1
India, Ahmedabad	190	4.0
Kuwait (Kuwaitis)	28	3.7
France, Martinique	30	3.2
Israel (non-Jews)	27	2.4
Algeria, Setif	22	1.6
China, Qidong	45	1.5
The Gambia	7	1.4
Mali, Bamako	7	1.0

suggests quite similar rates in successive birth cohorts born before 1925. For cohorts born after that, rates decreased in successive birth cohorts.

In Japan, both the truncated and overall age-adjusted mortality rates have been increasing rapidly since 1955. Birth-cohort examination shows a rapid increase in rates in successive birth cohorts for all age groups examined, particularly those aged over 50.

In Czechoslovakia, a consistent increasing trend was observed for both truncated and overall age-adjusted mortality rates since 1955. Birth-cohort examination suggests a slow but steady increase in rates in successive birth cohorts for age groups over 40.

In Poland, both the truncated and overall age-adjusted mortality rates increased rapidly after 1955 and peaked in 1977. There then followed a decline between 1978 and 1981. Since that time an increase in rates has again occurred. Birth-cohort examination shows an increase in rates in successive birth cohorts. However, the rates in different age groups have shown inconsistent changes in the latter time period.

In Germany, although the overall age-adjusted mortality rates remained relatively stable between 1968 and 1988, the truncated rates have been decreasing since the early 1970s. Birth-cohort examination indicates a slight increase in rates in successive birth cohorts until 1920 and a decreasing trend for cohorts born thereafter.

In Denmark, there has been a small increase in the overall age-adjusted mortality rates of ovarian cancer between 1955 and 1972, and thereafter a small decrease. Although subject to greater variation, this pattern is also evident in the truncated rates. Examination of rates by median year of birth shows no systematic change by birth cohort.

In Italy, both the truncated and overall age-adjusted mortality rates have been increasing rapidly since 1955. Examination by birth cohorts shows an increase in rates in successive birth cohorts for almost all the age groups examined.

In the United Kingdom, the truncated rates of ovarian cancer remained relatively stable until 1978. Since then , a small decrease in rates has occurred. The overall age-adjusted mortality rates, however, showed a slight increase before 1970 and remained relatively stable thereafter. Consequently, examination of rates by birth cohorts suggests an increase in rates in successive birth cohorts until the 1920 birth cohort, and a decrease for cohorts born thereafter.

In Australia, neither the truncated nor the overall age-adjusted mortality rates showed clear time trends before 1965, but they started to decline thereafter. Birth-cohort examination shows a relatively stable rate in successive birth cohorts for those born before 1930, and a rapid decrease thereafter.

Temporal trends in survival

Interpretation of mortality trends should also include discussion of temporal trends in survival. Most data available on this topic are from special hospital series or clinical trials. In Denmark and Scotland there are population-based ovarian-cancer survival data available for over 20 years. In Denmark[5], the 5-year survival rate increased from 24.5% for women diagnosed in 1953–57 to 25.7% for women diagnosed in 1968–72 and to 29.4% in 1983–87. In Scotland, where the national cancer registration and follow-up are of similar quality to that of Denmark, survival rose from 26.5% in women diagnosed between 1968 and 1972 to 29.4% among women diagnosed between 1983 and 1987. These improvements in 5-year survival are thought to be as a result of the introduction of platinum-based drugs.

Analytical epidemiology

Epithelial ovarian cancer is the most common type of ovarian neoplasia[6]. This term encompasses a very wide and diverse range of pathological entities, although by grouping these under a limited number of headings (serous, mucinous endometrioid, clear-cell and undifferentiated), no single group stands out as being different from the rest with regard to epidemiology. As is seen for other female-hormone related cancers, the age–incidence curve tends to flatten off around the menopause.

The risk of ovarian cancer is increased approximately twofold in nulliparous women compared with parous women. An increased risk has been suggested for late age at first birth, early menarche and late menopause, but the evidence is inconsistent. Typical findings are those of Franceschi and colleagues[7] from a large study conducted in northern Italy. With the referent group being those women with a parity of 3 or higher, the risk rose to 2.1 (95% confidence interval (CI) 1.2–3.5) among nulliparous women. Those women who had a first birth after age 25 had a relative risk of 2.0 (95% CI 1.2–3.1) compared with the referent category of women who had a first birth before age 25. Girls who had a menarche at 11 years or younger had an increased risk of 1.5, which was not statistically significant, compared with those who had menarche after age 15 (referent category). Age at menopause was a very important factor in this study. Using women who had a menopause before age 45 as referent, the risk rose among women aged 45–49 at menopause (odds ratio (OR) 2.9, 95% CI 1.1–7.9) to a peak among women who had menopause after the age of 50 years (OR 4.7, 95% CI 1.8–11.5), suggesting that some ovarian component (the corpus luteum?) begins to secrete much higher levels of carcinogen after the age of 45.

At least 15 case–control studies have uniformly indicated that oral contraceptive use is protective against ovarian carcinogenesis[8]. The incidence of epithelial invasive cancer was reduced by approximately 30% in ever users of oral contraceptives, and to a greater extent in long-term users: 5 or more years of use was associated with a 50% reduction in risk, while the relative risk for users of 97 months duration, or more, was only 0.3 (95% CI 0.1–0.7)[9]. The protective effect of oral contraceptives persists for 10 or more years after its use is discontinued and becomes apparent several years after beginning use. Reduced risks of ovarian cancer have been observed for all major histological types of ovarian cancer and among users in both developing and developed countries. The little information available suggests that the effects of oral contraceptives appear to be similar for both malignant and borderline malignant epithelial tumors. Thus, on a population scale, combined oral contraceptives have probably been the major determinant of the (favorable) decrease in ovarian-cancer rates observed in several Western countries over the last 30 years. The open question is whether this effect, only seen so far at premenopausal ages, will continue to protect against ovarian cancer at postmenopausal ages.

Among gravid women, a reported history of infertility has been associated with an odds ratio of 0.86 (95% CI 0.61–1.2) from a meta-analysis[10,11]. When analysis was made according to drug use for infertility (or, more correctly, subfertility), there were differences between those who reported drug treatment (OR 1.4, 95% CI 0.52–3.6) and those who did not (OR 0.84, 95% CI 0.58–1.2): these odds ratios were based on eight cases and 10 controls. Among nulligravid women, the overall odds ratio associated with a history of infertility was 2.1 (95% CI 1.0–4.2). When this nulligravid population was limited to women who reported drug treatment but remained non-pregnant, the odds ratio rose dramatically to 27.0 (95% CI 2.3–315.6), although it is important to note that this was based on only 12 cases and one control. Further research on this potentially vital topic is urgently needed or we may be accused in the future of not heeding the warning signs. Among subfertile women who reported no drug treatment, the odds ratio was 1.6 (95% CI 0.74–3.3) based on 22 cases and 22 controls.

These results are of considerable interest but deserve to be interpreted cautiously. The 12 studies entered into this meta-analysis were considered after they had been analyzed and published, and there was no opportunity for co-ordination in either study design or exposure assessment. Infertility was based on a report from the women that they had been told by a physician that they were infertile: the definition of infertile encompasses both a reduced ability to conceive and to maintain a pregnancy and they may have different etiologies. The findings are based on relatively small numbers of cases and controls in some strata in which the bases of the diagnosis are unknown.

Subsequently, the potential association of ovarian-cancer risk with a history of infertility was investigated in a study in Italy. Based on 195 epithelial ovarian cancers and 1339 controls, fewer ovarian-cancer cases reported use of fertility drugs than controls (OR 0.7, 95% CI 0.2–3.3). Among nulligravid women, five (out of 177) control women compared with zero (out of 36) cancer cases reported having ever used fertility drugs[12]. These null findings were also essentially similar to those reported in a similar study from Toronto[13].

These findings constitute a good basis for the development of a study hypothesis but require confirmation before being accepted as causal. A prospective study designed to explore the hypothesis is proposed in the UK and corresponding studies are under way in France and Australia.

Nutrition and diet remain open issues in ovarian-cancer epidemiology. The American Cancer Society One Million Study showed an elevated risk of ovarian cancer among obese women[14], but the evidence from case–control studies is largely negative, possibly on account of loss of weight secondary to the neoplastic process. Ecological studies found positive correlations with fats, proteins and calories, although these are less strong than for endometrial cancer. Case–control studies showed a possible association with total fat intake and some protection by green vegetables, but further research is required in the area, particularly because diet may be more amenable to intervention than reproductive or menstrual history. The protective effects of fruits and vegetables seen widely for many forms of cancer seem weaker or absent for ovarian cancer[15]. *In vitro* work on the inhibitory effects of various retinoic acid derivatives has been reported by Bast and colleagues[16].

Lactose has been proposed on biological grounds to be potentially associated with the risk of ovarian cancer. A recent large case–control study from Canada has found that neither lactose intolerance nor average daily intake of lactose or free galactose was associated with the risk of ovarian cancer. Lactose intake or intolerance did not appear to modify the protective effects of parity and oral-contraceptive use[17].

There is no evidence that cigarette smoking affects the risk of ovarian cancer in women of any age[18]. Four studies have investigated the association between ovarian-cancer risk and alcohol consumption. No study has demonstrated an increased risk of ovarian cancer among alcohol drinkers, with two studies suggesting a protective effect of heavy alcohol consumption against ovarian cancer in young women[19].

In all seven case–control studies which examined coffee intake, users had an increased risk of ovarian cancer although the elevation in risk was statistically significant in only two studies[20]. Comparing users with non-users, the odds ratio was between 1.1 and 1.3 in five studies, 1.4 in a further study and 1.9 in the remaining study. A Mantel–Haenszel analysis produced a (conservative) estimate of the pooled odds ratio of 1.3 (95% CI 1.1–1.5). Although the overall analysis reveals a marginal, significant increase in risk of ovarian cancer, bias from unidentified sources or chance cannot yet be ruled out[20].

Occupational factors have been investigated in a cross-sectional study of 159 000 women in Torino[21]. Metal, wood and clothing manufacturers showed a significantly increased risk of ovarian cancer.

Risk factors for benign ovarian teratomas, histologically confirmed in women aged below 65 years, have been investigated in a case–control study conducted in Milan[22]. Four of 77 cases and two of 231 controls reported a history of infertility, the corresponding odds ratio being 8.3 (95% CI 1.3–54). This gives some support to the association found of infertility with malignant tumors of the ovary. However, there was no clear association between parity and the risk of benign ovarian teratoma: in comparison with nulliparae, the estimated relative risks were

1.1 and 0.7 respectively for women reporting one or two or more births. No relation emerged between marital status, age at menarche, menstrual-cycle pattern, menopausal status, abortion history, age at first pregnancy, oral-contraceptive use and risk of benign ovarian teratomas[22]. These findings differ markedly from those found with malignant disease.

Biological and epidemiological interactions

The normal ovary is a complex structure which is primarily designed to make available a mature follicle such that fertilization of the latter can take place after the follicle is released from the ovary. In addition to ovulation, the main role of the ovary is to synthesize and secrete the female sex steroids: estradiol and progesterone. The principal reproductive function of the sex steroids is to prepare the endometrium for implantation of the fertilized egg and then maintain the pregnancy, once established. In evolutionary terms, the healthy woman was designed to be pregnant. Given that ovulation does not occur in women who are breast-feeding, one can argue that ovulation was designed to occur as rarely as once every 2 years. This would give a lifetime value of about 20 ovulations (i.e. 10 per ovary) and, therefore, only this number of subsequent repairs of the surface ovarian epithelium. In contrast, a woman who goes through life with normal menstrual cycles, but does not become pregnant, is likely to undergo 480 ovulations and repairs (240 per ovary). Since the vast majority of ovarian cancers are epithelial cancers, the working hypothesis is that ovarian cancer arises because of promotion of transformed epithelial cells during the course of the repair of surface epithelium damaged by ovulation. The rapid increase in relative risk as women move from menopause before 45 years to menopause after 50 years would suggest that the major carcinogens that cause such transformation may be locally produced by some ovarian component (e.g. corpus luteum). Work on point mutations in p53 has provided strong evidence that ovarian cancer is monoclonal, rather than arising from many different transformations of surface epithelial cells (or inclusions).

To explore the possibilities of prevention of ovarian cancer through endocrine manipulations, it is first necessary to review the endocrine control of the functional ovary. Follicular maturation is under the control of the gonadotropins, follicle-stimulating hormone (FSH) and luteinizing hormone (LH). These glycoproteins act through the plasma membrane receptors on their target cells. Simplistically, in the follicular phase of the ovarian cycle, FSH can be said to prime the maturing follicle (an event begun prior to the previous menstruation). Concurrently, LH acts on the theca cells to induce androgen synthesis. The androgens are secreted across to the neighbouring granulosa cells, where they are converted to estrogens by the enzyme aromatase. Aromatase action is stimulated by FSH in a process which is activated by the active androgen-receptor complex[23,24]. The LH surge that promotes ovulation involves local release of prostaglandins, together with FSH- and LH-induced release of plasminogen activator[25]. The plasmin, released by the action of plasminogen activator (uPA), is thought to mediate the release of the oocyte from the follicle wall[25]. This whole process appears to be under the control of transforming growth factor-β (TGF-β), and a critical part of the malignant transformation may relate to a changed response of uPA-secreting cells to TGF-β[26]. The role of uPA, as an important controlling element in the process of invasion, is now well established not only in ovarian cancer, but also in breast and many other cancers[27,28].

A further action of FSH on the granulosa cells is to induce synthesis of LH receptors. Thus, once ovulation is successfully completed, the granulosa cells can give rise to the corpus luteum which, under the continued action of LH, synthesizes and secretes the progesterone. Although the principal role of progesterone is to induce differentiation of, and invagination into, the endometrial epithelial cells, there is a secondary role of progesterone in the ovary itself. This action is, of course, mediated by the progesterone receptor.

Progesterone-receptor (PR) activity in the ovary is unusual. In most reproductive tissues, estrogens act through their receptor (ER) to induce synthesis of PR. However, PR is found in the ovary often in the absence of ER[29]. Indeed, it is thought that activated PR actually primes the differentiation of the epithelial cells. Breakdown of this control may be another step in the malignant process since ovarian cancer is associated with a decrease in PR and an increase in ER[30].

The role of paracrine agents, such as TGF-β, has already been alluded to. Normal ovarian thecal cells synthesize and secrete TGF-α (an analog of epidermal growth factor (EGF) which binds to and activates the EGF receptor with similar affinity to EGF). Since both thecal and granulosa cells have adequate EGF receptors[31] it is assumed that TGF-α causes growth responses in both cell types. Normal ovarian surface epithelium also stains strongly for both EGF and its receptor[31]. This supports the hypothesis that the postovulation repair mechanism is, at least in part, EGF-driven. Interestingly, TGF-α levels are detectable in almost all ovarian epithelial-cell cancers (over 90%) and very much elevated in some[32], suggesting loss of normal growth control. However, EGF receptor is only detected in about 45% of ovarian epithelial-cell cancers[33] so that EGF/TGF-α-induced growth promotion is not the only mechanism in ovarian cancer.

Transforming growth factor-β is also synthesized and secreted by the thecal cells. However, thecal cells do not appear to have TGF-β receptors and the main target is thought to be the granulosa cells, although ovarian-cancer cells in culture show marked growth inhibition by TGF-β, leading to the concept that a balance of control by TGF-α and -β may regulate the progression of some ovarian cancers[16,34]. A dose-dependent effect of LH on ovarian-cancer cells *in vitro* has shown that the inhibitory process is blocked if anti-TGF-β antibody is added prior to LH (the TGF-β-neutralizing antibody also gives growth stimulation in the control cells, suggesting that this ovarian-cancer cell line (OAW 42) is normally down-regulated by TGF-β).

Ovarian cancer is complex because of the large number of histological cell types that may be transformed. Even if attention is confined to epithelial cancers, classification is difficult. However, Malkasian and colleagues[35] have concluded (from a study of 1938 women) that the behavior of different cell types was similar when compared stage for stage and grade for grade. For example, mucinous cystadenocarcinomas tended to be low-grade and low-stage whereas serous cystadenocarcinomas tended to be high-grade and high-stage. Nevertheless, Stage-1 Grade-1 survival at 20 years was very similar for serous and mucinous tumors. Our own studies have failed to demonstrate any dramatic differences among the different histological subgroups of ovarian cancers in terms of content of either growth factors or their receptors[32,33].

There are differences in the incidence of ER and PR according to histological type[30,36]. If the tumor contains both functional ER and PR then the survival chance is better irrespective of cell type[30,37]. Unfortunately, ER and PR are only found together in about 20% of ovarian cancers and so ER-mediated approaches to therapy have, at best, limited application. Almost all ovarian cancers contain androgen receptor (AR). This may be a consequence for the requirement of AR to mediate the FSH-induced aromatase conversion of androgens to estrogens in the granulosa cells. Aromatase activity is retained in only about one-third of ovarian epithelial cell cancers[38,39]. Thus, if local estrogen synthesis and/or functional estrogen receptor is required for the early promotion of ovarian cancer, this requirement is lost by most tumors before they are clinically detectable.

About 90% of ovarian cancers also contain glucocorticoid receptors (GR)[40]. Ovarian-cancer cells grown in culture respond to the synthetic glucocorticoid dexamethasone[41]. The responses include 95% inhibition of uPA secretion, 50% inhibition of growth and pronounced morphological changes. The clinical significance of these *in vitro* observations is not clear since, *in vivo*, there is presumably a sustained, physiologically effective supply of glucocorticoid.

Prevention

Our baseline information is that:

(1) Most ovarian cancers are cancers of the surface epithelium or inclusions thereof;

(2) Procedures which reduce the numbers of ovulations are associated with a marked reduction in the risk of ovarian cancer.

Putting these two together, it follows that the repair mechanisms which are activated after ovulation may also be the mechanisms involved in the promotion of transformed cells into tumor. These mechanisms are thought, at least in part, to involve EGF receptor activation by either EGF or, more likely, TGF-α. Regulation of these growth factors by steroid hormones has been shown *in vitro* and the most effective known agent for reducing incidence of ovarian cancer is the contraceptive pill. However, it is not clear whether the effect of the pill is direct action of the steroids or is due to feedback onto the hypothalamic–pituitary axis, resulting in reduced levels of gonadotropins. Further, another anterior pituitary hormone, prolactin, may also have a role. Ovarian cancer is higher in subfertile patients and a proportion of these have hyperprolactinemia.

There may be as much as a fourfold increased risk of ovarian cancer for women who enter menopause after the age of 50, compared with women who become menopausal at 45 years. This suggests that the older the ovary, the more likely it is that the ovarian epithelial cells will contain transformations which, when promoted by postovulation growth repairs, will lead to ovarian cancer. Thus, prevention measures – application of agents to reduce cell division in surface epithelium – should be applied before the age of 45.

Possible additive endocrine/paracrine strategies include:

(1) Blocking gonadotropin secretion;

(2) Blocking EGF receptor function;

(3) Promoting apoptosis;

(4) Promoting selective TGF-β down-regulation of surface epithelium.

The contraceptive pill is the most obvious agent to use. However, some people may have clinical or ethical reasons for not wishing to go on the pill. An additional complication is that taking the pill in this late stage of reproductive life may raise the incidence of breast cancer. Because of the relative incidence rates, a small rise in incidence of breast cancer could give a net balance of an excess of total cancers, even if the reduction of ovarian cancer is large. Another approach might be use of luteinizing hormone-releasing hormone (LHRH) agonists, though there would be objections to giving such agents to 'well women' of 45 years of age. As our understanding of the cell biology of the ovary improves, so it may become more possible to select a specific intervention which does not have undesirable side-effects. This would tend to exclude strategies aimed at cell-signaling intermediates (e.g. EGF receptor-related tyrosine kinase has been shown to be elevated in platinum-resistant ovarian cancer cells[42]). Steroid and gonadotropin regulation of apoptosis in normal ovarian cells requires investigation[43].

The priority for prevention strategies should continue to revolve around the potential for oral-contraceptive use to halve (or more) the risk of ovarian cancer. There is a need to confirm that this protection continues in the long term, i.e. after use ends. It is also important to establish whether the protective effect is maintained after the menopause. Identification of the biological mechanisms underlying this association could serve to greatly increase the prospects for ovarian-cancer prevention.

Acknowledgements

The work described in this review is part of an ongoing collaboration with Peter Boyle and I am extremely grateful for his continued, valuable advice. I am very pleased to thank Ian Scott and Frank Sharp for their efforts to ensure that I understand something of the clinical problems of ovarian cancer and to Mike Wells for providing pathological guidance. I am delighted to thank all the members of my research group who have helped with our ovarian cancer work, especially Owen Owens and Andy Barbour.

References

1. Parkin, D. M., Ferlay, J. and Pisani, P. (1993). Estimates of the worldwide incidence of eighteen major cancers in 1985. *Int. J. Cancer*, **54**, 594–606

2. Simard, J., Tonin, P., Durocher, F. *et al.* (1994). Common origins of *BRCA1* mutations in Canadian breast and ovarian cancer families. *Nat. Genet.*, **8**, 392–8

3. MacCredie, M., Coates, M. and Grulich, A. (1994). Cancer incidence in migrants to New South Wales form the Middle East. *Cancer Causes Control*, **5**, 414–21

4. Hakulinen, T., Andersen, A. A., Malker, B., Pukkula, E., Schou, G. and Tulinius, H. (1986). Trends in cancer incidence in the Nordic countries. *Acta Pathol. Microbiol. Immunol. Scand.*, **94** (Suppl. 228)

5. Kruger, K. S. and Storm, H. H. (1993). Female genital organs. *Acta Pathol. Microbiol. Immunol. Scand.*, **101**, 107–21

6. Scully, R. E. (1985). Ovary. In Hempson, D. E. and Albores-Saaveba, J. (eds.) *Pathology of Incipient Neoplasia*, pp. 279–93. (Philadelphia: W. B. Saunders)

7. Franceschi, S., La Vecchia, C. and Negri E. (1994). Fertility drugs and risk of epithelial ovarian cancer in Italy. *Hum. Reprod.*, **9**, 1673–5

8. Stanford, J. L. (1991). Oral contraception and neoplasia of the ovary. *Contraception*, **43**, 543–56

9. Vessey, M. P. and Painter, R. (1995). Endometrial and ovarian cancer and oral contraceptives – findings in a large cohort study. *Br. J. Cancer*, **71**, 1340–2

10. Whittemore, A. S., Harris, R. and Intyre J. (1992). Collaborative Ovarian Cancer Group. Characteristics relating to ovarian cancer risk: collaborative analysis of 12 US case–control studies. II. Invasive ovarian cancers in white women. *Am. J. Epidemiol.*, **136**, 1184–203

11. Harris, R., Whittemore, A. S. and Intyre, J. (1992). Collaborative Ovarian Cancer Group. Characteristics relating to ovarian cancer risk: collaborative analysis of 12 US case–control studies. III. Epithelial tumors of low malignant potential in white women. *Am. J. Epidemiol.*, **136**, 1204–11

12. Franceschi, S., La Vecchia, C., Negri, E., Guarneri, S., Montella, M., Conti, E. and Parazzini, F. (1994). Fertility drugs and risk of epithelial ovarian cancer in Italy. *Hum. Reprod.*, **9**, 1673–5

13. Risch, H., Marret, L. D. and Howe, G. R. (1994). Parity, contraception, infertility and the risk of epithelial ovarian cancer. *Am. J. Epidemiol.*, **140**, 585–97

14. Lew, E. A. and Garfinkel, L. (1979). Variations in mortality by weight among 750 000 men and women. *J. Chronic Dis.*, **32**, 563–76

15. Steinmetz, K. A. and Potter, J. D. (1991). Vegetable, fruit, and cancer. I. Epidemiology. *Cancer Causes Control*, **2**, 325–58

16. Bast, R. C., Boyer, C. M., Xu, F. J., Weiner, J., Dabel, R. M., Havrilesky, L., Hurteau, J., Elbendary, A. and Burchuck, A. (1995). Cell growth regulation in human epthelial ovarian cancer. In Leake, R., Gore, M. and Ward, R. H. (eds.) *The Biology of Gynaecological Cancer*, pp. 119–27. (London: RCOG Press)

17. Risch, H., Jain, M., Marret, L. D. and Howe, G. R. (1994). Dietary lactose intake, lactose intolerance and the risk of epithelial ovarian cancer in southern Ontario. *Cancer Causes Control*, **5**, 540–8

18. IARC (International Agency for Research on Cancer) (1986). *Monographs on the Evaluation of the Carcinogenic Risk of Chemicals to Man*, Vol. 38, *Tobacco Smoking*. (Lyon: IARC)

19. IARC (International Agency for Research on Cancer) (1988). *Monographs on the Evaluation of Carcinogenic Risk to Humans*, Vol. 44, *Alcohol Drinking*. (Lyon: IARC)

20. IARC (International Agency for Research on Cancer) (1991). *Monographs on the Evaluation of Carcinogenic Risk to Humans*, Vol. 51, *Coffee, Tea, Mate, Methylxanthines (Caffeine, Theophylline, Theobromine) and Methylglyoxal*. (Lyon: IARC)

21. Costantini, A. S., Piratsu, R., Lagorio, S., Miligi, L. and Costa, G. (1994). Studies in cancer among female workers: methods and preliminary results from a record-linkage system in Italy. *J. Occup. Med.*, **36**, 1180–6

22. Parazzini, F., La Vecchia, C., Negri, E., Moroni, S. and Villa, A. (1995). Risk factors for benign ovarian teratomas. *Br. J. Cancer*, **71**, 644–6

23. Daniel, S. A. J. and Armstrong, D. T. (1980). Enhancement of FSH induced aromatase activity by androgens in cultured rat granulosa cells. *Endocrinology*, **107**, 1027–33

24. Hillier, S. G. and De Zwart, F. A. (1985). Evidence that granulosa cell aromatase induction/activation by follicle-stimulating hormones is an androgen receptor regulated process *in vitro*. *Endocrinology*, **109**, 1303–5

25. Beers, W. H., Strickland, S. and Reich, E. (1985). Ovarian plasminogen activator: relationship to ovulation and hormonal regulation. *Cell*, **6**, 387–94

26. Laiko, M. and Keski-Oja, J. (1989). Growth factors in the regulation of pericellular proteolysis: a review. *Cancer Res.*, **49**, 2533–53

27. Janicke, F., Scmitt, M., Hafter, R., Hollreider, A., Babic, R., Ulm, K. and Graeff, H. (1990). Urokinase-type plasminogen activator (uPA) antigen is a predictor of early relapse in breast cancer. *Fibrinolysis*, **4**, 69–78

28. Pedersen, H., Brunner, N., Francis, D., Osterlind, K., Ronne, E., Hoi-Hansen, H., Dano, K. and Grondahl-Hansen, J. (1994). Prognostic impact of urokinase receptor and type 1 plasminogen activator in squamous and large cell lung cancer tissues. *Cancer Res.*, **54**, 120–3

29. Soutter, W. P. and Leake, R. E. (1987). Steroid hormone receptors in gynaecological cancers. *Recent Adv. Obstet. Gynaecol.*, **15**, 175–94

30. Harding, M., Cowan, S., Hole, D., Davis, J., Kennedy, J. and Leake, R. E. (1990). Oestrogen and progesterone receptors in ovarian cancer. *Cancer*, **65**, 486–91

31. Scurry, J. P., Hammand, K. A., Astley, S. B., Leake, R. E. and Wells, M. (1994). Immunoreactivity of antibodies to epidermal growth factor, transforming growth factors alpha and beta and epidermal growth factor receptor in the premenopausal ovary. *Pathology*, **26**, 130–3

32. Owens, O. J., Stewart, C. and Leake, R. E. (1991). Growth factor concentration and distribution in ovarian cancer. *Br. J. Cancer*, **64**, 1177–81

33. Owens, O. J., Stewart, C., Brown, I. and Leake, R. E. (1991). Epidermal growth factor receptors in human ovarian cancer. *Br. J. Cancer*, **64**, 907–10

34. Hurteau, J., Rodriguez, G. C., Berchuck, A. and Bast, R. C. (1994). Transforming growth factor beta inhibits proliferation of human ovarian cancer cells obtained from ascites. *Cancer*, **74**, 93–9

35. Malkasian, G. D., Melton, L. J., O'Brian, P. C. and Greene, M. H. (1984). Prognostic significance of histologic classification and grading of epithelial malignancies of the ovary. *Am. J. Obstet. Gynecol.*, **149**, 274–84

36. Topilla, M., Tyler, J. P. P., Fay, R. and Hudson, C. (1986). Steroid receptors in human ovarian malignancy. A review of 4 years tissue collection. *Br. J. Obstet. Gynaecol.*, **93**, 986–92

37. Iversen, O. E., Skaarland, E. and Utaaker, E. (1980). Steroid receptor content in human ovarian tumors: survival of patients relative to steroid receptor content. *Gynecol. Oncol.*, **23**, 65–76

38. Kuknel, R., Dellemarre, J. F. M., Rao, B. R. and Stolk, J. G. (1986). Correlation of aromatase activity and steroid receptors in human ovarian carcinoma. *Anticancer Res.*, **6**, 889–92

39. Rao, B. and Slotman, B. J. (1991). Endocrine factors in common epithelial ovarian cancer. *Endocr. Rev.*, **12**, 175–87

40. Galli, M. C., De Giovanni, C., Nicoletti, G., Grilli, S., Nanni, P., Prodi, G., Gola, G., Rocchetta, R. and Orlandi, C. (1981). The occurrence of multiple steroid hormone receptors in disease-free and neoplastic human ovary. *Cancer*, **47**, 1297–302

41. Amin, W., Karlan, B. Y. and Littlefield, B. A. (1987). Glucocorticoid sensitivity of OVCA433 human ovarian carcinoma cells: inhibition of plasminogen activators, cell growth and morphological alterations. *Cancer Res.*, **47**, 6040–5

42. Leake, R., Barber, A., Owens, S., Langdon, S. and Miller, W. R. (1995). Growth factors and receptors in ovarian cancer. In Sharp, F., Mason, P., Blackett, T. and Berek, J. (eds.) *Ovarian Cancer 3*, pp.99–108. (London: Chapman & Hall)

43. Leake, R. E. (1995). Cell cycle. In Hillier, S., Kitchener, H. and Nielson, K. (eds.) *Scientific Essentials of Reproductive Medicine*, pp. 26–31. (London: W. B. Saunders)

Chemotherapy for ovarian cancer   30

J. S. Berek, M. Markman, W. P. McGuire, J. T. Thigpen and R. F. Ozols

Prognostic factors

Patients with limited disease are at low risk for recurrence if all of the following factors are present: low-grade disease, an intact ovarian capsule prior to surgery, no tumor on the external surface of the ovary, negative peritoneal cytology, no ascites and no extraovarian tumor. Patients with any one of the following are at high risk for recurrence: high-grade disease, pre-operative rupture of the ovarian capsule, tumor on the external surface of the ovary, positive peritoneal cytology, ascites or extraovarian tumor. As will be subsequently described, these categories will dictate further therapy after surgical resection[1,2].

The survival of patients with advanced disease correlates with the volume of disease. Patients with minimal residual disease (largest nodule < 0.5 cm diameter) at the time that the abdomen is opened (stages IIIa and IIIb) demonstrate the best survival. Within this subset, those who are free of gross disease (stage IIIa) achieve the best survival. Patients who have bulkier disease (stage IIIc) but reach minimal residual status as a result of surgery have a survival intermediate between the other two groups. Patients who have bulky disease (stage IIIc) that cannot be successfully bulk reduced and those with stage IV disease have the poorest survival[1,2].

Stages I and II

Approximately 15–20% of patients with ovarian cancer will be diagnosed when they have early-stage disease[3,4]. A comprehensive laparotomy is critical to evaluate all potential sites of disease including diaphragm, lymph nodes and peritoneal surfaces. After completion of such a laparotomy, patients are defined as either having low- or high-risk disease. Patients with low-risk disease have stages Ia and Ib tumors, which are well differentiated. These patients have a > 90% 5-year survival and do not require postoperative therapy[3]. High-risk, early-stage patients include all stage II, stage Ic and stage I patients with poorly differentiated tumors. In the United States, postoperative therapy has been routinely recommended with chemotherapy being the preferred modality. In the current Gynecologic Oncology Group (GOG) trial, there is a randomization to three to six cycles of carboplatin (dosed to an area under the curve (AUC) of 7.5) plus paclitaxel (175 mg/m^2) in a 3-h infusion. Recent studies from Europe have suggested that in some early-stage patients with high-risk features, a policy of observation until disease progression may produce the same long-term survival compared with immediate treatment. Frequently, patients are not adequately staged at the time of the initial surgical procedure. It remains uncertain as to what the optimum management is in this situation, and options include a relaparotomy to accurately stage the patient or to use chemotherapy based on the assumption that disease may be present that was not detected at the initial surgery.

Stages III and IV

The majority of patients with ovarian cancer will have International Federation of Obstetrics and Gynecology (FIGO) stages III and IV disease. Surgery remains a cornerstone of initial treatment with an attempt to remove as much disease as technically feasible. Patients who present with malignant pleural effusions are also usually candidates for maximal cytoreductive surgery even though they have extraperitoneal disease. However, patients with liver metastases or solid tumors outside the peritoneal cavity are not likely to benefit from cytoreductive surgery. Following surgery, patients should receive chemotherapy with the current state-of-the-art treatment consisting of paclitaxel together with a platinum compound (carboplatin or cisplatin). Clinical trials are currently in progress to evaluate different doses and schedules of paclitaxel with either cisplatin or carboplatin. Clinical trials are also investigating the use of high-dose chemotherapy, which requires hematological support. New agents with activity in recurrent disease have recently been identified, such as gemcitabine and topotecan, and their incorporation into the initial therapy of patients with ovarian cancer is under investigation.

The performance of a primary cytoreductive or debulking operation should be the standard of care for advanced ovarian cancer[5]. This is true for all stage III tumors and some selected stage IV (e.g. those with small pleural effusions only). Surgeries should be performed by those who are well trained in their performance, i.e. a gynecological oncologist, to maximize the probability of success. In women having undergone exploratory surgery without success, one can initiate chemotherapy and then attempt an interval debulking, which is associated with a prolonged survival compared with those who do not undergo such a procedure.

The European Organization for the Research and Treatment of Cancer (EORTC) study is the first prospective randomized trial to demonstrate that cytoreductive surgery improves outcome in patients with advanced ovarian cancer[6]. Previous retrospective studies and some meta-analyses failed to demonstrate that cytoreductive surgery had a significant impact on survival. In the European study, patients underwent an initial attempt at cytoreductive surgery and, if unsuccessful, they were eligible for this trial. They were treated with three cycles of chemotherapy and then randomized to interval debulking surgery followed by three cycles of chemotherapy or no interval surgery. The major difference from the trial currently in progress in

the United States is that paclitaxel and cisplatin are being used as the chemotherapy regimen instead of cyclophosphamide and cisplatin.

Based on a phase II study demonstrating the activity of paclitaxel in previously treated patients with ovarian cancer, the GOG performed a pivotal study in previously untreated patients with advanced ovarian cancer who were randomized to receive the prior standard regimen of cisplatin plus cyclophosphamide or cisplatin plus paclitaxel[7]. All patients received six cycles of chemotherapy and underwent clinical restaging followed by second-look laparotomy in those patients who were clinically disease-free. On the basis of the results of this study, cisplatin plus paclitaxel became the new standard regimen in the GOG.

Cisplatin plus paclitaxel had a superior response rate compared with cisplatin plus cyclophosphamide in patients with suboptimal stages III and IV ovarian cancer. In particular, the clinical complete remission (CCR) rate was improved by 20%.

Patients who achieved CCR were evaluated surgically by a second-look laparotomy. Although there was no significant difference in the percentage of negative second-look laparotomies between patients treated with or without paclitaxel, there was a markedly higher percentage of patients who had microscopic residual disease in those treated with paclitaxel (14% *vs.* 4%). The survival of patients with microscopic positive residual disease at second-look laparotomy is almost as favorable as that for patients who achieve a negative second look.

There was a 5-month improvement in median progression-free survival (PFS) for patients treated with the cisplatin plus paclitaxel regimen compared with those receiving cisplatin plus cyclophosphamide. In ovarian cancer, an improvement in PFS is usually associated with a concomitant improvement in long-term survival.

The median survival for patients treated with cisplatin plus cyclophosphamide was 24 months. In contrast, patients who received cisplatin plus paclitaxel had an improvement in median survival to 38 months. It is particularly noteworthy that this improvement was achieved in patients who had suboptimal stages III and IV ovarian cancer. It is anticipated that paclitaxel plus platinum chemotherapy may have an even more significant impact on survival of patients with less disease at the time chemotherapy is initiated, i.e. optimal stage III ovarian cancer patients who have no residual tumor nodule > 1 cm.

Although GOG protocol 111 established the superiority of cisplatin plus paclitaxel, numerous questions remain regarding the optimum use of paclitaxel and a platinum compound in ovarian cancer. Preclinical studies have demonstrated that prolonged exposure of tumor cells to paclitaxel increases cell kill. Clinical trials are currently evaluating the relative role of 3-, 24-, and 96-h infusions of paclitaxel. The duration of treatment has an impact on the patterns of toxicity with the shorter durations having less myelosuppression but perhaps being associated with increased neurotoxicity. In prospective trials of patients with bulky stage III and stage IV disease, carboplatin plus cyclophosphamide are as effective as cisplatin plus cyclophosphamide but associated with less toxicity. Most clinical trials comparing carboplatin and cisplatin have similarly demonstrated equal efficacy, although some investigators feel that carboplatin may not be as effective as cisplatin in patients with small-volume stage III disease. This issue is being specifically addressed in GOG protocol 158.

In a bifactorial study, 401 patients with platinum-resistant ovarian cancer were randomized to receive either paclitaxel 135 mg/m^2 or 175 mg/m^2 every 3 weeks and then re-randomized to receive the paclitaxel as either a 3-h or a 24-h infusion[8]. Analysis showed no difference between either dose or schedule with respect to response, PFS, overall survival or toxicity except for significantly decreased leukopenia and neutropenia with the 3-h infusion. Thus, the study shows that, at least in the setting of second-line therapy, there is no advantage to the higher dose or longer schedule, and the toxicity profile favors the shorter infusion. One caveat was provided by an analysis of the four patient subgroups in that the higher dose given over 24 h yielded a response rate of 24%, whereas the other three subgroups produced response rates of 14–16%. Although this difference was not statistically significant, it at least leaves open the question of differences between doses and schedules. Whether these results can be extrapolated to front-line therapy remains to be seen.

A phase I trial demonstrated that paclitaxel could be combined with carboplatin with both drugs being administered in full therapeutic doses[9]. This was a highly active regimen that was well tolerated. The carboplatin dose was individualized for each patient based on the formula developed by Calvert: dose (mg) = (target AUC × GFR) + 25[2]. The creatinine clearance was used to substitute for glomerular filtration rate (GFR) and was either measured or calculated based on patients' serum creatinine.

In an effort to address the issues regarding the role of cisplatin versus carboplatin and the optimum schedule paclitaxel, the GOG is performing a prospective randomized trial in previously untreated patients with optimal stage III disease in which patients are randomized into two different regimens. Most patients receiving the cisplatin plus paclitaxel regimen require hospitalization for the 24-h infusion, whereas the carboplatin plus paclitaxel regimen group is an outpatient treatment. It is this group of patients in whom some investigators have felt that carboplatin may not be as effective as cisplatin (small-volume stage III disease). Furthermore, there is experimental evidence to suggest that longer infusions of paclitaxel may be superior to shorter infusions. Consequently, this prospective randomized trial will compare a shorter infusion of paclitaxel together with carboplatin versus a 24-h infusion of paclitaxel combined with cisplatin.

While shorter infusions of paclitaxel in combination with carboplatin offer the advantage of ease of ambulatory administration, preclinical and at least some clinical evidence suggests that duration of exposure of tumor cells to paclitaxel may be critical and that longer infusions may offer a clinical advantage. The only study of a prolonged infusion (96 h) to date in ovarian cancer showed no significant activity. The patient population, however, had received from two to seven prior regimens; hence, the results do not rule out a therapeutic advantage for a longer infusion. The GOG is currently evaluating a regimen that includes a prolonged infusion of paclitaxel plus cisplatin as front-line therapy for patients with bulky advanced disease compared with standard paclitaxel plus cisplatin. This trial is still actively accruing patients.

Dose-intensity issues

Preclinical and retrospective studies have suggested that dose intensity is an important factor in the optimum treatment of patients with ovarian cancer. Controversy existed regarding what is the optimum dose for the platinum compounds (cisplatin and carboplatin). Uncontrolled phase II trials have also suggested that higher doses of paclitaxel may be superior in previously treated patients with advanced disease[10]. Intraperitoneal chemotherapy produces higher levels in the peritoneal cavity and can be achieved via the intravenous route, but whether this results in a clinical advantage has been an area of controversy. Similarly, high-dose chemotherapy with hematological support has been frequently used in patients with recurrent ovarian cancer, although there is controversy as to whether there is any significant long-term benefit.

The potential value of a doubling of platinum dose intensity in the management of patients with advanced ovarian cancer has been evaluated in seven randomized clinical trials and two meta-analyses. The meta-analyses suggest a direct correlation between clinical benefit and cisplatin dose intensity up to a cisplatin dose of $15-25$ mg/m^2 per week with no benefit for further dose escalation. Five of the seven randomized trials show no advantage to either a doubling of pure platinum dose intensity (both regimens prescribe the same total dose with a difference in the time over which the total dose is achieved) or a doubling of dose intensity and total dose[2].

Two of the randomized trials show an advantage for increased dose intensity in combination with increased total dose, but these two trials are the smallest of the seven and have multiple problems in design and execution. The weight of evidence favors a dose-intensity curve in which escalation of platinum dose yields clinical improvement until a threshold is reached; beyond the threshold (cisplatin 25 mg/m^2 per week or its equivalent), no benefit results from further escalation.

The response rate observed with high-dose paclitaxel (250 mg/m^2) was higher than reported for most previous phase II trials evaluating lower doses. Consequently, a randomized trial of paclitaxel at two different doses with and without filgrastim (granulocyte colony-stimulating factor, GCSF) was performed by the GOG in previously treated patients with advanced ovarian cancer. Patients were randomized to receive paclitaxel at doses of 175 or 250 mg/m^2 with the latter dose requiring GCSF either at a 5- or 10-mg/kg per day subcutaneous dose over 24 h every 3 weeks. While the higher dose produced a higher clinical response rate (36% vs. 28%), PFS and overall survival were similar. Toxicity was also substantially increased in patients receiving the high-dose treatment. While it appears there is a modest dose–response effect in previously treated patients, there was no survival benefit for the high-dose therapy. It remains to be determined whether there similarly is a modest dose–response effect in previously untreated patients with advanced disease.

Intraperitoneal chemotherapy

Intraperitoneal chemotherapy is designed to increase the concentration of cytotoxic agents in contact with tumors for longer periods than possible with systemic drug delivery.

Phase II trials have confirmed that surgically defined responses can be observed with cisplatin-based intraperitoneal chemotherapy in individuals who have previously responded to systemic chemotherapy but persist in having very small-volume residual disease.

A randomized Intergroup Study has demonstrated that the use of intraperitoneal cisplatin as front-line therapy of small-volume advanced ovarian cancer results in improved survival compared with the same dose of cisplatin delivered systemically. There are numerous concerns about using intraperitoneal therapy, including the limited penetration of drugs directly into tissue, problems with drug distribution throughout the cavity, the toxicity of drugs for the peritoneal lining, the need to safely and conveniently access the cavity for treatment and the risk of intra-abdominal infections[11].

The GOG has performed a randomized trial comparing IV cisplatin and cyclophosphamide with IV cisplatin and paclitaxel and a third arm consisting of intraperitoneal cisplatin and IV carboplatin and paclitaxel in optimal stage III patients. The IV cisplatin and cyclophosphamide arm was dropped when the results of GOG protocol 111 became known. Consequently, the study serves as a confirmation to the previous Intergroup Study that demonstrated an advantage for intraperitoneal cisplatin.

A small number of phase I and phase II trials of high-dose chemotherapy, supported by either autologous bone-marrow transplantation or peripheral blood progenitor cells in patients with disease recurrent after initial chemotherapy, demonstrate the feasibility of such approaches and report high response rates (albeit with short durations of response except in those with minimal residual chemosensitive disease). These trials do not, however, establish a role for such an approach. The patient populations are highly selected for favorable features, fail to distinguish clearly between chemosensitive and chemoresistant patients and include no control group for comparison.

Available data do not support a role for stem cell-supported high-dose chemotherapy. Phase I and II trials in recurrent disease establish feasibility only, and provide no information on the relative merits of the approach. Settings in which the use of high-dose regimens have been suggested include front-line therapy for newly diagnosed patients, consolidation therapy for patients who have responded to front-line treatment and second-line treatment for recurrent disease. The short duration of responses in the last setting in phase II trials provides little support for further study of that clinical circumstance. For the first two settings, phase III trials will be required to establish a role, if any, for high-dose therapy. A phase III trial of high-dose consolidation therapy opened in August 1996 as an Intergroup Study. No phase III trial of high-dose therapy as initial treatment is currently planned. Until a phase III trial demonstrates the value of stem cell-supported high-dose chemotherapy, the use of such an approach should be confined to clinical trials.

Expected results

Common end-points in ovarian cancer include response rate, pathological complete response rate, PFS and overall survival. Results in bulky advanced disease reflect the use of paclitaxel plus cisplatin, whereas results in minimal residual advanced disease come from trials using cyclophosphamide plus cisplatin (in the absence of data from those patients with paclitaxel plus platinum regimens). The use of paclitaxel plus platinum regimens is expected to yield results in minimal residual disease proportionately better than those in bulky advanced disease.

Issues after surgery

After cytoreductive surgery and chemotherapy, approximately 70% of patients will be in CCR at which point their CA125 levels will be in the normal range, and there will be no evidence of disease by physical examination or by computer tomography (CT) scans. Unfortunately, disease in at least 50% of these patients will ultimately recur. Currently, there is no evidence that any form of maintenance therapy can prevent or delay recurrences in this group of patients. Clinical trials are in progress including high-dose chemotherapy with hematological support, intraperitoneal chemotherapy, immunotherapy or radioisotopes, maintenance systemic therapy and whole abdominal radiation therapy. The role of second-look surgery in patients who achieve CCR is also an area of controversy[12]. Therapy for patients with recurring disease will depend on their response to initial therapy and the duration of such a response. Patients who had a response to chemotherapy that lasted > 6 months are termed chemotherapy-sensitive and these patients have a higher likelihood of responding to subsequent salvage therapy than patients who are chemotherapy-resistant, who either did not respond to chemotherapy or had a short disease-free interval (DFI).

Second-look laparoscopy should not be routinely performed in patients with epithelial ovarian cancer. The operation should be reserved for carefully selected patients or those on restricted protocols. While second-look laparotomies provide useful prognostic information, it is unclear whether survival is subsequently affected by management that is determined by the findings of the second look.

Secondary cytoreductive surgery, which is defined as an operation to remove persistent or recurrent disease after chemotherapy, should be performed in carefully selected patients, particularly those who have had chemosensitive disease; those who have a long disease PFS until clinical relapse; and those for whom there is a potential to resect all of the residual disease. Studies have shown that when the residual disease has been completely removed, subsequent survival is augmented[13,14].

Follow-up

The optimum management of patients who achieve CCR remains to be established. Patients are frequently followed by CT scans and measurement of serum CA125 levels. There is no evidence that CT scans are useful in patients who are in CCR. Likewise, the optimum use of CA125 levels in this situation is controversial.

Frequently, CA125 levels begin to rise at a time when there is no other evidence of disease. The median time for radiographic/physical evidence of recurrence in a patient with a rising CA125 level is 4–6 months, although some patients will have no evidence of disease for many months and sometimes years. There is no evidence that immediate treatment of these patients with cytotoxic chemotherapy, at the time their CA125 level starts to rise, is beneficial. Many clinicians are currently using tamoxifen in this situation and reserving cytotoxic chemotherapy for when there is other clinical evidence of disease. There is no established role for immunoscanning. Patients who have ovarian cancer and are in CCR are at risk of developing other malignancies, in particular breast cancer, and should undergo routine mammograms. Hormone replacement therapy in premenopausal women at the completion of their chemotherapy is frequently administered to decrease the effects of surgical castration.

The treatment of patients who relapse after achieving a complete remission depends on the nature and duration of their initial response to induction chemotherapy. Patients who had a long DFI frequently respond to retreatment with the same drugs that were used as part of their initial chemotherapy. In contrast, patients who have a short (< 6 months) DFI usually exhibit resistance to those agents that were used as part of their initial therapy. Options for second-line treatment in this group of patients include oral etoposide, topotecan, gemcitabine, altretamine, ifosfamide and tamoxifen. In addition, these patients are appropriate candidates for phase II clinical trials. Patients who have a very long DFI can be treated with combination chemotherapy. However, in most situations, patients are sequentially treated with single agents.

It must be remembered that the objective response rate to any chemotherapeutic agent in this setting is no more than 10–25%, with responses generally lasting < 6–8 months. Therapy in the patient with refractory disease should be considered palliative in nature.

Summary

Surgery is important for accurately diagnosing the stage of ovarian cancer as well as in cytoreductive surgery to remove as much disease as feasible. After completion of a comprehensive laparotomy, if patients have early-stage disease, treatment recommendations are based on clinical and pathological features with some patients requiring no adjuvant treatment. For patients with advanced stage disease, cytoreductive surgery is followed by chemotherapy with paclitaxel plus platinum compound. Patients who respond to initial chemotherapy and in whom disease recurs can be retreated with paclitaxel or platinum compounds. When they stop responding to these agents, or if they had a very short initial response to induction chemotherapy or never responded at all to paclitaxel plus platinum, successful palliation can be achieved with a variety of agents including newer drugs such as topotecan and gemcitabine. These drugs may also be used in chemotherapy-sensitive patients when disease recurs.

Fallopian tube cancer

Most Fallopian tube cancers are serous carcinomas and spread in a pattern similar to ovarian cancer[2]. They appear to have a proclivity for spread to the retroperitoneal lymph nodes. In general, Fallopian tube cancers are treated just like ovarian epithelial tumors, i.e. surgery followed by combination chemotherapy with paclitaxel and platinum drug.

Peritoneal cancer

The lining of the entire peritoneal surface comprises cells that are identical to those that are from the epithelial surface of the ovaries. Tumors that primarily arise from the peritoneum can appear just like ovarian cancer and behave in a similar manner, i.e. with disseminated carcinomatosis. Histologically, they are typically identical to serous ovarian carcinomas. The prognosis may be slightly worse because most present with extensive carcinomatosis at the time of diagnosis. However, the treatment is the same as for ovarian cancer, i.e. debulking followed by combination chemotherapy[15].

Borderline tumors

Borderline tumors, which tend to occur more often than invasive cancers in premenopausal women, are typically early-stage and can be cured with an oophorectomy, or in some cases a cystectomy. The cure rate for stage I tumors is high at > 95%. Multifocal (stage III) tumors are rare. Most borderline tumors or low malignant-potential tumors are serous tumors. Mucinous tumors can have a bad outcome because of the association with pseudomyxoma peritonei. In general, borderline tumors do not later become invasive cancers in most patients[2].

In early-stage disease, since many of these arise in women who wish to preserve fertility, removal of the involved ovary or a cystectomy only need be performed. When there is late-stage disease, this should be resected; however, postoperative chemotherapy is not beneficial.

Germ-cell tumors

Premenarchal girls and adolescents are much more likely to have a germ-cell malignancy than an epithelial cancer. In these patients, conservation of fertility is essential. The correct surgery is to remove the primary tumor and to preserve the majority of the reproductive tract. Appropriate postoperative chemotherapy is given based on the operative findings.

The pathology of germ-cell tumor can be divided into dysgerminomas, nondysgerminomas and mixed germ cell tumors. The most common types of this uncommon tumor are the dysgerminoma (identical to the seminoma in the male) and the immature teratoma. Tumor markers (human chorionic gonadotropin (hCG), alpha-fetoprotein (AFP) and lactate dehydrogenase (LDH)) may be positive in these patients and should be followed during the postoperative period.

The appropriate management of dysgerminoma is conservative surgery and a staging laparotomy. In those patients with disease confined to one ovary, postoperative chemotherapy is typically not necessary as relapses are uncommon and can be also cured with subsequent chemotherapy. The bleomycin, etoposide and cisplatin (BEP) combination regimen is associated with a very high cure rate in advanced stage disease[16].

In patients with nondysgerminoma germ-cell tumors, postoperative chemotherapy with BEP should be given to all patients except those with stage I grade 1 immature teratoma who have been comprehensively staged and have disease confined to one ovary. The outcome is excellent in these patients properly staged and treated.

Acknowledgements

The authors gratefully acknowledge the supporters of the UCLA Women's Reproductive Cancer Program and the Jonsson Comprehensive Cancer Center of UCLA. This paper is reproduced with permission from The Solid Tumor Oncology Education Foundation.

References

1. Young, R. C., Perez, C. A. and Hoskins, W. V. (1993). Cancer of the ovary. In DeVita, Jr, Hellman, S. and Rosenberg, S. A. (eds.) *Cancer: Principles and Practice of Oncology*, 4th edn, Ch. 39. Philadelphia, PA: J. B. Lippincott Co.)

2. Berek, J. S. and Hacker, N. F. (eds.) (1994). *Practical Gynecologic Oncology*, 2nd edn. (Baltimore, MD: Williams and Wilkins)

3. Young, R. C., Walton, L. A., Ellenberg, S. S., *et al.*, (1990). Adjuvant therapy in stage I and stage II epithelial ovarian cancer: results of two prospective randomized trials. *N. Engl. J. Med.*, **322**, 1021–7

4. Young, R. C., Decker, D. G., Wharton, J. T., *et al.* (1983). Staging laparotomy in early ovarian cancer. *J. Am. Med. Assoc.*, **250**, 3072–6

5. Berek, J. S. (1995). Interval debulking of ovarian cancer – an interim measure (editorial). *N. Engl. J. Med.*, **332**, 675–7

6. van der Burg, M. E. L., van Lent, M., Buyse, M., *et al.* (1995). The effect of debulking surgery after induction chemotherapy on the prognosis in advanced epithelial ovarian cancer. *N. Engl. J. Med.*, **332**, 629–34

7. McGuire, W. P., Hoskins, W. J., Brady, M. F., Kucera, P. R., *et al.* (1996). Cyclophosphamide and cisplatin compared with paclitaxel and cisplatin in patients with stage III and stage IV ovarian cancer. *N. Engl. J. Med.*, **334**, 1–6

8. Eisenhauer, E. A., ten Bokkel Huinink, W. W., Swenerton, K. D., *et al.* (1994). European–Canadian randomized trial of paclitaxel in relapsed ovarian cancer: high-dose versus low-dose and long versus short infusion. *J. Clin. Oncol.*, **12**, 2654–66

9. Bookman, M. A., McGuire, W. P. III, Kilpatrick, D., *et al.* (1996). Carboplatin and paclitaxel in ovarian carcinoma: a phase I study of the Gynecologic Oncology Group. *J. Clin. Oncol.*, **14**, 1895–902

10. Rowinsky, E. K. (1996). Meta analysis of paclitaxel (P) dose-response and dose-intensity (DI) in recurrent or refractory ovarian cancer (OC) (abstract). *Proc. Am. Soc. Clin. Oncol.*, **15**, 284

11. Alberts, D. S., Liu, P. Y., Hannigan, E. V., *et al.* (1996). Intraperitoneal cisplatin plus intravenous cyclophosphamide versus intravenous cisplatin plus intravenous cyclophosphamide for stage III ovarian cancer. *N. Engl. J. Med.*, **335**, 1950–5

12. Berek, J. S. (1992). Second-look versus second-nature (editorial). *Gynecol. Oncol.*, **44**, 1–2

13. Berek, J. S., Hacker, N. F., Lagasse, L. D., Nieberg, R. K. and Elashoff, R. M. (1983). Survival of patients following secondary cytoreductive surgery in ovarian cancer. *Obstet. Gynecol.*, **61**, 189–93

14. Hoskins, W. J., Rubin, S. C., Dulaney, E., *et al.* (1989). Influence of secondary cytoreduction at the time of second-look laparotomy on the survival of patients with epithelial ovarian carcinoma. *Gynecol. Oncol.*, **34**, 365–71

15. Fowler, J. M., Nieberg, R. K., Schooler, T. A. and Berek, J. S. (1994). Peritoneal adenocarcinoma (serous) of Müllerian type: a subgroup of women presenting with peritoneal carcinomatosis. *Int. J. Gynecol. Cancer*, **4**, 43–51

16. Williams, S., Blessing, J., Liao, S.- Y., Ball, H. and Hanjani, P. (1994). Adjuvant therapy of ovarian germ cell tumors with cisplatin, etoposide, and bleomycin: a trial of the Gynecologic Oncology Group. *J. Clin. Oncol.*, **12**, 701–6

Breast cancer and combined oral contraceptives: results from the Collaborative Group on Hormonal Factors in Breast Cancer

31

V. Beral and G. Reeves

Background

The Collaborative Group on Hormonal Factors in Breast Cancer was set up in January 1992. Its aims are:

(1) To obtain simple data from all epidemiological studies of female breast cancer and hormonal factors, including hormonal contraceptives, hormone replacement therapy and reproductive factors;

(2) To carry out analyses of the relationship of these factors with breast cancer risk and present the results separately for each study using, as far as possible, similar definitions for important factors;

(3) To combine the results from all studies, if appropriate; and

(4) To publish, in the name of all collaborators, the results of these analyses.

Data on individual women from each participating study are contributed to the Secretariat, based at the Imperial Cancer Research Fund Cancer Epidemiology Unit in Oxford. All data are checked and analyzed centrally.

Preliminary results were presented and discussed at meetings of collaborators in September 1993 and in March 1995. Draft reports were then prepared and circulated to all collaborators for comment, and redrafted in the light of their comments.

Participating studies

Studies were eligible for participation if they included at least 100 women with breast cancer and had obtained information from individual women on their use of hormonal contraceptives and on their reproductive history. Data were contributed from 54 of the 65 eligible studies that were identified from computer searches, literature reviews and discussion with colleagues. The main reason that the other studies did not participate was that their original data could not be retrieved. Only one research group declined participation. The 54 studies together included 53 000 women with breast cancer and 100 000 women without breast cancer from 25 countries. These studies contain about 90% of the worldwide information on the relationship between breast cancer and the use of hormonal contraceptives.

The women and their use of hormonal contraceptives

The median age of the women with breast cancer was 50 years, and the mean year of their cancer diagnosis was 1985. Approximately half of the women had used hormonal contraceptives, the vast majority having used combined oral contraceptives. Only 0.8% of the women had used progestogen-only oral contraceptives and 1.5% of the women had used injectable progestogens. The median duration of use of combined oral contraceptives was 3 years and 15% of users had used them for 10 or more years. Approximately half of the women had begun using combined oral contraceptives before 1970, and about a third had their cancer diagnosed 20 or more years after they had begun use. Approximately half of the women last used combined oral contraceptives after 1975 and half had used them in the 10 years before their cancer was diagnosed; 13% were using oral contraceptives at the time that their cancer was diagnosed.

The main results for combined oral contraceptives

A summary of the main findings on breast cancer risk in association with the use of combined oral contraceptives was published in the *Lancet* in June 1996[1]. A more detailed report was published in *Contraception* in September 1996[2]. There were two main results:

(1) While women are taking combined oral contraceptives, and in the 10 years after stopping, there is a small, but definite, increase in the relative risk of having breast cancer diagnosed; and

(2) Ten or more years after stopping the use of combined oral contraceptives, there is no increase in the relative risk of having breast cancer diagnosed compared with women who had never used such contraceptives.

In addition, the cancers diagnosed in women who had used combined oral contraceptives were less advanced clinically than the cancers diagnosed in women who had never used combined oral contraceptives. This applied at all times since last oral contraceptive use (Figure 1).

The main findings did not vary markedly across different studies or study designs, nor across women with different background risks of breast cancer. Nor did the findings vary significantly according to the duration of use or the hormone type or dose of the oral contraceptives that had been used[1,2].

Estimated number of excess breast cancers diagnosed among women who use combined oral contraceptives.

Because breast cancer is rare in young women, and the incidence increases sharply with age, the number of excess cancers diagnosed among women who are taking oral contraceptives or who ceased to take them in the last 10 years tends to be small, but increases with increasing age (Figure 2).

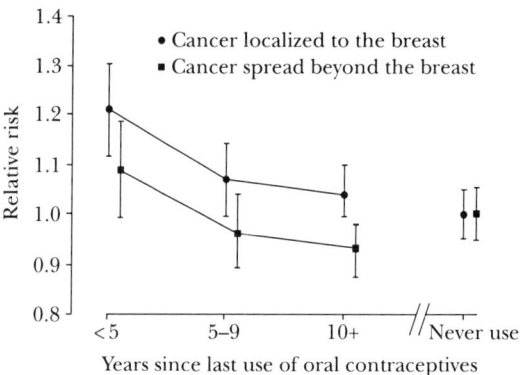

Figure 1 Relative risk of breast cancer according to time since last use of oral contraceptives and extent of tumor spread. (From reference 3)

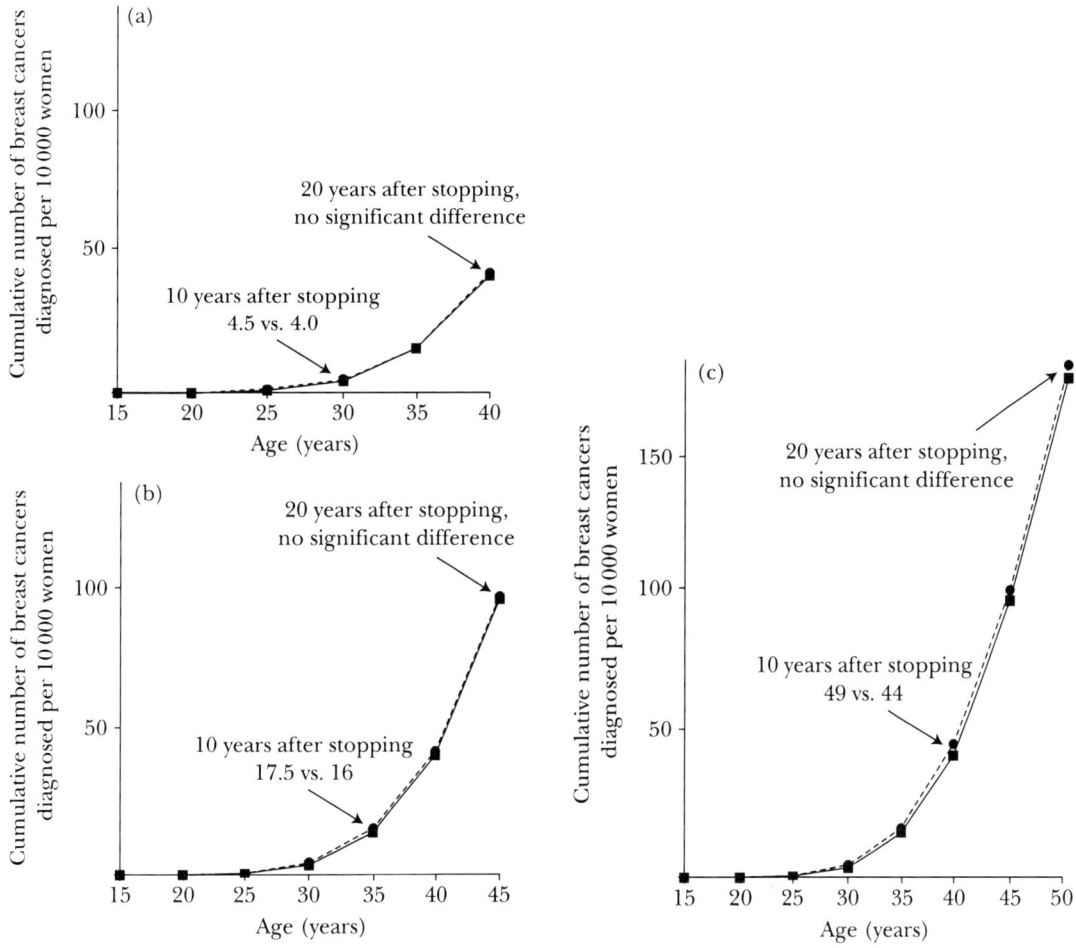

Figure 2 Estimated cumulative number of breast cancers diagnosed in never-users (—) and in women who used oral contraceptives (- - -) at various ages: (a) age 16–19 years; (b) age 20–24 years; (c) age 25–29 years. (From reference 1)

References

1. Collaborative Group on Hormonal Factors in Breast cancer (1996). Breast cancer and hormonal contraceptives: collaborative reanalysis of individual data on 53 297 women with breast cancer and 100 239 women without breast cancer from 54 epidemiological studies. *Lancet*, **347**, 1713–27

2. Collaborative Group on Hormonal Factors in Breast Cancer (1996). Breast cancer and hormonal contraceptives: further results. *Contraception*, **54** (Suppl. 3), 1–106S

3. Beral, V., Reeves, G., Bull, D. and Peto, R. on behalf of the Collaborative Group on Hormonal Factors in Breast Cancer (1996). Breast cancer and hormone exposure. *Lancet*, **348**, 683

32

The role of meta-analysis in gynecological decision-making

S. Daya

In trying to provide optimal care for patients, clinicians regularly face questions about the efficacy of a particular therapy or disease preventive strategy, the accuracy and interpretation of a diagnostic test, the effect associated with exposure to a putatively harmful agent, the course and prognosis of disease in a specific patient, and the cost-effectiveness of a new intervention. The standard approaches in trying to answer these questions include consulting a colleague who may be aware of recent advances in the particular area of concern and referring to textbooks or reviews. Unfortunately, textbooks are usually not up-to-date because of the time it takes to publish them. Similarly, reviews are usually narrative summaries of the author's opinions about a particular subject and may be biased in their conclusions by the selection and review of studies that support the authors' beliefs rather than reflecting all the available evidence.

The literature, on the other hand, is continuously accumulating new information generated from research. However, the demands of a busy practice make it increasingly difficult to keep abreast of the field, especially when there are at least 19 new articles available daily to general physicians[1]. Even the most enthusiastic clinician does not spend more than a few hours a week trying to keep up with new information, much of which is not valid or relevant to clinical practice. Reviewing the literature should be undertaken as an exercise in scientific inquiry and be done in a manner that avoids bias.

Systematic reviews

One approach to this problem is to look for systematic reviews on a particular subject. Such reviews involve taking the large and unmanageable amount of information from a complete search of the literature and reducing it into concise summaries that are easy to access. A systematic review is an efficient method of integrating existing data and information into rational and appropriate decision-making. The review also establishes whether scientific findings are consistent and can be generalized across populations, settings and treatment variations, or whether findings vary significantly by particular subsets[2]. In this manner, the busy clinician can keep abreast of the primary literature in a given field and maintain the appropriate focus for clinical care.

Another important reason for using systematic reviews is to avoid erroneous conclusions that can be made by consulting single studies which often use inadequate numbers of subjects to make confident inferences. For example, to demonstrate a clinically important difference of 5% between a control event rate of 15% and an experimental event rate of 20%, a sample of approximately 1450 subjects is required to give the study sufficient power to avoid type I and type II errors with probabilities of 0.95 and 0.8 respectively. Trials of this size are often difficult to conduct in gynecology and investigators often resort to smaller trials with the hope that useful information will be obtained. The evidence from such smaller trials may be pooled using the principles of meta-analysis so that an overall, summary effect measure can be calculated.

The steps involved in a systematic review include the formation of a specific research question, a search strategy to identify and select relevant studies, an assessment of study validity, the extraction and statistical pooling (i.e. meta-analysis) of data and summarizing the results so that appropriate inferences can be made. Thus, it is the quantitative approach to reviewing the literature that forms the basis of the systematic review; the meta-analysis provides a summary measure of the effect size.

There are two approaches to collecting data for a meta-analysis. The first approach utilizes published data from well-designed controlled trials. These data are extracted as aggregate data (expressed as proportions) on subjects in each trial and then pooled. An alternative approach is to obtain individual data for every subject enrolled in each controlled trial and then pool them as if they were participants in one large trial. Whether the information on the participants in the relevant trials should be collected as aggregate data per trial or as individual data per subject is the focus of much discussion and will be highlighted in this paper using relevant examples.

Problem of heterogeneity

In contrast to single trials, a meta-analysis attempts to achieve more objectivity, precision and external validity by including all the best available evidence from trials that address a particular problem. However, because of the broader objective of a systematic review, the trials included usually encompass a variety of specific treatment regimens, types of patient and outcomes[3]. Such variability may result in both clinical and statistical heterogeneity.

Statistical heterogeneity is observed when the effect size from each trial varies not only in magnitude (which is expected) but also in direction. Thus, in some studies, the intervention may have a positive effect while in others, it may have a negative effect. Such heterogeneity can be evaluated statistically by determining whether the individual effect size is significantly different from the overall, summary effect size obtained by pooling the data. Statistical heterogeneity may be caused by known clinical or methodological differences among trials or it may be related to unknown or unrecorded trial characteristics[3]. Formal testing for statistical heterogeneity should be performed before pooling the data. However, it should be emphasized that such testing has less power and may fail to detect even moderate amounts of heterogeneity. In the absence of statistical heterogeneity, pooling of data is undertaken using a fixed effects method. In contrast, when there is significant heterogeneity there are two options available reflecting the prevailing schools of thought; one approach is to not pool the data unless sources of heterogeneity can be identified and removed, and the other approach is to pool the data using a random effects method. The fixed and random effects methods often produce similar summary effects but vary in the precision of these estimates.

Clinical heterogeneity is expected to produce some degree of statistical heterogeneity and should be specified in advance[4]. This problem is magnified when there are many clinical differences but only a small number of trials available. Subgroups with similar clinical characteristics should be analyzed together to reduce the amount of heterogeneity.

Statistical heterogeneity may be caused by other factors. Publication bias[5] remains a cause for concern because of the potential for preferential publication of trials with positive results and rejection or non-submission for publication of those with a null effect. Differences in methodological quality[6] and early termination of clinical trials[7] are also potential sources of heterogeneity. Finally, heterogeneity may be observed owing to chance.

Although the statistical test for heterogeneity is important, the guiding principle for any meta-analysis is to investigate the influences of the specific clinical differences among studies, and to try to minimize the variability where possible by selecting only those studies that are relevant to the research question.

Examples

The use of meta-analysis in gynecological decision-making will be illustrated using two examples, namely, universal antibiotic prophylaxis for induced abortion and immunotherapy for recurrent abortion.

Universal antibiotic prophylaxis for induced abortion

The incidence of postabortal upper genital tract infection varies from 5 to 20% and can produce long-term sequelae such as chronic pelvic pain, dyspareunia and infertility[8]. The routine use of antibiotics at the time of surgical abortion to reduce the likelihood of upper genital tract infection is controversial, even though many trials to evaluate the efficacy of this approach have been conducted. Some trials have shown a beneficial effect whereas in others, a significant effect of treatment was not demonstrated although a trend towards prevention was observed[8]. Therefore, the objective of the study was to determine whether antibiotics given in the peri-abortal period were effective in reducing the likelihood of upper genital tract infections.

The authors performed a literature search of the Medline database covering the period of January 1966 to September 1994. Trials selected for review were restricted to randomized controlled trials comparing antibiotics with placebo in women undergoing therapeutic abortion by surgical curettage before 16 weeks' gestation. The outcome of interest was the incidence, within 6 weeks of the procedure, of upper genital tract infection diagnosed by standardized, objective criteria. Twelve out of 21 trials screened met the selection criteria for inclusion in the analysis.

For each trial, the relative risk (RR) and its 95% confidence interval (CI) were calculated from the data (Figure 1). The summary RR estimate was calculated using the fixed effects method of Mantel–Haenszel after a test of homogeneity of treatment effect showed no significant heterogeneity. Subgroup analysis in each stratum was performed after stratifying the data into risk groups for post-abortal infection. Risk factors included a history of pelvic inflammatory disease (PID), a positive preoperative culture for chlamydia trachomatis and bacterial vaginosis.

The overall RR for developing postabortal upper genital tract infection with antibiotic therapy was 0.58 (95% CI, 0.47–0.71). Among high-risk women, the overall RR was 0.50 (0.35–0.72) and in the low-risk group it was 0.64 (0.49–0.85). The RR with each antecedent factor within each of the two risk groups is shown in Figure 2. The lowest RR (0.22; 95% CI, 0.11–0.42) was among women drawn from a population with a low incidence (5.6%) of postabortal infection. Those with a mid-range incidence (10–16%) had a RR of 0.70 (95% CI, 0.56–0.88) and those with a high incidence (20–23%) had a RR of 0.26 (95% CI, 0.08–0.80).

A cumulative meta-analysis demonstrated that clear evidence of efficacy of peri-abortal antibiotics was already present by 1987, suggesting that any subsequent trials would not have

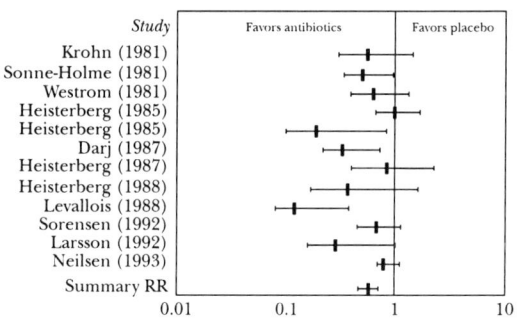

Relative risk of upper genital tract infection

Figure 1 Efficacy of antibiotic use for prophylaxis against upper genital tract infection

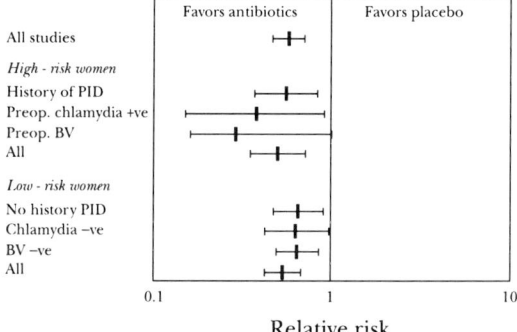

Relative risk

Figure 2 Risk factors for postabortal genital tract infection and effect of antibiotic prophylaxis. PID, pelvic inflammatory disease; Preop., preoperative; BV, bacterial vaginosis

been necessary had a meta-analysis been done at that time.

From the evidence in the literature, it can be seen quite clearly that the use of antibiotics at the time of a surgical abortion reduces the infection rate in all groups of women. In the high-risk group of women (with a postabortal infection prevalence of 20%), a RR of 0.50 implies an average relative risk reduction of 50% (to an infection prevalence of 10%), indicating that, for every 10 high-risk women so treated, one case of postabortal infection would be prevented. In the low-risk group (prevalence of infection 8%), the RR was 0.64 producing an average relative risk reduction of 36% (to an infection prevalence of 2.9%), giving a number needed to treat of 35.

A policy of routine use of antibiotics would produce significant health benefits that could be translated into significant economic savings to society[8].

Immunotherapy for recurrent abortion

Spontaneous abortion is a fairly common event that occurs in approximately 10–15% of pregnancies. In a small proportion of women, the losses are repetitive and can result from a variety of factors. In others, the repeated abortions are a manifestation of failure in the normal allo-immune recognition process that appears to be necessary to ensure pregnancy success. In this group of women, recurrent abortion is viewed as a partner-specific problem that may be immunologically modifiable by exposing the female to paternal antigens via a non-uterine route[9]. The resulting antibodies would be specific and induce the appropriate protective immune response at the maternal–fetal site.

This theory led to the use of leukocytes from the male partner or from unrelated donors for immunization of the female. The initial trial of paternal leukocyte immunization demonstrated a beneficial effect, with a significant reduction in the rate of miscarriage compared to placebo. However, subsequent trials were unable to substantiate this observation and led to the controversy that still persists. These conflicting

observations have been explained, in part, on the basis of inadequate sample sizes, heterogeneity of study samples among trials and the effect of co-intervention[10].

A search of the literature for randomized controlled trials comparing leukocyte immunization with placebo or no treatment produced five trials, the results of which are summarized by the odds ratio (OR) and its 95% CI as shown in Figure 3. There was no significant heterogeneity of treatment effect, and the common OR, calculated by statistically pooling the data using the fixed effects method of Mantel–Haenszel, was 2.13 (95% CI, 1.24–3.64). Although this meta-analysis demonstrated a beneficial effect of immunotherapy, the controversy persisted with a call for more studies, some of which are currently in progress.

To address this disagreement, a worldwide collaborative meta-analysis was organized with 15 centers participating in the study. The approach was to conduct a meta-analysis of randomized controlled studies using data from individual patients who had been identified as participants in the trials. A case-record form with 140 variables was completed for each patient. The forms were collated and the data extracted and analyzed by two separate groups of investigators. Although the independent analyses used different definitions and statistical methods, the results were remarkably similar[11]. The ratios of the number of live births in the treatment group to the number in the control group were 1.16 (95% CI, 1.01–1.34; $p = 0.03$)

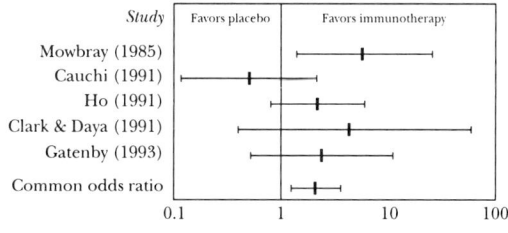

Figure 3 Efficacy of leukocyte immunization in the treatment of unexplained recurrent spontaneous abortion

and 1.21 (95% CI, 1.04–1.37; $p = 0.02$) for the two analyses. The absolute treatment effect was 8% and 10%, respectively.

This relatively low treatment effect may be accounted for by variability among trials in the diagnostic tests used to select patients for treatment, and the inclusion of couples in which the female partner had autoimmune abnormalities, pre-exisiting antipaternal leukocyte antibodies or a previous successful pregnancy.

A subgroup evaluation was performed after restricting the analysis to the data from women with unexplained primary recurrent abortion (i.e. three or more spontaneous abortions and no previous pregnancy beyond 20 weeks' gestation) and in whom there was no evidence of antipaternal antibody[12]. This analysis was conducted using data from each center and from individual patient data. In the meta-analysis by center, immunotherapy significantly improved the live birth rate (OR = 1.94; 95% CI, 1.20–3.12). In the meta-analysis by patient, the likelihood of a successful outcome was also significantly better with treatment (RR = 1.46, 95% CI, 1.19–1.69). The absolute treatment effect was 16.3% (i.e. > 50% higher than that obtained in the initial analysis).

A further subgroup analysis was performed after restricting the data to those from double-blind trials because of the knowledge that lack of blinding can bias the outcome of the trial. The overall OR obtained was 2.42 (95% CI, 1.31–4.47; $p = 0.005$) in favor of immunotherapy[9]. The absolute treatment effect was 21% indicating that, for every five women treated with immunization, one successful outcome can be expected.

This meta-analysis (either by 'center' or by 'patient') demonstrates that immunotherapy with leukocytes is efficacious in women with unexplained recurrent abortion. By restricting treatment to a specific group of women with recurrent abortion, the success rate can be optimized. The challenge that now awaits is to develop better diagnostic tests to identify those women with alloimmune recognition failure in whom the therapy has the best chance of success.

Summary

Meta-analysis is a powerful statistical tool that provides a quantitative overall estimate of effect size using evidence from published trials with the highest methodological quality. Using this approach to systematic reviews, a more reliable, generalizable and accurate estimate of the effect of treatment can be produced. This information becomes very relevant in guiding clinicians in the care of their patients. In this paper, examples from two different areas in gynecology were chosen to illustrate the principles. Subgroup analyses within a meta-analysis may provide more appropriate information from which to make inferences. The importance of selecting trials with high methodological quality cannot be emphasized enough. The overall goal is to obtain the best estimates of the effect of treatment by minimizing bias as much as possible. Only then can clinical care be optimized.

References

1. Davidoff, F., Haynes, B., Sackett, D. and Smith, R. (1995). Evidence-based medicine. A new journal to help doctors identify new information they need. *Br. Med. J.*, **310**, 1085–6
2. Mulrow, C. D. (1994). Rationale for systematic reviews. *Br. Med. J.*, **309**, 597–9
3. Thompson, S. G. (1994). Why sources of heterogeneity in meta-analysis should be investigated. *Br. Med. J.*, **309**, 1351–5
4. Oxman, A. D. and Guyatt, G. H. (1992). A consumer's guide to subgroup analyses. *Ann. Intern. Med.*, **116**, 78–84
5. Easterbrook, P. J., Berlin, J. A., Gopalan, R. and Matthews, D. R. (1991). Publication bias in clinical research. *Lancet*, **337**, 867–72
6. Schulz, K. F., Chalmers, I., Haynes, R. J. and Altman, D. G. (1995). Empirical evidence of bias: dimensions of methodological quality are

associated with estimates of treatment effects in 250 controlled trials from 33 meta-analyses. *J. Am. Med. Assoc.*, **273**, 408–12

7. Hughes, M. D., Freeman, L. S. and Pocock, S. J. (1992). The impact of stopping rules on heterogeneity of results in overviews of clinical trials. *Biometrics*, **48**, 41–53

8. Sawaya, G. F., Grady, D., Kerlikowske, K. and Grimes, D. A. (1996). Antibiotics at the time of induced abortion: the case for universal prophylaxis based on a meta-analysis. *Obstet. Gynecol.*, **87**, 884–90

9. Daya, S. (1997). Immunotherapy for unexplained recurrent spontaneous abortion. *Infertil. Reprod. Med. Clin. North Am.*, **8**, 65–77

10. Clark, D. A. and Daya, S. (1991). Trials and tubulation in the treatment of recurrent spontaneous abortion. *Am. J. Reprod. Immunol.*, **25**, 18–24

11. The Recurrent Miscarriage Immunotherapy Trialists Group. (1994). World wide collaborative observational study and meta-analysis on allogenic leukocyte immunotherapy for recurrent spontaneous abortion. *Am. J. Reprod. Immunol.*, **32**, 55–72

12. Daya, S., Gunby, J. and the Recurrent Miscarriage Immunotherapy Trialists Group (1994). The effectiveness of allogeneic leukocyte immunization in unexplained primary recurrent spontaneous abortion. *Am. J. Reprod. Immunol.*, **32**, 294–302

There is no place for electronic fetal monitoring in low-risk pregnancy

33

J. Yam, S. Arulkumaran and S. Chua

Introduction

Intermittent auscultation of the fetal heart rate (FHR) and continuous electronic fetal heart rate monitoring are the most popular methods of intrapartum fetal surveillance. It is recommended that, in the first stage of labor, intermittent auscultation of the fetal heart rate every 15 min for a duration of 1 min during and soon after a contraction, and auscultation after every other contraction or every 5 min in the second stage, may identify fetuses at risk.

Cardiotocography was incorporated in clinical obstetrics with the hope of reducing intrapartum mortality and morbidity. It still remains the 'gold standard' of intrapartum fetal monitoring. The development of technology which has reduced the cost of the equipment, together with a shortage of trained and experienced midwives to provide optimal standards of intermittent auscultation, has made continuous electronic fetal monitoring (EFM) a norm in many labor wards in developed countries. However, debate is still unsettled regarding the benefits of EFM as opposed to intermittent auscultation in low-risk labor. If it benefits high-risk labor, it should benefit low-risk labor, but the cost-effectiveness and possibility of increasing the Cesarean section rate without any substantial fetal benefits argue against its use in low-risk pregnancy. The Dublin randomized study consisted of 13 000 women; one half had EFM while the other had intermittent auscultation. The results did not show any significant difference in terms of perinatal mortality and morbidity[1]. However, high-risk groups like those with thick meconium, a majority of preterm pregnancies and those who had rapid labor were not included in

the study. Another large study had adequate numbers to debate this issue (35 000 women), but it compared the results of routine or universal EFM with selective fetal monitoring[2]. More recently, a smaller study compared the use of intermittent auscultation with EFM in detecting fetal hypoxia in parturients with low or moderate risk factors for fetal distress[3]. The results of these studies point to the fact that in low-risk labor, intermittent auscultation is as good as EFM in detecting fetal hypoxia.

Meta-analysis of the trials of the liberal use of intrapartum EFM vs. intermittent auscultation shows that EFM, with or without adjunctive fetal acid–base assessment, is associated with a significant increase in Cesarean delivery and instrumental vaginal delivery for fetal distress[4,5]. This increase in operative delivery is not associated with improved neonatal morbidity or mortality, except in cases when labor ceases to be 'physiological'. The meta-analyses show that in labors associated with the use of oxytocin for induction or augmentation of labor, and in prolonged labor, there were more infants with neonatal seizures in the intermittent auscultation group compared to the more intensively monitored group. Thus, the cost- effectiveness and possibility of increasing the Cesarean section rate without any substantial fetal benefits argue against the use of EFM in low-risk pregnancy.

In spite of such studies, continuous EFM is practiced as routine in many labor wards because antenatal risk classification into high and low risk, to select those who need monitoring, is often considered insufficient to predict fetal compromise appearing in labor[6]. Even after rigorous selection based on a known antenatal risk classification system, fetal morbidity and mortality tend to occur in the so-called low-risk population[7]. It is also known that the incidence of acidosis at birth is not very different between the low- and high-risk groups[8]. In addition, there is a tendency in the medical profession to use technology because it is available and not because it is necessary. In order to move away from this technological imperative and to use the technology of electronic fetal monitoring appropriately, a new system may have to be developed to identify those who are at risk in labor. The admission test[9,10] may help to identify those cases at risk in labor. EFM should be offered to those selected to be at risk based on high risk factors or admission test, and in those where intermittent auscultation cannot be practiced satisfactorily.

The admission test

A desirable way to screen patients admitted in labor would be to assess the ability of the fetus to withstand the functional stress of uterine contractions of early labor. A short recording of the fetal heart rate immediately after admission in early labor – the admission test – might select those fetuses with hypoxia present on admission or those who are likely to become hypoxic in the next few hours of labor.

The 'admission test' is a small strip of electronic FHR recording on admission in early labor. If during the recording time one or two contractions are observed, these will act as a stress to the fetus. If no FHR changes are observed with these contractions (stress) and the trace was reactive and normal, the risk of fetal hypoxia other than due to acute events is low in the next few hours of labor[10]. The duration of an admission test can be as short as 5 or 10 min if it is possible to identify the baseline rate, baseline variability, two accelerations and two contractions with no FHR changes.

The results of the first admission test study[9] are given in Table 1. In this study involving 1041 fetuses, fetal distress was considered to be present when FHR changes with or without fetal

Table 1 Results of the admission test in relation to the incidence of fetal distress

Admission test	Fetal distress
Reactive, $n = 982$ (94.3%)	13 (1.3%)
Equivocal, $n = 49$ (4.7%)	5 (10.2%)
Ominous, $n = 10$ (1.0%)	4 (40.0%)

scalp blood sampling led to operative delivery or the fetus was born normally but with an Apgar score < 7 at 5 min. Of the 13 who developed fetal distress with a reactive admission test, ten developed fetal distress only 5 h after admission. Of the three with a reactive admission test and who developed fetal distress in less than 5 h, one had cord prolapse (delivered by Cesarean section in good condition) and the other two delivered normally but were preterm, had low Apgar scores, and needed minimal resuscitation. There was one intrapartum still birth and one neonatal death in the group who had an ominous admission test. The auscultation chart in the case of the fresh still birth showed a steady observation of 140 bpm for 2 h at the end of which the fetal heart was not audible. The result of the admission test was not disclosed to the clinician and if known may have helped to prevent this occurrence. There is debate about whether intervention at this stage may result in a neurologically handicapped baby. This is not the case in most instances with timely intervention.

The results of the admission test suggest that, barring acute events, it may be a good predictor of fetal condition at the time of admission and during the next few hours of labor in term fetuses labelled as low-risk. Based on these results, if the admission test is reactive, intermittent electronic fetal monitoring for 10–20 min every 2–3 h and auscultation every 20–30 min may suffice. If the admission test is normal, a gradually developing hypoxia will be reflected by a rising FHR and should be picked up by auscultation[11]. When there is an increase in baseline FHR on auscultation, a small strip of electronic recording should be performed to verify the other abnormal features like absence of accelerations and reduction in the baseline variability associated with hypoxia.

Such practice should not cause problems because it is known that, if the FHR trace is reactive in labor in an averagely-grown fetus at term with clear amniotic fluid, it takes some time for fetal acidosis to develop from the onset of abnormal/suspicious FHR changes. It was estimated that in these situations, for 50% of fetuses to get acidotic, it took 115 min with repeated late decelerations, 145 min with repeated variable decelerations, and 185 min with a flat trace (baseline variability < 5 bpm)[12]. If the fetus develops abnormal FHR changes soon after a reactive admission test, it would take some time before the fetus becomes hypoxic and acidotic, and the changes in the FHR rate on intermittent auscultation should signify this probability. When suspicion arises on intermittent auscultation, it can be verified by a small strip of continuous recording by EFM. If the trace is found to be abnormal, a diagnosis of fetal acidosis can be made by fetal scalp blood sampling, or likely acidosis can be excluded by fetal stimulation tests.

Problems with electronic fetal monitoring

Electronic fetal monitoring has become popular because of the possible on-line documentation, easy application of the equipment, and because of the additional information obtained about the fetal heart rate and uterine contractions. In busy units with a less than optimal number of midwives provide desirable standards of intermittent auscultation, EFM may be an appropriate alternative for intrapartum fetal surveillance. Furthermore, concerns about litigation[13,14] have contributed to the widespread use of EFM, even in low-risk pregnancies.

However, the potential benefits of EFM must be weighed against the potential problems associated both with the accurate interpretation of an FHR trace and the increased operative interventions for fetal distress. Interpretation of a suspicious trace may be difficult and adequate training and education are necessary for all

personnel involved in intrapartum fetal surveillance. Furthermore, interpretation of EFM traces may vary greatly among practitioners. The clinical picture of the patient (age, parity, past obstetric history, and obstetric factors such as intrauterine growth retardation, prolonged pregnancy, presence of meconium, stage and rate of progress of labor) should also be taken into account when deciding on the action to be taken. In centers where EFM is available, problems may arise due to poor understanding of the FHR pattern and inappropriate or delayed action because of lack of consideration of the clinical picture[15].

Another problem with EFM is the high proportion of 'abnormal' recordings with a relatively low incidence of abnormal outcome. FHR changes of some form can be seen in 60% of all cases in an unselected population, indicating that these changes are not specific to hypoxia[16]; even if most of these changes are innocuous, they can cause anxiety. The risk of fetal acidosis is small when the trace is reactive; the predictive value of a normal EFM trace for a normal pH is estimated to be 98%[6,17]. Alternatively, fetal acidosis is not a consistent finding when ominous FHR changes are seen[17–19]. In two studies when an FHR pattern was ominous, only 50–65% of the newborns were found to be depressed as judged by the Apgar score[20,21], i.e. a 35–50% false prediction. Other workers[17,22] estimated the ability of an abnormal EFM trace to predict a low pH to be as low as 11% and around 50% at best.

In the case of the adult, many parameters are available, the adult is more resilient, and caregivers are knowledgeable about alterations in parameters. In the case of the fetus, the practitioner has only a limited number of indicators of fetal wellbeing or compromise, and interpretation of the information available varies. As the fetus is easily vulnerable to hypoxia, there may be over-intervention to save a few babies who are likely to be hypoxic. This leads to a significant increase in Cesarean delivery and instrumental vaginal delivery for fetal distress without any proven decrease in neonatal morbidity or mortality.

Meta-analyses of randomized trials have shown a reduction in neonatal convulsions in the EFM group[1,23,24]. However, the studies available have no power to demonstrate a reduction in other parameters like mortality and cerebral palsy. There is an exponential increase in the sample size needed if one is to study the intervention–benefit ratio as the prevalence of adverse outcomes becomes smaller. About 6000 cases are needed to show differences in Apgar scores, but 42 000 cases are needed to show differences in encephalopathy[25].

Despite the lack of evidence for fetal benefit from electronic fetal monitoring, the associated possibility of increased operative delivery, and the discomfort of being strapped down to a bed by transducers, there are many women, together with their midwives and obstetricians, who prefer to have electronic fetal monitoring in labor, even in low-risk labor. Preliminary results of an ongoing survey of the preferences of obstetricians, midwives and patients for the use of continuous EFM in low-risk labor, both in

Singapore and in some Western countries, attest to this.

Conclusion

Electronic fetal monitoring has become an accepted standard of care in intrapartum fetal surveillance. However, there are important questions regarding the accuracy and reliability of electronic fetal monitoring in discriminating accurately between pregnancies with and without fetal distress. It is also questionable whether the use of this technology in low-risk labors results in a significantly improved outcome for the baby when compared with intermittent auscultation.

Considering its uncertain benefits, with its attendant maternal risks and costs, an admission test, followed by intermittent electronic monitoring every 2–3 h with auscultation in between, may be adequate and appropriate in low-risk pregnancy.

References

1. MacDonald, D., Grant, A., Sheridan-Pereira, M., Boylan, P. and Chalmers, I. (1985). The Dublin randomized controlled trial of intrapartum fetal heart rate monitoring. *Am. J. Obstet. Gynecol.*, **52**, 524–39

2. Leveno, K. J., Cunningham, F. G., Nelson, S., Roark, M., Williams, M. L., Guzick, D., Dowling, S., Rosenfeld, C. R. and Buckley, A. (1986). A prospective comparison of selective and universal electronic fetal monitoring in 34 995 pregnancies. *N. Eng. J. Med.*, **315**, 615–19

3. Herbst, A. (1994). Intermittent versus continuous electronic monitoring in labour: a randomised study. *Br. J. Obstet. Gynaecol.*, **101**, 663–8

4. Neilson, J. P. (1995). EFM vs. intermittent auscultation in labour (revised 1994). In Keirse, M. J. N. C., Renfrew, M. J., Neilson, J. P. and Crowther, C. (eds.) *Pregnancy and Childbirth Module*. In *The Cochrane Pregnancy and Childbirth Database*, Issue 2. (Oxford: The Cochrane Collaboration). Available from BMJ Publishing Group, London

5. Neilson, J. P. (1995). Fetal blood sampling as adjunct to heart rate monitoring (revised 1994). In Keirse, M. J. N. C., Renfrew, M. J., Neilson, J. P. and Crowther, C. (eds.) *Pregnancy and Childbirth Module*. In *The Cochrane Pregnancy and Childbirth Database*, Issue 2. (Oxford: The Cochrane Collaboration, Update Software). Available from BMJ Publishing Group, London

6. Ingemarsson, E. (1981). Routine electronic fetal monitoring during labour. *Acta Obstet. Gynaecol. Scand. (Suppl.)*, **99**, 1–29

7. Hobel, C. J., Hyvarinen, M. A., Okada, D. M. and Oh, W. (1973). Prenatal and intrapartum high risk screening. I. Prediction of the high risk neonate. *Am. J. Obstet. Gynecol.*, **117**, 1–9

8. Arulkumaran, S., Gibb, D. F. and Ratnam, S. S. (1983). Experience with a selective intrapartum fetal monitoring policy. *Singapore J. Obstet. Gynaecol.*, **14**, 47–51

9. Ingemarsson, I., Arulkumaran, S., Ingemarsson, E., Tamby Raja, R. L. and Ratnam, S. S. (1986). Admission test: a screening test for fetal distress in labor. *Obstet. Gynecol.*, **68**, 800–6

10. Ingemarsson, I., Arulkumaran, S., Paul, R. H., Ingemarsson, E., Tamby Raja, R. L. and Ratnam, S. S. (1988). Fetal acoustic stimulation in early labor in patients screened with the admission test. *Am. J. Obstet. Gynecol.*, **158**, 70–4

11. Gibb, D. M. F. and Arulkumaran, S. (1992). *Fetal Monitoring in Practice*, pp. 104–26. (Oxford: Butterworth Heinemann Ltd.)

12. Fleischer, A., Schulman, H., Jagani, N., Mitchell, J. and Randolph, G. (1982). The development of fetal acidosis in the presence of an abnormal fetal heart rate tracing. I. The average-for-gestational-age fetus. *Am. J. Obstet. Gynecol.*, **144**, 55–60

13. Prentice, A. and Lind, T. (1987). Fetal heart rate monitoring during labour: too frequent intervention, too little benefit? *Lancet*, **2**, 1375–7

14. Cunningham, A. S. (1987). Electronic fetal monitoring in labour. *J. R. Soc. Med.*, **80**, 783

15. Arulkumaran, S. and Chua, S. (1996). Cardiotocography in labour. *Curr. Obstet. Gynaecol.*, **6**, 182–8

16. Ingemarsson, E., Ingemarsson, I., Solum, T. and Westgren, M. (1980). A 1-year study of routine fetal heart rate monitoring during the first stage of labour. *Acta Obstet. Gynaecol. Scand.*, **59**, 297–300

17. Beard, R. W., Filshie, G. M., Knight, C. A. and Roberts, G. M. (1971). The significance of the changes in the continuous fetal heart rate in the first stage of labour. *J. Obstet. Gynaecol. Br. Commonw.*, **78**, 865–81

18. Katz, M., Mazor, M. and Insler, V. (1981). Fetal heart rate patterns and scalp pH as predictors of fetal distress. *Israel J. Med. Sci.*, **17**, 260–5

19. Zalor, R. W. and Quilligan, E. J. (1979). The influence of scalp sampling on the Cesarean section rate for fetal distress. *Am. J. Obstet. Gynecol.*, **135**, 239–46

20. Clarke, S. L., Gimovsky, M. L. and Miller, F. C. (1984). The scalp stimulation test: a clinical alternative to fetal scalp blood sampling. *Am. J. Obstet. Gynecol.*, **148**, 274–7

21. Tejani, N., Mann, L. I. and Bhakthavathsalan, A. (1976). Correlation of fetal heart rate patterns and fetal pH with neonatal outcome. *Obstet. Gynecol.*, **48**, 460–3

22. Sykes, G. S., Molloy, P. M., Johnson, P., Stirrat, G. M. and Turnbull, A. C. (1983). Fetal distress and the condition of the newborn infants. *Br. Med. J.*, **287**, 943–5

23. Renou, P., Chang, A., Anderson, I. *et al.* (1976). Controlled trial of fetal intensive care. *Am. J. Obstet. Gynecol.*, **126**, 470–6

24. Chalmers, I. (1979). Randomised controlled trials of intrapartum monitoring. In Thalhammer, O., Baumgarten, K. V. and Pollak, A. (eds.) *Perinatal Medicine*, pp. 260–5 (Stuttgart: George Thieme)

25. Mongelli, M., Chung, T. K. H. and Chang, A. M. Z. (1997). Intervention and benefit for conditions of very low prevalence. *Br. J. Obstet. Gynaecol.*, in press

Cesarean section in Brazil: benefits and issues

34

M. J. do A. Vasconcellos

Main reasons for Cesarean section

The rate of performance of Cesarean section throughout the world has been pointing to definite changes during the past decades. In developed countries, those rates are rising, and dividing the countries into groups:

(1) Countries with a substantial increase in Cesarean rate: United States, Canada and Italy;

(2) Countries with a slight increase in Cesarean rate: Slovakia, Scotland, Norway, Hungary, Poland, Japan and The Netherlands (6–7%); United Kingdom (steady at 12% for the past decade); Ireland (with an increase of 6% to 10% from 1973 to 1987);

(3) Countries with a declining Cesarean section rate: Australia, Denmark and Finland.

The United States[1] has been showing a rising tendency in Cesarean rate as can be seen from Table 1. Canada presents a similar situation to its neighbor although its rates are not so high.

In Italy, national data[2] have recorded a significant growth in Cesarean rate as seen from Table 2. In some regions, such as Lazio, the rate rose to 24.3% in 1987.

Statistics from the developing countries are not different. In India, current Cesarean rates are around 18–20%, whereas in 1960, the reported rate was around 1%[3].

There are several possibilities to explain this increase in Cesarean section rates. Primary Cesarean sections are carried out because of mechanical problems, such as cephalopelvic disproportion and malpresentation. With the development of fetal medicine, more interruptions have been performed because of fetal distress, antepartum hemorrhage and hypertensive diseases. As well as an increase in primary Cesarean rates, 15–45% of all childbirth occurs through abdominal incision, with an indication of repeat Cesarean section. It is easier to perform another Cesarean section than properly monitor labor in a pregnant patient with a prior uterine scar.

In the early days of Cesarean section its indication was related to mechanical problems of childbirth, such as transverse presentation and cephalopelvic disproportion. With the increasing safety of obstetric surgery, Cesarean section became more and more frequent, and today repeat Cesarean, fetal distress, breech presentation, pre-eclampsia and antepartum hemorrhage are the most common reasons for abdominal obstetric surgery.

Table 1 Cesarean rates in the United States from 1965–88. Adapted from reference 1

Year	Cesarean section (%)
1965	4.5
1970	5.5
1975	10.4
1980	16.5
1988	24.7

Table 2 Cesarean rates in Italy from 1980–87. Adapted from reference 2

Year	Cesarean section (%)
1980	4.2
1983	14.5
1987	17.5

The American consensus of 1987 considered dystocia to be the leading reason for Cesarean section, followed by repeat Cesarean, fetal distress and breech presentation. Statistics show that only 3–5% of the patients with prior Cesarean were submitted to vaginal delivery. If these data are compared with data from Norway (43%) or Hungary (32%), it becomes clear that the American rates are very low[4].

Economic incentives are also responsible for the augment of Cesarean rate. The chances of being submitted to a Cesarean section are 20% higher in patients who have private health insurance. In California, Cesarean has been indicated in 29% of patients with private health insurance, in 23% of those assisted by public health insurance and in 16% of indigents. In New York, Cesarean rates are three times higher for patients who pay a private insurance company.

Another reason for high rates of Cesarean section is the low use of forceps in vaginal delivery. The Netherlands, Italy and Slovakia show a high incidence of forceps use and coincidentally lower Cesarean delivery rate, as opposed to Canada, Australia, Hungary and Israel[5].

In Germany, obstetricians are the specialists more likely to be sued, and for that reason insurance annuities are more expensive, as can be noted from Table 3[6].

Incidence of Cesarean section in Brazil

The incidence of Cesarean section in Brazil has been increasing at a faster rate than in the developed countries. Official rates are the highest, and the degree of mortality and lethality resulting from the abdominal incision is startling.

The Health Ministry of Brazil has published statistics on the incidence of Cesarean in the country in 1995, comparing the different age ranges. These numbers come from the hospitals that are part of the Unified Health Assistance. Unfortunately, the Cesarean rates for hospitals that assist health insurance companies, and for

medical insurance and obstetrical private clinics are not available, but it is known *ex officio* that the rate of Cesarean is about 60–70%. Therefore, any analysis that is to be carried out of the rate of Cesarean section should be performed taking into consideration two realities: analysis of private data is almost impossible, for not only is there no concern with recording of data, but also the cases that result in death are concealed.

Officially available material defines the lethality rate of Cesarean section. In 1995, 2 822 394 vaginal deliveries were performed by the Unified Health Assistance. Table 4 gives the incidence of vaginal and Cesarean deliveries with their relative percentages. Cesarean deliveries accounted for 32.45%.

Table 5 gives the mortality rates for vaginal and Cesarean deliveries in patients of the Unified Health Assistance in 1995.

Figure 1 shows the distribution by age range of the 366 maternal deaths resulting from vaginal childbirth, and the 580 deaths resulting from Cesarean section in 1995. Mortality rates are three times higher in Cesarean childbirth. Another important remark is that most cases occurred when the patient was between 25 and

Table 3 Insurance cost evolution in Germany for each specialty[5]

Specialty	1981 expenses (DM/year)	1991 expenses (DM/year)
Anesthesiology	9 480	11 600
Internal medicine	4 200	13 700
Urology	7 250	14 650
Radiology	10 300	15 600
Orthopedics	12 100	17 200
Surgery	21 000	26 250
Obstetrics/gynecology	12 000	75 000

Table 4 Percentages of Cesarean and vaginal deliveries that occurred in 1995 and were assisted by Unified Health Assistance in Brazil. Source: Ministry of Health of Brazil

Deliveries	Absolute number	%
Total	2 822 394	100.00
Vaginal	1 906 340	67.55
Cesarean	916 054	32.45

234

40 years old. This fact should be enough to establish a health-care policy aiming at the decline of the number of Cesareans.

Table 6 gives a comparison between vaginal and Cesarean deliveries that did not result in maternal death.

Reasons for the excessive number of Cesareans

(1) The correct diagnosis of labor will play a decisive role in the indication of Cesarean for a first gestation. If the diagnosis is incorrect, several procedures will be adopted which may include the indication of unnecessary Cesarean. Labor should be diagnosed by the currently more experienced health-care professional. Admission should be indicated only once labor has really started, for an early admission could turn into a source of anxiety for the patient, the family and consequently for the obstetrician. The patient should be properly informed of several details like the length of labor, which might take 12 h[7].

(2) Electronic fetal monitoring may lead to the increase in Cesarean rates: the use of monitoring should be well performed and interpreted.

(3) In the case of breech presentation, Cesarean tends always to be performed, irrespective of parity. Breech delivery should be better taught. The rule in most services is to indicate Cesarean for a fetus of estimated weight greater than 4000 g and less than 2500 g.

(4) Accepting that in the case of hypertension interruption is better for the newborn, the recognition of the pathophysiology of the complication allows for higher rates of interruption.

(5) Insufficient payment of the health-care professional may lead to an increase in Cesarean rate. High rates are observed in private entities where the need for not wasting time is associated with derisive payment.

(6) Lack of proper education of the specialist, beginning at the university stage, may lead to an increase in Cesarean rate.

Table 5 Mortality rate resulting from vaginal and Cesarean deliveries in 1995 in patients assisted by Unified Health Assistance of Brazil. Source: Ministry of Health of Brazil

Mortality	n	Rate
Total	946	33.5/100 000
Mortality vaginal delivery	366	19.1/100 000
Mortality Cesarean delivery	580	63.3/100 000

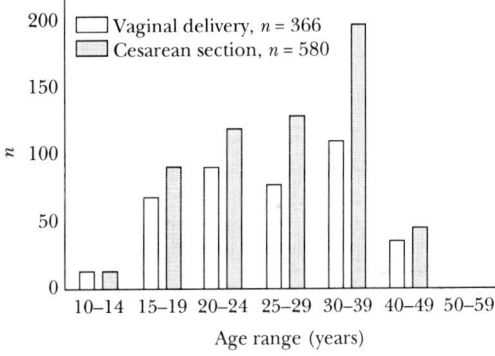

Figure 1 Distribution of childbirths assisted by Unified Health Assistance of Brazil in 1995, in vaginal and Cesarean delivery rates according to age ranges; occurrences where there was maternal death. Source: Ministry of Health of Brazil

Table 6 Distribution of childbirths assisted by Unified Health Assistance of Brazil in 1995, in vaginal and Cesarean delivery rates according to age ranges; occurrences where there was no maternal death. Source: Ministry of Health of Brazil

Age range (years)	Vaginal delivery (n (%))	Cesarean delivery (n (%))
10–14	20 324 (1.06%)	7 958 (0.86%)
15–19	486 656 (25.53%)	174 674 (19.08%)
20–24	629 374 (33.02%)	286 770 (31.32%)
25–29	402 314 (21.10%)	231 103 (25.24%)
30–39	326 597 (17.13%)	195 871 (21.39%)
40–49	39 816 (2.08%)	18 755 (2.04%)
50–59	893 (0.04%)	343 (0.03%)

(7) There may be fear of medical error in vaginal delivery, resulting from inexperience with vaginal childbirth. The current situation leads to the conclusion that the obstetrician will not be sued for having performed a Cesarean but, by not performing it, his chances of being sued are greater.

(8) Lack of proper equipment for fetal and maternal monitoring results in forcing the professional to turn to Cesarean section.

(9) There are astounding differences between daytime and night-time quality of assistance.

Proposals to reduce Cesarean section rates

(1) Education of the health-care professional and of the population through information provided by the media about the advantages of vaginal delivery is paramount. The pregnant woman should be taught to question the reason for the obstetrical indication of Cesarean.

(2) The health-care professional should be educated by improving vaginal delivery awareness at medical schools and in postgraduate courses.

(3) There should be consultants available to evaluate indications, if possible with more than two points of view about each case.

(4) Correct diagnosis of labor should be performed, always done by the currently most experienced professional.

(5) There should exist protocols to be followed in the case of indication of Cesarean section, preferably sponsored by representative entities of the specialty.

(6) Changes to judicial implications, that are currently extremely aggressive towards the obstetrician, should be made.

(7) Vaginal childbirth should be encouraged through institutional procedures, including pecuniary incentives.

(8) Health-care professionals ought to be able to admit that well-monitored vaginal delivery is possible after a Cesarean section, since the previous indication is not repeated.

(9) It should also be admitted that modern fetal monitoring is not at the service of Cesarean, but at the service of safe vaginal delivery.

(10) There should exist a mandatory communication for private clinics, through the creation of a single document for civil records.

References

1. Meyers, S. and Glescher, N. G. (1990). US Caesarean section rate – good news or bad? *N. Engl. J. Med.*, **323**, 200
2. Signorelli, C., Elliot, P., Cattaruzza, M. S. and Osborn, J. (1991). Trends in Caesarean section in Italy – an examination of national data 1980–85. *Int. J. Epidemiol.*, **20**, 712–16
3. Rao, K. B. (1995). Global aspects of a rising Caesarean section rate. *Women's Health Today*, **3**, 59–62
4. Hickel, E. J. (1995). The safety of Caesarean section. *Women's Health Today*, **3**, 65–70
5. Stephenson, P. A., Bakoula, C., Hemminki, E., Stembera, Z., Tiba, J., Verbrugge, H. P., Zupan, J., Wagner, M. G., Karugas, M., Pizacani, B., Pineault, R., Tuimala, R., Houd, S. and Lomas, J. (1993). Patterns of use of obstetric interventions in 12 countries. *Pediatr. Perinat. Epidemiol.*, **7**, 45–54
6. Savage, W. and Francome, C. (1993). British Caesarean section rates: have we reached a plateau? *Br. J. Obstet. Gynaecol.*, **100**, 493–6
7. Stronge, J. M. (1995). Strategies for reducing the Caesarean section rate. *Women's Health Today*, **3**, 55–8

What does 'optimal' Cesarean section rate mean?   35

G. P. Mandruzzato

According to the *WebsterDictionary*, 'optimum' is the greatest number or degree, or the most favorable condition. When dealing with the problem of the Cesarean section (CS) rate and its increase, we cannot indicate absolute numbers but try to find a compromise. Practically, the 'optimal' CS rate should be the 'minimal' one offering the best clinical outcome in terms of neonatal and maternal morbidity and mortality. A rational approach should be based on the evaluation of the efficacy of CS management under various clinical conditions, in which CS is believed to be necessary or beneficial for the health of the baby, the mother or both.

In recent times, the main indications for CS have remained almost unaltered and are mainly represented by dystocia, breech presentation, previous CS and fetal distress. With regard to these four conditions, by improving diagnostic accuracy and management a certain reduction of CS rate can be expected; but this reduction will be very little. In fact, the large increase of CS rate observed in recent years seems to be principally related to non-clinical factors. Socioeconomic aspects are likely to influence the CS rate and, also, the physician's attitude plays an important role[1,2]. The importance of economic factors is clear when analyzing the situation in Europe. The highest rate of CS is recorded in Western Europe (13.7%), is intermediate in Central European countries (8.77%) and is much lower in Eastern Europe (3.53%). Among the three groups, large differences exist and the highest CS rate is recorded in Italy (22.74%).

This picture is very crude, and does not offer the possibility of drawing conclusions that indicate the reasons for these large differences,

or how to find a way of attaining an 'optimal' CS rate.

In order to draw upon more detailed information, the Italian situation has been analyzed. As in the majority of countries, a large increase in CS rate between 1980 and 1991 was also recorded in Italy (Table 1). In 12 years, the CS rate doubled, while in the same period the number of liveborns per year reduced by about 12%. In the year 1991, the total number of liveborns was 562 787 and 13% of the births took place in private institutions (Table 2). The CS rate in public hospitals during this period was 21.5%, and in private hospitals 28.5%. As a consequence, the odds ratio to have a CS for an Italian woman was 1.32 when choosing to deliver in a private hospital. Subsequently, the situation has been separately analyzed for each of the 20 Italian regions (Table 3). Large differences exist for the total number of live deliveries per year among the regions: the lowest was recorded in Valle d'Aosta (967) and the largest in Campania (81 003). The percentage of births in private

Table 1 Trend of Cesarean section (CS) rate in Italy

Year	Liveborns (n)	CS (%)
1980	640 401	11.2
1981	623 103	12.7
1982	619 097	13.2
1983	601 928	14.5
1984	587 871	15.7
1985	577 345	15.8
1986	555 445	15.7
1987	551 539	17.5
1988	569 698	19.1
1989	560 688	19.9
1990	568 855	21.2
1991	562 787	22.4

hospitals was also largely different among the regions: in three regions (Basilicata, Umbria and Valle d'Aosta), this figure was practically zero. The mean rate of births in private hospitals was 13%; a lower value than this was found in 12 regions, while in five regions (Lazio, Campania, Calabria, Sicily and Sardinia), higher values were recorded. The odds ratio to have a CS, except in three cases, was always higher in private hospitals reaching a peak of 2.05 in Piemonte, followed by Abruzzo (1.95) and Molise (1.81).

In Table 4, the CS rate is presented together with the perinatal mortality rate in each region. The perinatal mortality rate in Italy in the year 1991 was 10.4 per thousand. The lowest peri-natal mortality was observed in Friuli Venezia Giulia, where the CS rate in 1991 was 17%. The highest perinatal mortality rate was observed in Calabria (16.1/1000), where the CS rate was the lowest in Italy (16.3%). At the same time, it is possible to observe that the region with the highest CS rate (Basilicata 29.6%) had a peri-natal mortality rate of 14.2/1000, inferior only to Calabria.

As more detailed data are available for Friuli Venezia Giulia, particular attention has been devoted to their analysis. In the years 1992 and 1993, the total number of deliveries was 17 904, and the CS rate was, respectively, 19.1% and 17.4% (Table 5). In Friuli Venezia Giulia, there are 15 hospitals attending deliveries and only

Table 2 Data for Cesarean section (CS) in Italy, 1991

Total liveborns (n)	Births in private hospitals (%)	Total CS (%)	CS in public hospitals (%)	CS in private hospitals (%)	OR in private hospitals
562 787	13	22.4	21.5	28.5	1.32

OR, odds ratio for CS

Table 3 Cesarean section (CS) rate in Italian regions, 1991

Region	Liveborns (n)	Births in private hospitals (%)	Total CS rate (%)	CS rate in public hospitals (%)	CS rate in private hospitals (%)	OR
Piemonte	33 511	4.4	23.9	22.9	47.1	2.05
Valle d'Aosta	967	0.1	26.5	26.5	—	—
Lombardia	76 595	3.5	20.0	19.8	29.3	1.48
Trentino	9 681	6.3	17.7	17.9	16.6	0.93
Veneto	37 665	1.4	19.3	19.3	22.7	1.18
Friuli Venezia Giulia	9 090	5.5	17.0	17.1	18.3	1.07
Liguria	11 512	1.3	23.1	23.1	35.6	1.54
Emilia Romagna	28 788	8.5	23.3	22.8	29.4	1.29
Toscana	26 395	2.6	18.0	18.0	21.3	1.18
Umbria	6 651	0.0	21.4	21.6	—	—
Marche	12 338	9.4	23.9	23.7	27.4	1.16
Lazio	50 261	13.1	28.7	26.9	37.9	1.41
Abruzzo	12 032	6.1	22.0	20.8	40.7	1.95
Molise	3 268	0.6	21.1	21.0	38.1	1.81
Campania	81 003	41.7	24.4	21.9	28.2	1.29
Puglia	50 190	10.8	22.7	23.4	17.9	0.27
Basilicata	6 274	0.0	29.6	29.8	—	—
Calabria	24 384	21.9	16.3	14.2	24.1	1.70
Sicilia	65 494	13.4	24.1	22.8	33.3	1.46
Sardegna	16 688	14.1	16.9	17.6	13.6	0.77
Italy	562 787	13.0	22.4	21.5	28.5	1.32

OR, odds ratio for CS

two are private: Casa di cura di Pordenone and Casa di cura di Udine (Table 6). In those two institutions, 5.5% of the region's liveborn babies were delivered. As the mean CS rate in that period was 18.3%, it is easy to observe that six hospitals presented rates inferior to the mean.

In Table 7, the odds ratio for CS is considered according to the number of deliveries in each unit and whether public or private. The odds ratio is inversely proportional to the number of deliveries per year, being about double if the delivery took place in units attending less than 500 deliveries per year. The odds ratio for private hospitals is also higher (1.28) than that for public hospitals, and similar to that observed for all Italy (see Table 3).

Moreover, the CS rate has been recorded according to the day of the week and the hour of the day. Observing Table 8, it is possible to see that the CS rate during the weekend was lower compared with that for the other days. Looking at the distribution of CS rate according to the hour of the day, it is possible to see that, during the night, the CS rate was much lower

Table 4 Comparison of Cesarean section (CS) rate and perinatal mortality (PM) rate in Italian regions, 1991

Region	CS rate (%)	PM rate (per 1000)
Piemonte	23.9	9.5
Valle d'Aosta	26.5	8.3
Lombardia	20	7.8
Trentino	17.7	6.5
Veneto	19.3	7.8
Friuli Venezia Giulia	17	5.4
Liguria	23.1	9.1
Emilia Romagna	23.3	8.5
Toscana	18	8.8
Umbria	21.4	9.6
Marche	23.9	8
Lazio	28.7	9.8
Abruzzo	22	11
Molise	21.1	13.6
Campania	24.4	13.7
Puglia	22.7	12.3
Basilicata	29.6	14.2
Calabria	16.3	16.1
Sicilia	24.1	13.6
Sardegna	16.9	10

Table 5 Deliveries in Friuli Venezia Giulia (total deliveries = 17 904)

Year	Vaginal delivery		Cesarean section	
	n	%	n	%
1992	7472	80.9	1766	19.1
1993	7156	82.6	1510	17.4

Table 6 Cesarean section (CS) rate in hospitals, Friuli Venezia Giulia

Hospital	CS rate (%)	Births per year (n)
S. Daniele	11.7	630
Pordenone	12.4	1150
Monfalcone	14.1	400
S. Vito	17.1	540
Burlo Garafolo-Trieste	17.1	1860
Tolmezzo	17.5	320
Latisana	18.5	520
Palmanova	19.6	460
Gorizia	20.9	410
Spilimbergo	21.3	270
Casa di cura di Pordenone	21.3	380
Gemona	21.9	496
Cividale	24.9	285
Casa di cura di Udine	24.3	210
Policlinico Universita Udine	25.6	930

Table 7 Odds ratio (OR) for Cesarean section, Friuli Venezia Giulia

	OR
Number of deliveries per year	
1000–2000	1
500–999	1.47
499 or less	1.94
Hospital	
Public	1
Private	1.28

Table 8 Cesarean section (CS) rate according to day of the week, Friuli Venezia Giulia

Day	CS rate (%)
Sunday	7.9
Monday	14.3
Tuesday	16.5
Wednesday	14.9
Thursday	18.2
Friday	17.9
Saturday	10.3

6

Table 9 Cesarean section (CS) rate according to hour of the day, Friuli Venezia Giulia

Hour	CS rate (%)
00–01	13.9
01–02	6.3
02–03	10.1
03–04	5.7
04–05	7.6
05–06	8.1
06–07	9.0
07–08	8.3
08–09	29.3
09–10	29.5
10–11	34.2
11–12	31.2
12–13	29.4
13–14	22.1
14–15	18.4
15–16	12.8
16–17	17.0
17–18	15.4
18–19	18.4
19–20	21.4
20–21	14.2
21–22	12.4
22–23	13.0
23–24	14.3
Total	18.1

than that between 8 a.m. and 2 p.m. and 6 p.m. and 8 p.m. (Table 9).

Discussion

Data have been analyzed with regard to the whole of Europe, Italy and one Italian region, namely, Friuli Venezia Giulia.

Looking first at the CS rate in Europe and the differences recorded for Western, Central and Eastern Europe, the only apparent evidence is that the CS rate is directly proportional to the economic situation of the different parts of the continent. This very crude consideration does not offer possibilities for defining the reasons of the increase in CS rate and how to reach an 'optimal' figure.

Moving to analyze a more restricted area such as Italy, where the CS rate is the highest in Europe, the only clear evidence is that CS was more frequently performed in private than public hospitals. However, this is not always true because in three Italian regions the odds ratio for CS was lower in private hospitals. No correlation has been found between CS rate and perinatal mortality. The region presenting the highest perinatal mortality also had the lowest CS rate, but the region that had the highest CS rate had the second worst result in terms of perinatal mortality. Moreover, the lowest perinatal mortality rate was observed in one region (Friuli Venezia Giulia) where the CS rate was also at a minimal level.

The three aforementioned observations are clearly contradictory. A more detailed picture is available for Friuli Venezia Giulia, also offering the possibility to indicate some reasons for the CS rate and how a more 'optimal' number could be approached.

Again, the odds ratio for CS was higher in private hospitals compared with that for public hospitals. However, as the number of deliveries in private institutions was rather small, this fact does not very much influence the overall figure. Besides this fact, other evidence is clear: the CS rate was inversely proportional to the number of deliveries that were attended in the unit. Considering as 1 the odds ratio in hospitals with more than 1000 deliveries per year, it became 1.47 when the deliveries were between 500 and 999 per year and reached a peak of 1.94 when the number of deliveries was 499 or less.

This observation, together with those of the CS rate distribution according to day of the week and hour of the day, leads to the following consideration. As it is difficult to believe that biological or clinical conditions are reasons for this uneven distribution, it seems possible that, in smaller units, the level of assistance offered is not the same at any time of the day or night, or on any day of the week, therefore inducing an attitude to deliver some particular cases in the most favorable conditions. This consideration is also supported by looking at the rate of vaginal delivery after previous CS in the different hospitals. The rate of vaginal delivery in the smaller hospitals was less than the mean observed for the entire region (33%) (Table 10).

Table 10 Rate of vaginal deliveries in previous Cesarean section (CS), Friuli Venezia Giulia, 1992–93

Hospital	Vaginal deliveries		CS		Births per year
	n	%	n	%	
Monfalcone	21	65.6	11	34.4	400
S. Daniele	31	47.7	34	52.3	630
Pordenone	51	46.4	59	53.6	1150
Burlo	82	44.8	101	55.2	1860
Casa di cura di Pordenone	16	42.1	22	57.9	380
Policlinico Universita Udine	53	41.7	74	58.3	930
Palmanova	16	41.0	23	59.0	460
Tolmezzo	12	38.7	19	61.3	320
S. Vito	19	29.7	45	70.3	540
Spilimbergo	7	26.9	19	73.1	270
Gorizia	12	23.5	39	76.5	410
Gemona	5	8.6	53	91.4	496
Cividale	3	7.3	38	92.7	285
Latisana	4	6.7	56	93.3	520
Casa di cura di Udine	2	4.7	41	95.3	210
Mean regional rate of vaginal delivery		33.0			

As far as clinical conditions are concerned, it is possible to speculate, on the basis of Friuli Venezia Giulia data, what could be the magnitude of CS rate reduction by applying different kinds of management for two conditions: previous CS and breech presentation. If, in any hospital, the regional mean rate of vaginal delivery after previous CS could be attained, a 0.9% reduction of CS rate would be achieved. Breech presentations are delivered by CS in the large majority of cases, and its frequency is about 3%. Assuming that external cephalic version is successful in 40% of cases, allowing vaginal delivery, another 1.3% of CSs could be avoided. The total expected reduction in CS rate being 2.2% for the region, therefore, means that the overall CS rate could be reduced to 16.1%, based on the figures for 1992–93.

Conclusions

The definition of an 'optimal' CS rate is more than a puzzling problem. It can be easy to analyze casuistics coming from a single institution and to define possible solutions in order to reach this 'optimal' number. When faced with data from large areas such as Europe or smaller areas such as Italy, the only clear evidence is that non-clinical factors, primarily economic situations, are strictly linked to the CS rate and probably to its increase observed in recent years.

The possibility to realistically influence these aspects, at least in a short period of time, is small. On the contrary, a further increase in CS rate can be expected as the economic situation improves in some countries.

Returning to the concept that an 'optimal' CS rate can be defined as a compromise between the lowest possible number of CSs compatible with the best clinical outcome, some conclusions can be drawn from the Italian situation.

In one region (Friuli Venezia Giulia), the perinatal mortality rate is the lowest in Italy with the lowest CS rate of 18.3% for the period 1992–93. Analyzing some clinical indications for CS and possible alternative management, a reduction of 2.2% could be achieved, reducing the CS rate to 16.1%. This figure is close to that indicated by the World Health Organization (WHO), that suggests the CS rate should not exceed 15%. To achieve such a result requires better organization, particularly within the smaller obstetric units, and an educational program in order to modify some medical attitudes.

References

1. Gould, J. B., Davey, B. and Stafford, R. S. (1989). Socioeconomic differences in rates of cesarean section. *N. Engl. J. Med.*, **321**, 233–9

2. Goyert, G. L., Bottoms, S. F., Treadwell, M. C. and Nehra, P. C. (1989). The physician factor in cesarean birth rates. *N. Engl. J. Med.*, **320**, 706–9

Vaginal delivery after previous Cesarean section

36

S. Chua, S. Arulkumaran and W. L. Choo

Introduction

In the 1970s and early 1980s, Cesarean section rates rose rapidly, especially in the industrialized countries[1]. This appears to have given way to stabilization of the Cesarean section rate in the late 1980s and 1990s[1].

The population of women with a previous Cesarean section scar are at high risk of a repeat Cesarean section. It has been reported that 99% of women with a previous Cesarean section were delivered by repeat Cesarean section in American hospitals in 1974[2]. Previous Cesarean section is a major indication for Cesarean section in many other countries[3]. The contribution of this indication to the overall Cesarean section rates varies (Table 1)[1], and repeat Cesarean section may be performed in one in three births after a previous Cesarean section[4]. Underlying the national differences in contribution of previous Cesarean section were strong differences in attitudes to vaginal delivery after Cesarean section in the different countries[1]. To prevent this rapidly increasing Cesarean section rate, the different management policies of a woman with previous Cesarean section need to be assessed critically.

Table 1 Rates of vaginal delivery (%) after Cesarean section, 1980–90. From reference 1

	1980	*1985*	*1990*
Norway	56.9	53.8	56.2
Scotland	38.7	56.3	50.0
Sweden	40.7	47.4	52.9
United States	3.0	7.0	19.5

Trial of labor

The rate of a successful vaginal delivery after previous Cesarean section has been reported to vary from 38 to 93%[4–6]. Women for a trial of scar (trial of labor in women with a scarred uterus) should be carefully selected based on the events that led to the previous Cesarean section. The current pregnancy must also be assessed for feasibility of a trial of scar. Patient preference also plays an important role in decision making. About 40–50% of women eligible for trial of scar may opt to undergo repeat Cesarean section[7,8]. If we are able to allow more women a proper trial of scar instead of adhering to the concept of repeated Cesarean section, then the increase in Cesarean rates may be controlled.

Maternal mortality associated with Cesarean section can be up to 10 times that of a woman delivered vaginally[9]. Maternal morbidity is also increased after Cesarean section compared with vaginal delivery. While neither Cesarean section nor a trial of labor is risk-free, there is evidence that vaginal birth after Cesarean section is associated with a shorter hospital stay, fewer postpartum transfusions and a decreased incidence of postpartum maternal fever[10]. Despite that, many obstetricians prefer to deliver women by a repeat Cesarean section, even though the incidence of scar rupture is low[11–13].

The most serious risk associated with a trial of scar is the potential of scar rupture. However, the incidence of scar rupture has been reported to be as low as 0.3–1.7%[11–13]. Data also shows[14,15] that loss of integrity of a transverse low-segment incision (window, dehiscence, frank rupture) occurred as frequently in women without labor as in those allowed a trial of scar. Many series have shown that rupture of a transverse low-segment scar does not carry an increased fetal risk if appropriately managed. Today maternal mortality from rupture of a previous Cesarean scar is uncommon. Bloodless dehiscence is the most common form of loss of integrity of the lower-segment Cesarean scar. It has few clinical signs and usually does not cause significant morbidity and mortality. It is more often than not diagnosed at the time of abdominal delivery for some other indication such as failure to progress, or after vaginal delivery[16].

A review of the literature on vaginal birth after a previous Cesarean section has shown that rupture of a prior lower-segment uterine incision is often incomplete, as compared to spontaneous or traumatic rupture of an unscarred uterus which is often complete and may be catastrophic. It is this rupture of the unscarred uterus that is associated with high maternal and fetal mortality rates, and not rupture of post-Cesarean scars[17–19].

It is thus not surprising that 97% of consultants in the UK are in general agreement[20] with the recommendations of the Canadian policy statement that a trial of labor after a previous Cesarean section is recommended for women who meet the following criteria: one low transverse incision Cesarean section, a singleton vertex presentation and no absolute indication for Cesarean section in the present pregnancy[21].

The National Institute of Health[22] has also produced similar guidelines, although consultants in the United States are less aggressive in pursuing a vaginal delivery than their colleagues across the Atlantic. The National Institute of Health recommended that patients should be properly selected to permit a safe trial of labor. Patients who have had a previous classical inverted T incision, or low vertical incision, should be excluded. Informed consent must be obtained for a trial of labor. Labor should be performed in a hospital where appropriate facilities, services and staff are available for prompt emergency Cesarean section. Patients should be informed in advance about the limits of a particular institution's capabilities and the availability of other institutions capable of

offering this service. Patient participation plays a very important part in the management of a woman who has had a previous Cesarean section.

The American College of Obstetricians and Gynecologists has collected and analyzed several studies, and agrees that vaginal birth after Cesarean section is indicated in all women who have no contraindications as mentioned above, and who are agreeable to a trial of labor. Trial of labor should be conducted in a hospital which is equipped to handle intrapartum emergencies[23].

Selection of women for trial of labor

Number of previous incisions

While a trial of vaginal delivery after one previous Cesarean section in selected patients has become an accepted option with a success rate of 38–93%[4–6], a trial of scar in patients with more than one previous Cesarean section remains controversial. Whether the number of previous Cesarean section scars has any influence on uterine scar rupture is not known.

Several papers suggest that multiple scars rule out the possibility of vaginal delivery because of the increased risk of scar dehiscence and rupture[24,25]. Other authors believe that multiple scars should not be a contraindication to vaginal delivery[26–29]. In a recent trial of planned vaginal delivery after two previous Cesarean sections[29], the rates of vaginal delivery, scar dehiscence, uterine rupture and associated complications among 115 women with two previous Cesarean sections who underwent trial of labor were compared with those of 1006 women with two previous Cesarean sections who did not have a trial of labor. One hundred and three (89%) of the women who had a trial of labor were delivered vaginally. Prostaglandin was used for induction of labor in 37 women (32%) and augmentation of labor with oxytocin was required in 32 (28%) in the trial-of-labor group. One scar dehiscence (0.8%) was detected among the 115 women who had a trial of labor after two previous Cesarean sections, compared with seven (0.7%) among 1006 women with two previous Cesarean sections scheduled for elective Cesarean section over the same period of time. The woman who developed scar dehiscence during trial of labor had secondary arrest of labor, and the dehiscence was detected and repaired at Cesarean section. She subsequently went on to have two uncomplicated Cesarean sections. Cesarean hysterectomy was performed on one patient (0.8%) in the trial-of-labour group because of atonic postpartum hemorrhage at Cesarean section for secondary arrest in labor. Fifteen (1.4%) hysterectomies were performed in women scheduled for elective repeat section, eight for atonic postpartum hemorrhage and seven for placenta accreta. There was one maternal death among the women scheduled for elective repeat section. The authors concluded that a trial of labor in selected women with two previous Cesarean sections appears to be a reasonable option.

Type of scar

The incidence of uterine rupture is increased 2–10 fold[6,11,17] in women with a previous classical Cesarean section; maternal and perinatal mortality is 5–10 times higher[17,30] when compared to women with previous lower segment Cesarean section. These patients should be excluded from trials of labor. The clinical picture is also less serious after a ruptured lower segment scar compared with a ruptured classical Cesarean section scar. In Dewhurst's series[30], two-thirds of women with a classical scar rupture were collapsed requiring transfusion and urgent treatment, compared with less than one-tenth of cases after a lower-segment scar rupture. In this review, there were five maternal deaths after 100 ruptured classical scars and no deaths with 55 ruptured lower-segment scars. In other reports, complete ruptures occurred more frequently in classical scars, and incomplete ruptures in the lower-segment scars[17]. Women with inverted T incisions, extensive lateral tears and perforations of the fundus are better excluded from trials of labor. Those with lower-segment transverse scars are the most suitable for a trial of

labor[3,12]. Limited data appears to support trial of scar for patients with previous vertical incisions confined to the lower segment of the uterus[31,32].

Indication for previous Cesarean section

In selecting women with a previous Cesarean section for a trial of vaginal delivery, the indication for the previous Cesarean section has traditionally been a significant factor. Some studies specifically exclude women with previous Cesarean section for a recurrent cause, such as cephalopelvic disproportion, from trial of labor because of fear of scar rupture, but others include them[4,24,28,33–37].

In a recent large multicenter study, women who had the primary Cesarean section for cephalopelvic disproportion or failure to progress were found to be less likely to deliver vaginally, but were still successful in two-thirds of cases[10]. Many authors[33,36,37] have shown that the vaginal delivery rates for women with a previous lower-segment Cesarean section for recurrent indications like cephalopelvic disproportion and no progress of labor, were not significantly different from those of women with previous Cesarean section done for non-recurrent indications. Exclusion of women from a trial of labor after a previous lower-segment Cesarean section for cephalopelvic disproportion or failure to progress is not justified. In some of these women failure to progress in the previous labor could have been due to malposition (relative cephalopelvic disproportion). With normal position and adequate uterine activity, vaginal delivery may be achieved safely. Feto-pelvic disproportion will have to be excluded in the present pregnancy before a trial of labor is permitted. To assess the adequacy of the pelvis for vaginal delivery, clinical pelvimetry or X-ray pelvimetry for a less subjective assessment can be carried out[11,14,38]. However, the reliability of routine antepartum X-ray pelvimetry for deciding the route of delivery has recently been questioned[39,40]. Routine X-ray pelvimetry in women with a previous Cesarean section may increase the elective Cesarean section rate without assuring vaginal delivery in women considered for a trial of labor[39].

The fetal size is estimated by considering the gestational age, size of patient, size of fetal head and clinical experience and knowledge of fetal weight at different gestations. Ultrasound estimation of fetal weight may be useful. A trial of labor may still be given to a patient with a bigger baby than the previous ones if the labor is progressing well without any evidence of fetal distress[3,41]. In a case–control study there were no significant differences in maternal and perinatal morbidity for women who underwent a trial of scar and delivered infants > 4000 g compared to those who delivered infants < 4000 g[41]. Maternal and perinatal morbidity were also similar when women who delivered macrosomic infants after trial of scar were compared with women who delivered macrosomic infants without a previous history of Cesarean section[41].

Facilities available for trial of labor

To conduct a trial of labor, fetal monitoring, blood transfusion, anesthetic and pediatric facilities should be available. During labor, scar rupture can present with clinical symptoms and signs of bleeding per vaginum, tenderness over the scar or abnormal fetal heart rate pattern. Acute fetal bradycardia may be a sign of scar rupture, and if it is > 10 min duration from whatever cause, it is likely to be associated with severe acidosis and hence needs delivery by Cesarean section within 10–15 min of decision[42]. A code of 'immediate' Cesarean section should be used to indicate the urgency of the situation to the theater staff and anesthetist.

The woman and her partner should be properly counseled regarding the benefits and risks of the trial of labor and how the trial will be performed. Informed consent should be obtained.

Use of oxytocin

The reluctance to use oxytocin to augment labor in women with a previous Cesarean scar is because of the fear of uterine rupture or dehiscence. As a result, a trial of labor may be abandoned prematurely in women with inadequate uterine contractions. Recent studies have shown that judicious use of oxytocin and careful monitoring in labor do not result in an increased risk of rupture, or any change in maternal or perinatal outcome[13,15,36,43–46].

Uterine activity profiles in women with a Cesarean scar and poor progress of labor have been described[46]. In 63 women with one previous Cesarean section who did not progress in labor due to poor uterine activity but with no clinical evidence of cephalopelvic disproportion, labor was augmented using oxytocin. Following augmentation, 78% delivered vaginally and the rest needed Cesarean section. The study showed that there was no difference in the frequency of uterine contractions, amplitude of uterine contractions and uterine activity integral, between the vaginal delivery group and the Cesarean section group before augmentation. After augmentation, the frequency, amplitude and uterine activity were significantly but similarly elevated in the two groups. The median uterine activities in these two groups were higher than in the women with previous Cesarean sections who had normal progress of labor without oxytocic augmentation and vaginal delivery. The women who delivered vaginally after augmentation dilated at a rate of 1.5 cm/h, whilst the women ending in a Cesarean section dilated only at the rate of 0.3 cm/h. All Cesarean sections were for cephalopelvic disproportion, and the mean birthweight of babies born by Cesarean section (3598 g) was significantly heavier than that of babies born vaginally (3230 g). Presumably, the heavier babies had cephalopelvic disproportion and failed to progress despite adequate uterine activity for a sufficient length of time. The authors concluded that satisfactory cervical dilatation in the presence of optimum uterine activity for the next few hours after augmentation would be an important factor in predicting the mode of delivery.

In a previous study, the same authors studied the characteristics and outcome of labor in 1158 nulliparae and 1360 multiparae who had no previous Cesarean scar. Of these, 220 nulliparae and 99 multiparae had dysfunctional first stage of labor[47]. The majority (65.5% of nulliparae and 83.3% of multiparae) with dysfunctional labor responded with satisfactory progress within the first 4 h of augmentation. The Cesarean section rate was low (1.3%) in this group who had satisfactory progress, and the neonatal outcome was good. In nulliparae who did not show satisfactory progress in the first 3–4 h with oxytocic augmentation, the Cesarean section rate was 49% despite a 15-h labor. In multiparae, the Cesarean section rate in those who did not respond satisfactorily to augmentation was 66% despite 14 h of labor.

Women with previous Cesarean section and dysfunctional labor can be subjected to judicious oxytocin augmentation. The rate of progress of labor during the first 3–4 h after augmentation appears to indicate the likely outcome and hence should help in the decision about whether to continue oxytocin. Scar rupture has been reported with prolonged infusion of oxytocin for > 6 h despite poor progress of labor[16]. Despite reports of scar dehiscence with oxytocin use, the benefits of oxytocin appear to outweigh the risks, provided the patient is monitored appropriately.

Symptoms and signs of scar rupture: monitoring in labor

Many studies have shown that the classical symptoms and signs described with scar rupture, such as scar pain or tenderness, bleeding per vaginum, maternal tachycardia and hypotension, are poor indicators of a rupture as they often occur late and after severe degrees of rupture[16,48]. Fetal distress manifested by changes in the cardiotocograph is not an uncommon finding with scar rupture[48]. Early fetal heart rate changes associated with scar dehiscence include variable decelerations with progressive fetal tachycardia and loss of baseline variability at the onset. This may progress to more severe variable decelerations and ultimately to terminal fetal bradycardia and intrauterine death. These findings suggest that continuous fetal heart rate monitoring may provide early signs of scar rup-

ture, compared with other clinical symptoms and signs which may develop later with further loss of scar integrity[16].

Beckley and colleagues[49] analyzed 10 cases of scar rupture in labor after a previous lower segment Cesarean section. All the women were monitored with continuous electronic fetal heart rate recording and intrauterine pressure measurements. In four cases, recordings showed a marked fall in uterine activity because of clipping off of pressure peaks, and these features occurred before fetal heart rate changes were identified. In another report of nine cases of scar rupture[16], three cases showed reduction of uterine activity and one showed fetal bradycardia.

Sudden reduction of uterine pressure may be an early warning sign of scar rupture. However, when external tocography is used, loosening of the belt or a change in position of the woman may account for reduction in uterine activity[16]. However, intrauterine pressure monitoring should not be a substitute, nor an over-riding factor in overall clinical appraisal of the woman during a trial of labor. It should not in itself be regarded as a 'safeguard' against scar rupture, and the decision to continue labor, especially when augmentation of labor with oxytocin is necessary, should be based on assessment of progress of labor and the fetal heart rate pattern.

Cesarean section statistics in Singapore

The Cesarean section rate in Singapore has increased from 14.7% in 1980 to 27.2% in 1995 (Table 2). This rise in the Cesarean section rate is also found in most other countries.

The repeat Cesarean section rate in patients with a previous Cesarean section in our department during the period of January 1990 to December 1996 was analyzed. There were 2460 pregnancies with a previous Cesarean section. Of these, 11.6% underwent an elective repeat Cesarean section, and 15.5% had an emergency Cesarean section. Of those who had a trial of scar after one previous Cesarean section, 72.9%

Table 2 Cesarean section rates and perinatal mortality rates in Singapore, 1980–95. The figures in parentheses are the rates for the University department

	1980	1986	1990	1995
Cesarean section rate (%)	14.7 (9.7)	18.5 (13.5)	21.9 (12.2)	27.2 (16.9)
Perinatal mortality rate (per 1000 births)	13.4 (12.2)	10.2 (7.9)	7.3 (6.9)	4.3 (5.5)

Prepared by the Epidemiology and Disease Control Department, Ministry of Health Headquarters, Singapore

delivered vaginally. There were five emergency Cesarean sections carried out for impending scar rupture; all scars were noted to be intact during the operation. There were three scar ruptures. In two of these women, cardiotocographic changes, which progressed over time from a reactive fetal heart rate trace to fetal tachycardia and severe variable decelerations and ultimately fetal bradycardia, prompted the decision for operation. There were no maternal signs and symptoms in labor. In the third woman, fetal tachycardia and prolonged (> 90 s) and severe (> 60 bts/min) variable decelerations were present in the late first stage. She progressed to a normal vaginal delivery. Post-delivery, she developed signs and symptoms of an acute abdomen. At laparotomy, repair of the scar dehiscence was performed and post-operative recovery was uneventful. In all three women, the babies were delivered in good condition with Apgar scores ≥ 8 at 5 min. Oxytocin was used for augmentation of labor in all three women who had scar dehiscence/rupture.

Medicolegal aspects

Many clinicians are reluctant to give a trial of labor due to the fear of medicolegal consequences in cases of scar rupture.

It is important to:

(1) Carefully select the women for a trial of labor;

(2) Explain clearly to both the woman and her husband the conduct of the trial of labor, its benefits and risks, and document the discussion;

(3) Conduct the labor in a fully equipped center, preferably with continuous electronic fetal heart rate monitoring and, where facilities permit, intrauterine pressure monitoring;

(4) Have facilities and training for emergency intervention when required;

(5) Act promptly when the situation demands.

Conclusion

In properly selected cases, vaginal delivery is the best and safest form of obstetric management. The incidence of scar rupture is low, and maternal and fetal morbidity are not common or serious when such trials of labor are appropriately managed.

References

1. Notozon, F. C., Cnattiys, S., Bergsjo, P., Cole, S., Taffel, S., Irgens, L. and Daltveit, A. K. (1994). Cesarean section delivery in the 1980s: international comparison by indication. *Am. J. Obstet. Gynecol.*, **170**, 495–504

2. Saldana, L., Schulman, H. and Reuss, L. (1979). Management of pregnancy after Cesarean section. *Am. J. Obstet. Gynecol.*, **135**, 555–61

3. Bolaji, I. I. and Meehan, F. P. (1993). Post-Caesarean section delivery. *Eur. J. Obstet. Gynaecol.*, **51**, 181–92

4. ACOG Practice Patterns (1996). Vaginal delivery after previous cesarean birth. *Int. J. Gynecol. Obstet.*, **52**, 90–8

5. Meehan, F., Moolgaoker, A. and Stallworthy, J. (1972). Vaginal delivery under caudal analgaesia after Caesarean section and other major uterine surgery. *Br. Med. J.*, **2**, 740

6. Wilson, A. L. (1951). Labor and delivery after cesarean section. *Am. J. Obstet. Gynecol.*, **62**, 1225–33

7. Hueston, W. J. and Rudy, M. (1994). Factors preceding elective repeat cesarean delivery. *Obstet. Gynecol.*, **83**, 741–4

8. Joseph, G. F. Jr, Stedman, C. M. and Robichaux, A. G. (1991). Vaginal birth after cesarean section: the impact of patient resistance to a trial of labor. *Am. J. Obstet. Gynecol.*, **164**, 1441–4

9. Ritchie, J. W. K. (1986). Obstetric operations and procedures. In *Dewhurst's Textbook of Obstetrics and Gynaecology for Postgraduates*, 4th edn. pp. 428–41 (Oxford: Blackwell Scientific Publications)

10. Flamm, B. L., Goings, J. R., Liu, Y. and Wolde-Tsadik, G. (1994). Elective repeat cesarean delivery versus trial of labor: a prospective multicenter study. *Obstet. Gynecol.*, **83**, 927–32

11. Lavin, J. P., Stephens, R. S., Miodovnik, M. and Barden, T. P. (1982). Vaginal delivery in patients with a prior cesarean section. *Obstet. Gynecol.*, **59**, 135–47

12. Nielsen, T. F., Ljungblad, U. and Hagberg, H. (1989). Rupture and dehiscence of cesarean section scar during pregnancy and delivery. *Am. J. Obstet. Gynecol.*, **160**, 569–73

13. Flamm, B. L., Naoman, L. A., Thomas, S. J., Fallon, D. and Yoshida, M. M. (1990). Vaginal birth after Cesarean delivery: results of a 5-year multicenter collaborative study. *Obstet. Gynecol.*, **76**, 750–3

14. Gibbs, C. (1980). Planned vaginal delivery following cesarean section. *Clin. Obstet. Gynecol.*, **23**, 507–15

15. Clark, S. L. (1988). Rupture of scarred uterus. *Obstet. Gynecol. Clin. N. Am.*, **15**, 737–44

16. Arulkumaran, S., Chua, S. and Ratnam, S. S. (1992). Symptoms and signs with scar rupture – value of uterine activity measurements. *Aust. NZ J. Obstet. Gynaecol.*, **32**, 208–12

17. Muller, P. F., Heiser, W. and Graham, W. (1961). Repeat Cesarean section. *Am. J. Obstet. Gynecol.*, **81**, 867–76

18. Schrinsky, D. L. and Benson, R. L. (1978). Rupture of the pregnant uterus. A review. *Obstet. Gynecol. Surv.*, **33**, 217–32

19. Golan, A., Sandbank, O. and Rubin, A. (1980). Rupture of the pregnant uterus. *Obstet. Gynecol.*, **56**, 549–59

20. Roberts, L. J., Beardsworth, S. A. and Trew, G. (1994). Labour following Caesarean section: current practice in the United Kingdom. *Br. J. Obstet. Gynaecol.*, **101**, 153–5

21. Panel and Planning Committee of the National Consensus Conference on Aspects of Cesarean Birth (1996). Indications for cesarean section: final statement of the panels of the National Consensus Conference on aspects of cesarean birth. *Can. Med. Assoc. J.*, **134**, 1348–52

22. NIH Consensus Development Task Force (1981). NIH Consensus Development Task Force statement on cesarean childbirth. *Am. J. Obstet. Gynecol.*, **139**, 902–9

23. ACOG Practice Patterns (1995). Vaginal delivery after a previous Cesarean section. *Int. J. Obstet. Gynecol.*, **52**, 90–8

24. Tahilramaney, M. P., Boucher, M., Eglinton Garry, S., Beall, M. and Phelan, J. P. (1984). Previous cesarean section and trial of labor; factors related to uterine dehiscence. *J. Reprod. Med.*, **29(1)**, 17–21

25. Pedowitz, B. and Schwartz, R. M. (1987). The true incidence of silent rupture of cesarean section scar. A prospective analysis of 403 cases. *Am. J. Obstet. Gynecol.*, **74**, 1071–81

26. Meier, P. R. and Porreco, R. P. (1982). Trial of labor following cesarean section: a two-year experience. *Am. J. Obstet. Gynecol.*, **144**, 671–8

27. Porreco, R. P. and Meier, P. R. (1983). Trial of labor in patients with multiple cesarean section. *J. Reprod. Med.*, **28**, 770–2

28. Phelan, J. P., Clark, S. L., Diaz, F. and Paul, R. H. (1987). Vaginal birth after cesarean section. *Am. J. Obstet. Gynecol.*, **157**, 1510–15

29. Chaltopadhyay, S. K., Sherbeeni, M. M. and Anokute, C. C. (1994). Planned vaginal delivery after two previous Caesarean sections. *Br. J. Obstet. Gynaecol.*, **101**, 498–500

30. Dewhurst, C. L. (1957). The ruptured Caesarean section scar. *J. Obstet. Gynaecol. Br. Commonw.*, **64**, 113–18

31. Pichkart, M. G., Martin, J. N. Jr, Maydrech, E. F., Blake, P. G., Martin, R. W., Perry, K. G. Jr *et al.* (1992). Vaginal birth after cesarean delivery: are there useful and valid predictors of success or failure? *Am. J. Obstet. Gynecol.*, **166**, 1811–15

32. Stovall, T. G., Shaver, D. C., Solomon, S. K. and Anderson, G. D. (1987). Trial of labor in previous cesarean section patients, excluding classical cesarean sections. *Obstet. Gynecol.*, **70**, 713–17

33. Seitchik, J. and Rao, V. R. R. (1982). Cesarean delivery in nulliparous women for failed oxytocin-augmented labor. Route of delivery in sub-

sequent pregnancy. *Am. J. Obstet. Gynecol.*, **143**, 393

34. Benedetti, T. J., Platt, L. D. and Druzin, M. (1982). Vaginal delivery after previous cesarean section for a non-recurrent cause. *Am. J. Obstet. Gynecol.*, **112**, 358–9

35. Clark, S. L., Eglinton, G. S., Beall, M. and Phelan, J. P. (1984). Effect of indication for previous cesarean section on subsequent delivery outcome in patients undergoing a trial of labor. *J. Reprod. Med.*, **29**(1), 22–5

36. Chua, S., Arulkumaran, S., Piara Singh and Ratnam, S. S. (1989). Trial of labour after previous Caesarean section: obstetric outcome. *Aust. NZ J. Obstet. Gynaecol.*, **29**, 12–17

37. Miller, M. and Leader, R. (1992). Vaginal delivery after Caesarean section. *Aust. NZ J. Obstet. Gynaecol.*, **32**, 213–16

38. Nielson, T. F., Hokegard, K.-H. and Moldin, P. G. (1985). X-ray pelvimetry and trial of labor after previous Cesarean section. *Acta Obstet. Gynecol. Scand.*, **64**, 485–90

39. Thubisi, M., Ebrahim, A., Moodug, J. and Shweni, P. M. (1993). Vaginal delivery after previous Cesarean section. Is pelvimetry necessary? *Br. J. Obstet. Gynecol.*, **100**, 421–4

40. Krishnamurthy, S., Fairlie, F., Cameron, A. D., Walker, J. J. and Mackenzie, J. R. (1991). The role of postnatal X-ray pelvimetry after Caesarean section in the management of subsequent delivery. *Br. J. Obstet. Gynaecol.*, **98**, 716–18

41. Flamm, B. L. and Goings, J. R. (1989). Vaginal birth after Cesarean section: is suspected fetal macrosomia a contraindication? *Obstet. Gynecol.*, **74**, 694–7

42. Ingermasson, I., Arulkumaran, S. and Ratnam, S. S. (1985). Bolus injection of terbutaline in labor. Effect on fetal pH in cases with prolonged bradycardia. *Am. J. Obstet. Gynecol.*, **153**, 859–65

43. Horenstein, J. M., Eglinton, S. G., Thilramaney, M. P., Boucher, M. and Phelan, J. P. (1984). Oxytocin use during a trial of labor in patients with previous cesarean section. *J. Reprod. Med.*, **29**(1), 26–30

44. Flamm, B., Goings, J., Fulbright, N.-J. *et al.* (1987). Oxytocin during labor after previous cesarean section. Results of a multicenter study. *Obstet. Gynecol.*, **70**, 709–12

45. Horenstein, J. M. and Phelan, J. P. (1985). Previous cesarean section – risks and benefits of oxytocin usage in trial of labor. *Am. J. Obstet. Gynecol.*, **151**, 564–9

46. Arulkumaran, S., Ingermasson, I. and Ratnam, S. S. (1989). Oxytocin augmentation in dysfunctional labour after previous Caesarean section. *Br. J. Obstet. Gynecol.*, **96**, 939–41

47. Arulkumaran, S. Koh, C. H., Ingermasson, I. and Ratnam, S. S. (1987). Augmentation of labour – mode of delivery related to cervimetric progress. *Aust. NZ J. Obstet. Gynaecol.*, **27**, 304–8

48. Leung, A. S., Leung, E. K. and Paul, R. H. (1993). Uterine rupture after previous cesarean delivery: maternal and fetal consequences. *Am. J. Obstet. Gynecol.*, **169**, 945–50

49. Beckley, S., Gee, H. and Newton, J. R. (1991). Scar rupture in labour after previous lower uterine segment Caesarean section: the role of uterine activity measurement. *Br. J. Obstet. Gynaecol.*, **98**, 265–9

Cervical cancer screening in Denmark: can cervical cancer screening be cost-effective? 37

E. Lynge

Introduction

The effect of screening with Pap smears for cervical cancer has never been tested in a randomized trial, and evidence of its effectiveness comes only from observational studies.

The debate in the early 1980s on the optimal interval for screening clearly illustrated the lack of firm data. In 1981 in the United States, the American Cancer Society recommended screening every 3 years rather than annually. This view was opposed by the American College of Obstetricians and Gynecologists. A panel of experts then reached a compromise, which effectively left the decision to the doctor[1].

Population-based data on cancer incidence from the mid-1950s are available for all the Nordic countries. An analysis of these data from the early 1980s showed a marked decline in the incidence of invasive cervical cancer in Iceland, Sweden, Finland and Denmark starting in the mid-1960s when nationwide or regional (as in Denmark) organized screening was introduced. In the screening programs, invitations were issued every 3rd or 5th year to all women within a given region and a given age group. The incidence of invasive cervical cancer continued to increase in Norway where organized screening existed only in a single region[2]. These observational data clearly indicated that organized cervical cancer screening was an effective tool in reducing the incidence of invasive cervical cancer.

The screening programs in the Nordic countries followed different schemes. One interesting aspect was that the effective Finnish program was based on women being invited to have a smear taken by a midwife every 5th year. In the early 1980s, the opinion on the optimal screening interval thus varied from screening annually to screening every 5th year; these policies had marked differences in their economic implications.

To improve the basis for decision-making, a multicenter study was undertaken by the International Agency for Research on Cancer (IARC) Working Group on Evaluation of Cervical Cancer Screening Programmes[3]. Data were collected from ten regional populations involved in both population-based screening and cancer registration for 20 years. The idea behind the IARC study was to follow cohorts of women with negative smears and measure their incidence of invasive cervical cancer in relation to the time elapsed since the last negative smear. This observed incidence was then compared with the expected incidence, given that no screening had taken place.

The key results from the IARC study published in 1986 showed that annual screening of women aged 35–64 years could be expected to lead to a 94% reduction in the incidence of invasive squamous cell cervical cancer, screening every 3rd year to a 91% reduction and screening every 5th year to an 84% reduction[3].

Cervical cancer screening in Denmark before 1986

Pap smears were introduced in gynecology departments in Copenhagen in the 1950s[4]. A population-based screening program for women aged 30–45 started in the small municipality of Frederiksberg in 1962[5], and for all hospitalized women in Copenhagen in 1964[6]. Population-based screening programs started in three major regions in 1967–68; in Copenhagen municipality[7], in Copenhagen county[8] and in Maribo county[9].

In 1969, the National Health Insurance Scheme agreed to pay for all smears taken by general practitioners independent of whether or not these smears were taken as part of an organized program[4]. This happened despite the fact that a working group under the National Board of Health concluded at the same time that cervical cancer screening should be organized in population-based programs in order to be effective[10].

National screening recommendations from 1986

In the 1980s, Denmark had one of the highest rates of cervical cancer incidence in Europe. In 1983–87, the age-standardized incidence using the World Standard Population was 15.9 per 100 000, only exceeded by 22.5 in the German Democratic Republic, 16.3–23.8 in Poland, 17.8 in Vila Nova de Gaia, Portugal, 16.0 in County Cluj, Romania, 16.1 in Mersey, UK and 16.5 in Yorkshire, UK[11].

In 1986, the total number of smears taken in Denmark could in theory cover screening of all women aged 20–59 years every second year, but only 25% of women were actually covered by organized screening programs.

A new working group under the National Board of Health came up with the following recommendations[12]:

(1) All women should be offered a smear every 3rd year;

(2) The program should be aimed at women aged 23–59 years;

(3) Women aged 60–74 years should also be invited once;

(4) Smears should be taken by general practitioners; and

(5) A co-ordinated program should be set up with invitations to women not already screened by their general practitioner or elsewhere.

Based on the results of the IARC study, screening was recommended every 3rd year. The program should be aimed at women aged 23–59 years. The lower age limit was set as a compromise between the widespread use of screening of very young women and the epidemiological evidence indicating that screening should start at around the age of 30. The annual number of cases of invasive cervical cancer in women aged 20–24 was around five. Women above the age of 60 were less likely to have been covered by the widespread spontaneous screening, and 40% of the invasive cervical cancers occurred in women above the age of 60. It was also therefore recommended to offer screening, once, to women aged 60–74.

All Danish citizens are registered with a general practitioner, and to achieve an optimal co-ordination it was decided that smears should be taken by the general practitioners. To avoid widespread spontaneous screening running in parallel with the organized programs, it was decided to register all smears in computerized data bases which would be checked before invitations were issued. A woman would be invited to have a smear taken 3 years after the previous smear was taken.

Development 1986–97

Health care is now organized by 15 regions in Denmark. When the new screening recommendations were issued in 1986, none of the then 16 regions had programs fully in accordance with the guidelines, and only 25% of women aged 23–59 years were covered by an organized program.

Five years later, only one region, the Fyn county, had fully implemented the new guidelines. Five regions, the Copenhagen and Frederiksberg municipalities, and the Frederiksborg, Roskilde and Århus counties, had implemented the guidelines apart from inviting women above the age of 60 for screening. The organization elsewhere was hampered for several reasons, including resistance from private pathologists towards the transfer of smears to hospitals, prolonged negotiations with the general practitioners concerning payment and administrative problems with data legislation. The experiences from Fyn county showed that forming a multidisciplinary local steering committee highly facilitated the organization process. In 1991, only 57% of women aged 23–59 and only 9% of women aged 60–74 were invited for screening. This was clearly not satisfactory. The regions had already a widespread spontaneous screening activity, and a campaign was therefore started to convince the regions about the benefits of organizing this activity.

Comparison between regions in the late 1980s with and without organized screening showed that 85–90% of women aged 30–49 were screened with organized programs, but only 65–70% without. With organized screening, 20–25% of young women aged 15–22 were screened, but in regions without organization the numbers reached 50–60%. Vestsjælland county, for example, did not have an organized program, but took as many smears per woman as Bornholm county with an organized program. In Vestsjælland county, 14% of the smears were taken from women below the age of 23, and 28% of women aged 23–75 were screened more often than every 3rd year, which meant that 42% of the resources were used outside the national guidelines[13].

The organized screening was seen to be beneficial in comparison with the spontaneous screening. The introduction of organized screening programs by some of the Danish regions at different points in time and with different age intervals could be seen as a 'natural experiment'. The incidence and mortality data, defined by a 5-year age group (between 30 and 59 years), a 5-year time period (between 1968 and 1987) and region, was coded according to whether organized screening did not exist (the baseline), whether organized screening was introduced during the last 0–2 years, or was introduced 3 or more years ago. For the latter group, the relative risk of cervical cancer incidence was 0.77 (95% confidence interval 0.69–0.86) and the relative risk of cervical cancer mortality was 0.75 (95% confidence interval 0.61–0.92) when compared with the baseline[14].

The campaign was successful. In 1997, 90% of women aged 23–59 and 46% of women aged 60–74 are covered by organized screening programs[15]. Only two regions, Copenhagen county and Ringkøbing county, have still to make substantial progress. In Copenhagen county, only women aged 25–45 are invited for screening and in Ringkøbing county a program covering women aged 35–49 stopped recently due to computer problems. At a conference organized by the Danish Cancer Society in December 1996, attention was drawn anew to the benefits of organized screening[16]. Following this, proposals on organized screening covering women aged 23–59 will be presented by the health administrators to the politicians in both the Copenhagen and Ringkøbing counties during the autumn of 1997 (personal communication, Health Administrations of Copenhagen and Ringkøbing counties). Thus, 12 years after the national guidelines were issued, nationwide coverage of organized screening in Denmark is finally being approached.

Both the incidence of, and the mortality from, cervical cancer has decreased in Denmark to an age-standardized incidence rate of 12.6 per 100 000 (World Standard Population) and an age-standardized mortality rate of 4.1 per 100 000 (World Standard Population).

Quality assurance

While much energy has been devoted during recent years to organization, less emphasis has been given to quality assurance at the national level. The European Guidelines on Quality Assurance in Cervical Cancer Screening[17] have not been implemented in Denmark. Whether we at present actually get the maximum benefit from our investment is thus open to question. Three problems are illustrated below.

Participation

In the 1990s, participation rates above 80% were reached in Fyn[18] and Bornholm[19] counties. The participation rate has been somewhat lower in Århus county (75%)[20], and even lower in the Copenhagen municipality, where 70% is the best estimate[21]. The Danish participation rates for urban areas are thus not impressive, compared with, for example, a national coverage in the United Kingdom of 85.7% in 1994–95[22].

Follow-up and treatment guidelines

Seven regions in Denmark have published their follow-up and treatment guidelines. Comparison of these guidelines clearly shows that there is not a national consensus on, for example, the appropriate follow-up of smears with atypical cells. A follow-up with a new smear is recommended after 6–12 months in Nordjylland county[23], and after 3 months in Vestsjælland[24], Viborg[25], Ribe[26] and Storstrøm[27] counties, whereas direct referral to colposcopy is recommended in Fyn[28] and Ringkøbing[29] counties. Guidelines are published for about half of the screening regions but may cover a much broader range of actual follow-up practice.

Lack of follow-up of positive smears

It is possible to check in the pathology registers if a woman with a positive smear has been followed up. This was studied in the Copenhagen municipality and the Bornholm county for 1991–93. In this study, the definition of a positive smear did not include the systemized nomenclature of medicine (SNOMED) codes for atypical smears. A follow-up was defined as the presence of a new registration in the pathology register of either a histological or a cytological investigation on the uterine cervix. The data from the Copenhagen municipality included only women with positive smears following invitation, as the SNOMED codes are known for only these smears.

In Copenhagen, of 314 women with a positive smear, 84% were followed up within the first 3 months. However, for 7% of women, no follow-up was registered within the first 6 months after screening had taken place[21]. In Bornholm, of 81 women with a positive smear, 63% were followed up within the first 3 months, but for 5% more than 12 months elapsed before the follow-up, and no follow-up was registered within the first 13 months after screening had taken place for 6% of the women[19].

A thorough search for further information concerning the eight women without follow-up from Bornholm found that one 39-year-old woman who had been a non-participant in previous screening programs, presented with symptoms in 1993 and died of cervical cancer in the same year. One 40-year-old woman died of lung cancer within a year after her positive smear. Three women were diagnosed with carcinoma *in situ* and one with atypical cells at the next screening round. One woman had a moderate dysplasia diagnosed before being screened again, and no further information could be found for the last woman. This small study clearly indicated that repeated invitations for cervical screening after 3 years had been an important 'safety net'.

Conclusion

Analysis of the cost-effectiveness of cervical cancer screening in Denmark with certain assumptions indicated that screening of 23–59-year-old women every 3rd year will result in 4500 saved years of life at the cost of 34 000 DKr per saved year[30,31]. These results were based on predictions for a 36-year period and an annual discount rate of 5%. Screening of 25–59-year-old women every 4th year would be slightly more cost effective with 3900 saved years of life at the cost of 25 000 DKr per saved year.

As the incidence of cervical cancer is decreasing in Denmark, there is no doubt that we should move towards a longer screening interval than the presently recommended 3 years.

However, before changes are made in the Danish recommendations, more detailed data on the actual performance of the currently running screening programs are warranted.

References

1. Editorial (1981). Intervals between Pap tests: a compromise. *World Health Farum*, **2**, 533–40
2. Hakama, M. (1982). Trends in the incidence of cervical cancer in the Nordic countries. In Magnus, K. (ed.) *Trends in Cancer Incidence*. (Washington: Hemisphere publishing)
3. IARC Working Group on Evaluation of Cervical Cancer Screening Programmes (1986). Screening for squamous cervical cancer: duration of low risk after negative results of cervical cytology and its implication for screening policies. *Br. Med. J.*, **293**, 659–64
4. Lynge, E. (1982). Vaginalcytologiske undersøgelser i Danmark. *Ugeskr. Læg.*, **144**, 124–9
5. Koch, F. (1966). *The Population Screening for Cervical Carcinoma in the Borough of Frederiksberg 1962–63*. (Disp.). (Copenhagen: Munksgaard)
6. Kærn, T., Bredahl, E. and Schäffer, B. (1969). Cytologisk screening i graviditeten for cervixcancer. Diagnostiske og terapeutiske konsekvenser. *Ugeskr. Læg.*, **131**, 922–8
7. Københavns Kommunes Sundhedsdirektorat (1979). *Vaginalcytologiske Undersøgelser af Ikke-hospitaliserede Kvinder i Københavns Kommune 1972–75*. (Copenhagen: Københavns Kommune)
8. Københavns Amtskommune Sundhedsdirektoratet (1977). *Beretning om Forløbet og Resultaterne af de Forebyggende Cancerundersøgelser af Ikke-hospitaliserede Kvinder i Københavns amt i 4 års Perioden 1968/72*. (Copenhagen: Københavns Amtskommune)
9. Berget, A. (1979). Influence of population screening on morbidity and mortality of cancer of the uterine cervix in Maribo amt. *Dan. Med. Bull.*, **26**, 91–100
10. Indenrigsministeriet (1971). *Betænkning Vedrørende Forebyggelse af Livmoderhalskræft. Afgivet af det af Indenrigsministeriet den 27. Maj 1969 Nedsatte Udvalg*. (Copenhagen: Indenrigsministeriet)
11. Parkin, D. M., Muir, C. S., Whelan, S. L., Gao, Y. T., Ferlay, J. and Powell, J. (eds.) International Agency for Research on Cancer (1992). *Cancer Incidence in Five Continents*, Vol. VI, no. 120. (Lyon: IARC Scientific Publications)
12. Underudvalget Vedrørende livmoderhalskræftundersøgelse (1986). *Forebyggende undersøgelser mod livmoderhalskræft*. (Copenhagen: Sundhedsstyrelsen)
13. Lynge, E., Poll, P., Larsen, J., Schultz, H. and Thommesen, N. (1992). Screening mod livmoderhalskræft i Storstrøms, Vestsjællands og Bornholms amtskommuner 1979–1989. *Ugeskr. Læg.*, **154**, 1335–8
14. Lynge, E., Engholm, G. and Madsen, M. (1992). Organiseret screenings betydning for udviklingen af livmoderhalskræft i Danmark i 1968–1987. *Ugeskr. Læg.*, **154**, 1330–4
15. Lynge, E., Arffmann, E., Behnfeld, L., Byrjalsen, C., Glenthøj, A., Hølund, B., Knudsen, E. S., Knudsen, J. L., Olesen, F., Poll, P. A., Rasmussen, B. B., Rasmussen, J., Sonne, A. and Øtoft, E. (1996). Forebyggende undersøgelser mod livmoderhalskræft i Danmark. Status i 1995. Planer for 1996. *Ugeskr. Læg.*, **158**, 4916–19
16. Kræftens Bekæmpelse (1996). *Konference om Screening for Livmoderhalskræft 10. December 1996*. (Copenhagen: Kræftens Bekæmpelse)
17. Coleman, D., Day, N., Douglas, G., Farmery, E., Lynge, E., Philip, J. and Segnan, N. (1993). European guidelines for quality assurance in cervical cancer screening. *Eur. J. Cancer*, **29A** (Suppl. 4), 38
18. Hølund, B., Jeune, B. and Jørgensen, F. (no year). *Befolkningsundersøgelsen Mod Livmoderhalskræft i Fyns Amt*. (Fyns Amt: Odense Universitetshospital)
19. Lynge, E. (1977). *Screening Mod Livmoderhalskræft i Bornholms Amtskommune 1987–90 og 1990–93*. (Copenhagen: Kommunedata A/S, Kræftens Bekæmpelse)
20. Larsen, L. P. S. and Olesen, F. (1996). Karakteristik af "ikkedeltagere" i organiseret screeningsundersøgelse mod livmoderhalskræft. *Ugeskr. Læg.*, **158**, 2987–91
21. Lynge, E., Carstensen, B. and Vang, A. (1994). *Screening Mod Livmoderhalskræft i Københavns Kommune i Perioden 1.7.1987–31.12.1990 og Perioden 1.1.1991–31.12.1993*, Direktoratet. (Copenhagen: Københavns Sundhedsvæsen)
22. NHS Cervical Screening Programme (1996). *Cervical screening. A pocket guide*. (Sheffield: NHS Cervical Screening Programme)
23. Kræftens Bekæmpelse (1994). *Forebyggende Undersøgelse Mod Livmoderhalskræft i Nordjyllands Amt*. (Nordjyllands Amt: Kræftens Bekæmpelse)
24. Kræftens Bekæmpelse (1996). *Forebyggende Undersøgelse Mod Livmoderhalskræft i Vestsjællands Amt*. (Vestsjællands Amt: Kræftens Bekæmpelse)
25. Kræftens Bekæmpelse (1993). *Forebyggende Undersøgelse Mod Livmoderhalskræft i Viborg Amt*. (Viborg Amt: Kræftens Bekæmpelse)
26. Kræftens Bekæmpelse (1995). *Forebyggende Undersøgelse Mod Livmoderhalskræft i Ribe Amt*. (Ribe Amt: Kræftens Bekæmpelse)

27. Kræftens Bekæmpelse (1994). *Forebyggende Undersøgelse Mod Livmoderhalskræft i Storstrøms Amt.* (Storstrøms Amt: Kræftens Bekæmpelse)

28. Kræftens Bekæmpelse (1994). *Forebyggende Undersøgelse Mod Livmoderhalskræft i Fyns Amt.* (Fyns Amt: Kræftens Bekæmpelse)

29. Kræftens Bekæmpelse (1993). *Forebyggende Undersøgelse Mod Livmoderhalskræft i Ringkjøbing Amt.* (Ringkjøbing Amtskommune: Kræftens Bekæmpelse)

30. Gyrd-Hansen, D., Hølund, B. and Andersen, P. (1996). Omkostninger og effekter af alternative screeningsprogrammer mod livmoderhalskræft. *Ugeskr. Læg.*, **158**, 4912–5

31. Søgaard, J. and Gyrd-Hansen, D. (1997). *Omkostningskonsekvenser og Omkostningseffektanalyse af Indførelse af Mammografiscreening i Danmark. Foreløbige Resultater Baseret på Udenlandske Erfaringer. I: Sundhedstyrelsen. Statusrapport fra Sundhedstyrelsens Følgegruppe Vedr. Brystkræft.* (Copenhagen: Sundhedsstyrelsen)

Risks and benefits of hormone therapy   *38*

C. B. Hammond

Introduction

It is clear that we live in an aging society. Women in the United States today can anticipate a life expectancy of approximately 80 years (Table 1)[1]. It is also interesting to study the slow and progressive lengthening of life expectancy that has occurred over the past century, as contrasted by gender and ethnicity[2]. The death rate for men is higher than for women at all ages. It is higher in African–Americans than in whites for both sexes. While there are many reasons for the changing demographics of death, it is obvious that women have lagged behind men by 10 years or more in the incidence of coronary artery disease and by 20 years in the incidence of sudden death due to coronary events. On the other hand, it may be speculated that, as cigarette smoking continues to increase among women, and that, as the number of women in the workforce increases, their body weight increases, cholesterol control reduces and

regular exercise decreases, it is likely that the gender difference in premature death may narrow. What is important for today is to explore the differences that cause the discordance in death rates and to determine, if possible, how much of a role hormonal replacement therapy can play in prolonging healthy and functional life for women.

Fries[3] has published interesting information regarding life span and life expectancy. Life span is the biological limit to life, the maximum obtainable age by a member of a species. There is a statistical variance from this for an individual but, overall, life span is finite. Despite the general feeling that life span is increasing, it is not. What is increasing is life expectancy. Thus, the number of older people is increasing but should eventually reach a fixed limit. The percentage of a typical life span spent in older age is increasing, as we have nearly eliminated premature death. Diseases such as cancer and circulatory diseases are now the leading causes of death. The reason for these changes is not an epidemic of such problems, but purely a reflection of our success in virtually eradicating previously fatal infectious diseases. In the United States we are now in an era characterized by diminution of function: fading eyesight and hearing, impaired cognitive function and memory, and decreased strength and stamina are all occurring in significantly increasing rates among an aging population. That we will eventually die is certain. What we hope to do is postpone illness and compress morbidity. We would like to live relatively healthy and long lives, and then compress our illnesses into a short period of time just before our deaths, somewhere just beyond the age of 80

Table 1 Female life expectancy at birth and at age 65, US, 1900–2050 (from reference 1)

| Year | Life expectancy (years) | |
	At birth	At age 65
1900	48.3	12.2
1950	71.7	15.0
1960	73.1	15.8
1970	74.8	17.0
1980	77.4	18.3
1985	78.2	18.6
1990	79.2	19.5
2000	80.5	20.5
2010	81.5	21.2
2020	82.0	21.7
2030	82.5	22.1
2040	83.1	22.6
2050	83.6	23.1

(Figure 1)[4]. Ideally, disease is something not treated, but rather prevented or postponed. It is the present author's belief that hormonal replacement therapy, while probably not suitable for everyone, is a very useful technique to assist in this prevention or postponement.

This paper addresses risks and benefits of hormonal therapy. However, such therapy cannot be considered in isolation, as it must include an enhanced educational effort for all physicians and, importantly, for their patients as we try to achieve the goals listed above. As women age after the menopause, one major consideration for their health maintenance should be the administration of hormonal replacement therapy. Generally, hormonal replacement therapy implies chronic treatment with estrogen. However, if the uterus is *in situ*, it also should include progestational agents. Androgens may also be used. The purpose of this paper is to explore the pros and cons of such therapy. While not stated, it should be understood that in this discussion the author's perspective also includes remedial education to enhance lifestyle changes that will benefit health. Thus, cessation of smoking, increase in regular exercise, reduction of obesity and maintenance of normal body weight, control of cholesterol, reduction of alcohol intake, regular exercise and other factors should be included as other primary mechanisms to enhance life and function. What is important to

consider is when that is all complete, how much hormonal therapy can either add to the function that is obtained or overcome unhealthy lifestyle issues that are continued. All of these factors: education, monitoring, change in lifestyle and hormonal therapy, should be presented to patients as they consider their options for the future[5].

This paper will ask a series of questions and try to provide information that will respond in relation to the impact of hormonal replacement therapy upon that particular issue. While this cannot be encyclopedic, it is perhaps the best way to try to discuss the protective benefits and potential risks of hormonal replacement therapy for the aging woman.

Is hormonal replacement therapy the most appropriate management for patients with hot flushes, and what are the alternatives?

Vasomotor hot flushes are a significant symptom for many women. As many as 85% of perimenopausal and postmenopausal women have hot flushes, and they often are disabling[4,6,7]. Sleep interruption is well documented, and cognitive function may be impaired[8]. Whether this is due to sleep deprivation or other mechanisms remains to be fully explained.

It is quite clear from the literature that replacing estrogen is the most efficient treatment for vasomotor hot flushes[9,10]. Whether the estrogen is replaced by oral, injectable, transdermal or other routes seems relatively unimportant if an adequate dosage is provided (Figures 2 and 3). Many patients may be eased off the medication after 1 or 2 years without recrudescence of hot flushes, although as many as 25% of patients may have them continue for years, if untreated.

There are other therapies that can be used for treatment of hot flushes, but none are as efficient as estrogen. Such therapies include progestin[11], either by depo or in oral forms (Figure 4), or clonidine[12], an antihypertensive. Data for Bellergal® and others show no better than the placebo effect.

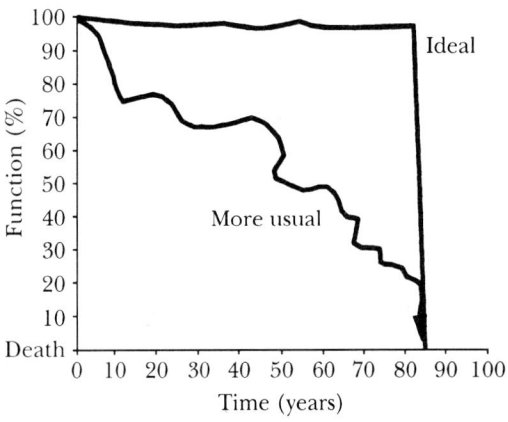

Figure 1 Functional ability versus age (adapted from reference 4)

Layering of clothing, avoidance of spicy foods, increase in the ingestion of phytoestrogens and other mechanisms have all been suggested to reduce the intensity of hot flushes, but suffer from a lack of well-documented studies.

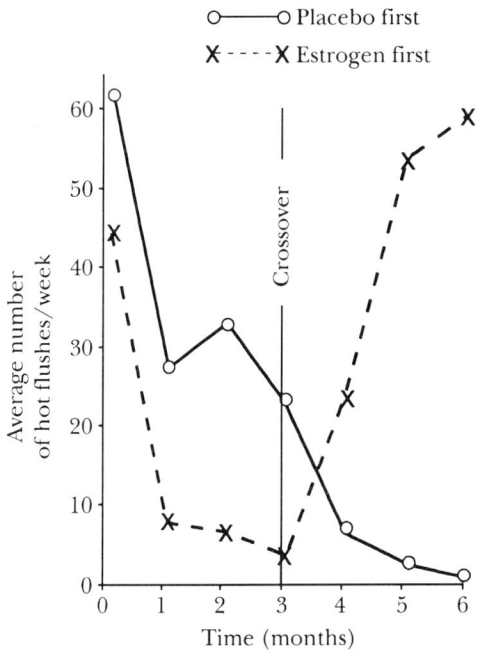

Figure 2 Hot flushes with and without oral estrogen (adapted from reference 9)

In the patient with significant vasomotor hot flushes, they seem to be of relatively little benefit.

What are appropriate therapies for the management of atrophic genital symptoms, and how long should they be continued?

Atrophic changes of the vulva and vagina, urethra and base of the bladder are well documented in women who are hypoestrogenic. Approximately 75% of women will show such changes, and nearly half of this number will have symptoms of sufficient magnitude for them to seek medical attention[4,13]. All are due to diminution of estrogen and atrophy of the associated structures. There is also an age-related atrophic change in the vulva which is additive. Common symptoms include burning and discomfort in the vagina, discomfort with coitus to the point of avoidance of intercourse and an abacteruric dysuria, frequency, urgency and nocturia which all may be explained by loss of estrogen[13].

Coital lubricants may be of some benefit in reduction of dyspareunia due to atrophic changes. Regular coitus is associated with diminution of shrinkage and atrophy of the

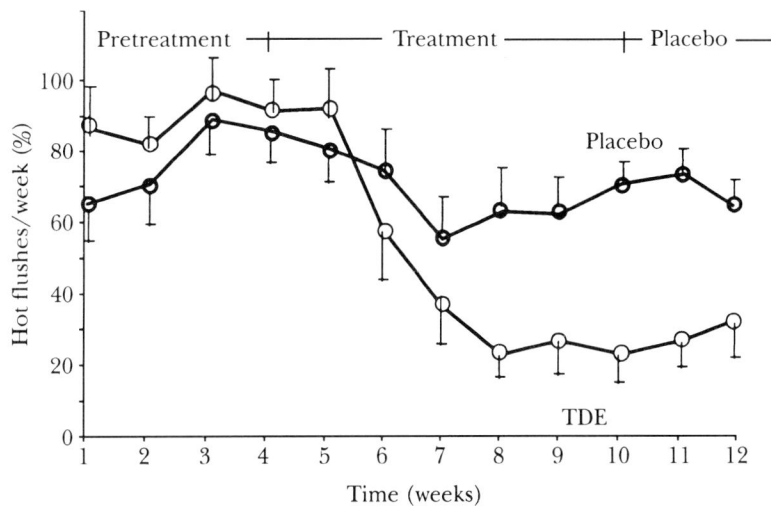

Figure 3 Total hot flushes with and without transdermal estradiol (TDE) (adapted from reference 10)

259

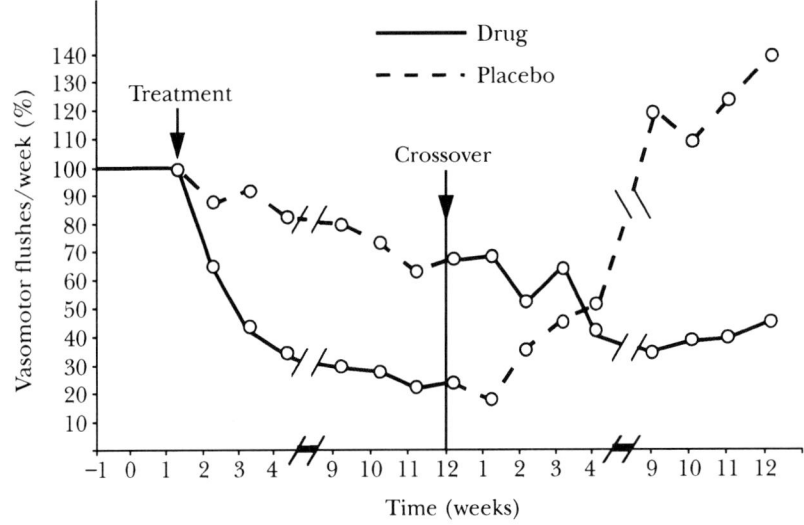

Figure 4 Effect of oral medroxyprogesterone acetate on hot flushes (adapted from reference 11)

vagina in this setting. However, the atrophic changes of the genitalia may preclude such activity. It appears that estrogen is the only specific therapy to help restore such structures to normalcy[14–17]. Relatively little estrogen is required for this, and it may be delivered by either a transvaginal or systemic route. It is likely that such therapy will be required for the remainder of a woman's life if the symptoms are sufficient to warrant therapy.

Interesting data exist to evaluate the role of hormonal replacement therapy by mechanisms that focus on central nervous-system (CNS) function and beyond that of vaginal atrophy (Figure 5). It does appear that estrogen and androgens possibly have functions in maintaining libido and effective normalcy, and impact positively on cognitive function in women[4,18–20].

Does hormonal replacement therapy modify the risk and course of osteoporosis?

Postmenopausal osteoporosis is a well-documented syndrome in which bone loss increases the fragility of bone causing atraumatic fracture to occur prematurely[21]. While there are many causes of bone-density loss other

than postmenopausal change related to hypo-estrogenism, the comments that follow presume that we are dealing only with the postmeno-pausal type of loss. Osteoporosis is a significant disease process that involves one in three women in the United States who will develop some complication of osteoporosis postmeno-pausally. This process is the cause of more than 1.3 million fractures each year, and most of the 250 000 hip fractures that occur in people over age 45 are due to osteoporosis. When one considers the loss of function, the cost of care and the increasing disability that is so commonly associated with loss of independence, it is obvious that postmenopausal osteoporosis is a major health risk in the United States[22].

In both sexes, maximal skeletal mass is obtained by approximately age 30. By age 50, both men and women have begun to experience generalized loss of bone. After menopause, bone density rapidly decreases in some women unless estrogen is replaced. By the age of 80, some untreated Caucasian women have lost 30–50% of their skeletal mass.

A woman's genetic background, lifestyle, dietary habits, co-existing endocrine diseases and age of her menopause are major factors that determine whether or not she will develop

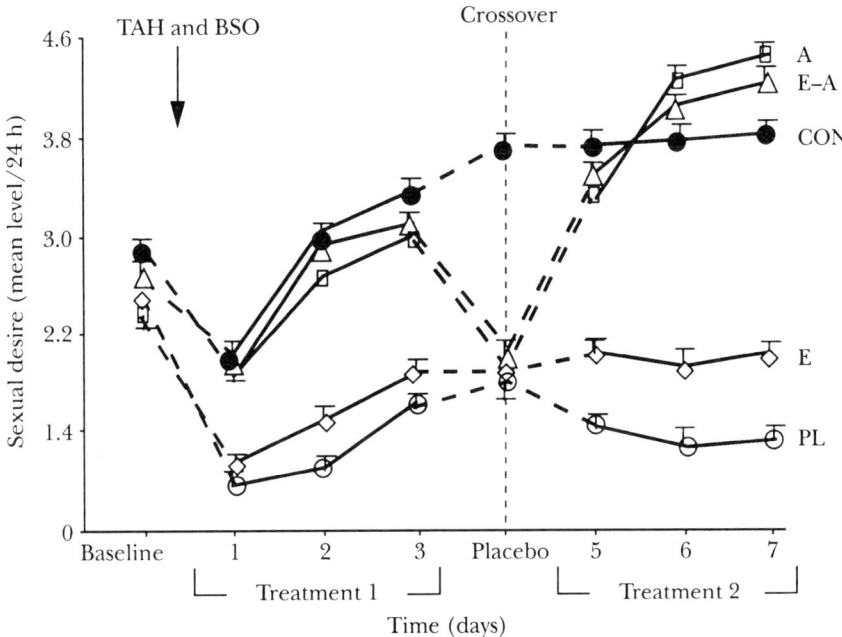

Figure 5 Sexual desire and steroid hormones (adapted from reference 18). TAH, total abdominal hysterectomy; BSO, bilateral salpingo-oophorectomy; A, androgen; E, estrogen; E–A, estrogen–androgen; PL, placebo; CON, control (hysterectomy)

osteoporosis. There now are tests which are available to precisely document bone density and, when used repetitively, can clearly identify the patient at extra risk for osteoporotic complications. However, such tests are relatively costly and require fairly sophisticated instrumentation. It is unlikely that the American population can be screened in such a fashion due to these cost issues.

It is quite obvious that an adequate calcium and vitamin D intake are important to bone health. Weight-bearing exercise is an additional requirement to maintain strong and healthy bones. However, it is the author's opinion that neither calcium supplementation nor exercise, either alone or together, are adequate to protect women from osteoporosis.

There are now three treatment methods to retard the development of osteoporosis. The first of these is estrogen, which has a well-documented database showing a protective effect when taken chronically, even in modest dosage (Figure 6)[23,24]. This has been true

regardless of route of administration and may provide a woman with long-term benefit as long as she continues to take the preparation. Also, there are data to suggest that even after significant bone loss has occurred, the implementation of estrogen therapy may benefit the woman by causing a cessation of loss, despite the fact that there is little, if any, appreciable gain after the estrogen therapy is begun. However, when estrogen therapy is withdrawn, loss of bone may occur. Thus, chronic therapy over a long time interval is important.

Alendronate, a member of the bisphosphonate family, has been shown to be a very useful drug in the treatment of patients who have osteoporosis or, potentially, to manage patients prophylactically who are at risk for this process. There are data to suggest that a bone-density increase may occur with alendronate therapy, rather than only maintenance of previously present levels (Figure 7)[25,26]. To date, there are few data regarding the combination of alendronate and estrogen, and there are

261

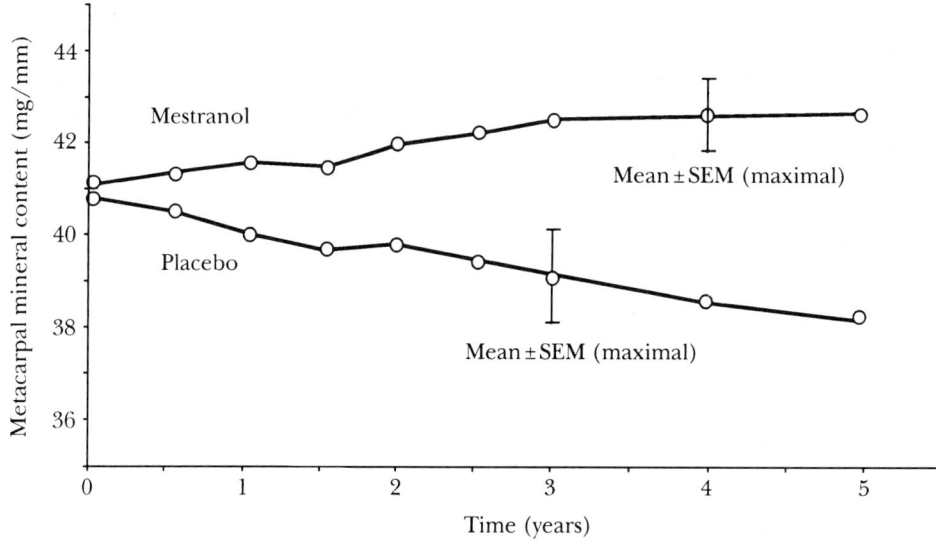

Figure 6 Effect of estrogen (mestranol 20 mg q.d.) on long-term maintenance of bone density in women after surgical menopause (adapted from reference 23)

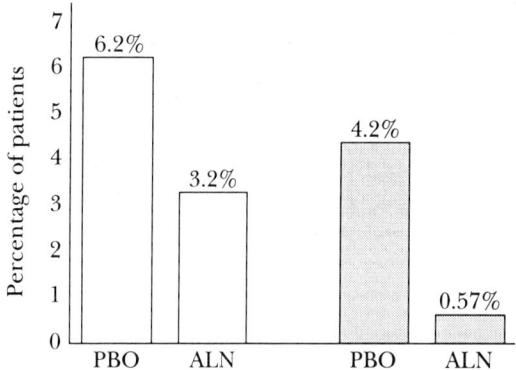

Figure 7 Reduction in incidence of vertebral fractures in women treated with alendronate (ALN). Risk of sustaining at least one fracture (white bars) was reduced by 48% among women treated with ALN compared with those receiving placebo (PBO) (3.2% vs. 6.2%; relative risk, 0.52; 95% confidence interval, 0.28–0.95; $p = 0.034$). Risk of sustaining two or more vertebral fractures (shaded bars) was reduced by 87% in ALN patients compared with PBO patients (0.57% vs. 4.2%; relative risk, 0.13; 95% confidence interval, 0.05–0.38; $p < 0.001$) (adapted from reference 26)

shown to be of benefit in selected patients with osteoporosis[27].

The present author's opinion is that patients who elect to take estrogen, either for control of acute symptoms or for protection against atherosclerotic cardiovascular disease or other reasons, probably do not need bone-density studies and probably will receive the prophylactic benefit to bone that their estrogen provides. However, if a patient elects not to take estrogen or should not take estrogen, then bone density studies would probably be appropriate. Dual energy X-ray absorptiometry (DEXA) or quantitative digital radiography (QDR) of the spine and hip are the studies that would currently be used. Then, alternative therapies could be considered, such as alendronate and nasal calcitonin, for such patients. Calcium supplementation, weight-bearing exercise and vitamin D should be considered for all patients.

side-effects from alendronate, such as an erosive esophagitis which may occur if patients are recumbent after taking the medication. No long-term data regarding the use of alendronate are available. Lastly, nasal calcitonin has been

Is there a role in cardiovascular disease for protection from hormonal replacement therapy?

Each year, more than 500 000 women in the United States die of cardiovascular disease, twice as many as those who die from all malignancies[28]. Many of these patients will dramatically benefit from improvement of lifestyle issues such as cessation of smoking, achievement of appropriate body weight, reduction of alcohol intake, control of hypertension and hyperlipidemia and an increase in aerobic exercise[29,30]. Each of these areas has been shown to improve prognosis and function for the postmenopausal patient as she faces an increase in the risk of cardiovascular atherosclerotic disease.

There are now considerable data to suggest that hormonal replacement therapy has a dramatic protective impact on cardiovascular disease in women. On the basis of angiographic studies, it appears that the risk ratio for coronary disease can be reduced to a level of 60–70% or more of that present in untreated women (Table 2). Table 3 gives the results of a number of earlier studies demonstrating the benefit of estrogen on myocardial infarction. Exciting data now exist to suggest mechanisms that include improvement of lipid profiles[28,33] and also by direct effect of estrogen upon the coronary wall[4]. Dilatation of the coronary vessel is enhanced in the presence of estrogen versus the hypoestrogenic state, and such therapy tends to have a significant duration of benefit[34]. There are data to document an enhanced survival of women who start hormonal replacement therapy after a coronary attack and even some data to suggest regression of the pre-existing atherosclerotic changes after estrogen treatment is begun[35-37].

Are there data to suggest that hormonal replacement therapy improves function of the aging brain?

It is the present author's opinion that there are exciting data to suggest that hormonal replacement therapy may be associated with a delay in the age of onset and an actual reduction in the incidence of Alzheimer's syndrome[31,38-40]. These data are probably not yet conclusive, but the several studies published to date provide significant clues that this may be true. There are receptors for estrogen in appropriate areas of the brain involved with this disease, and there are certainly experiments of nature in addition to the presently limited studies showing such a benefit. Hopefully future studies will show an actual protective effect.

Table 2 Estrogen therapy and reduced angiographically demonstrated cardiovascular disease (from reference 31)

Study	n	Relative risk	p
Sullivan et al. (1988)	2188	0.40	0.022
Gruchow et al. (1988)	933	0.59	< 0.01
McFarland et al. (1989)	345	0.50	< 0.01
Hong et al. (1992)	90	0.13	< 0.001

Table 3 Estrogen therapy and reduced cardiovascular disease (reproduced with permission from reference 32)

Study	n	Relative risk
Henderson (1985)	7 610	0.8
Wilson (1985)	1 234	1.9
Stampfer (1985)	32 317	0.3
Petitti (1986)	16 638	0.5
Bush (1987)	2 270	0.3
Criqui (1988)	1 868	0.7

Is hormonal replacement therapy associated with an increased risk of breast cancer?

There are many epidemiological, endocrinological, clinical, pathological and experimental data that, when considered together, provide evidence that ovarian hormones play some role in the various stages of development of breast cancer. Additionally, a few studies have suggested that hormonal replacement therapy is associated with an increase in the risk of this disease[41-44]. All have been debated, and based on the population studies in the literature, Spicer and Pike have projected an increase in breast cancer of 1–2% per year of estrogen use (Figure 8)[45]. Many other investigators have chal-

Table 4 Estrogen therapy and breast cancer: meta-analysis data

Meta-analysis	Number of studies	Relative risk	95% confidence interval
Armstrong[46]	23	1.01	0.95–1.08
Bates[47]	11	1.03	0.87–1.17
Dupont and Page[48]	28	1.08	0.96–1.2
Sillero-Arenas et al[49]	27	1.06	1.00–1.18
Sternberg et al[50]	16	1.3	1.2–1.6

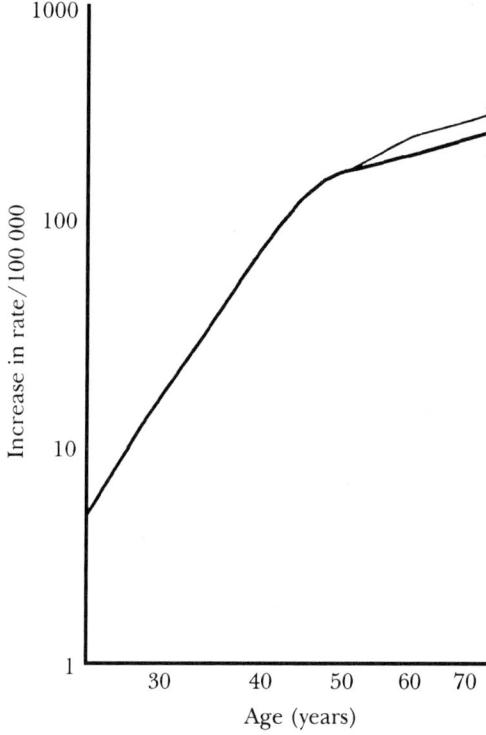

Figure 8 Breast cancer and estrogen therapy (adapted from reference 45). A, patients on estrogen replacement therapy; B, patients not on estrogen replacement therapy

lenged these data and suggested that their studies have shown no increase (Table 4)[46–52].

In the present author's opinion, the addition of progestin to estrogen therapy neither increases nor decreases the risk of breast cancer, although the addition of progestin of an adequate duration and dosage will probably negate the vast majority of risk associated with estrogen as a causative factor in endometrial adenocarcinoma[53]. Indeed, these are difficult questions to answer with absolute certainty, but it is likely that if taking replacement estrogen increases the risk of breast cancer, it must do so to a very limited degree. On the other hand are the significant benefits already presented in regard to cardiovascular disease and osteoporosis.

Summary

This paper attempts to point out what the present author considers to be the primary benefits and risks associated with hormonal replacement therapy. Such therapy is probably not suitable for every patient. However, every patient should be made aware of the risks and benefits, and these risks and benefits should be individualized as much as possible. A woman needs appropriate education regarding the disease states, alternative treatments and alternative methods of lifestyle adjustment that will benefit her health to a maximum degree. She can then make an informed, individualized decision. In such a fashion, she will be able to successfully traverse the interval from menopause to death in the healthiest and most normally functional way possible.

References

1. Evans, W. J., Evans, M. I. and Hajj, S. N. (1993). The aging population. In Hajj, S. N. and Evans, W. J. (eds.). *Clinical Postreproductive Endocrinology*, p. 3. (Connecticut, CT: Appleton and Lange)

2. National Center for Health Statistics (1994). *Health, United States, 1993*, p. 91. (Hyattsville, M: Public Health Service)

3. Fries, H. T. (1980). Natural death and compression of morbidity. *N. Engl. J. Med.*, **303**, 130

4. Hammond, C. B. (1994). Menopause and hormone replacement therapy: an overview. *Obstet. Gynecol.*, **87**(Suppl. 2), 2s–15s

5. Speroff, L. (1994). The menopause, a signal for the future. In Lobo, R. A. (ed.) *Treatment of the Postmenopausal Woman: Basic and Clinical Aspects*, pp. 1–8. (New York: Raven Press)

6. Kronenberg, F. (1994). Hot flushes. In Lobo, R. A. (ed.) *Treatment of the Postmenopausal Woman: Basic and Clinical Aspects*, pp. 97–117. (New York: Raven Press)

7. Aksel, S., Schomberg, D. W. and Tyrey, L. (1976). Vasomotor symptoms, serum estrogens and gonadotropin levels in menopause. *Am. J. Obstet. Gynecol.*, **126**, 165–9

8. Erlik, Y., Tataryn, I. V. and Meldrum, D. R. (1981). Association of waking episodes with menopausal hot flushes. *J. Am. Med. Assoc.*, **245**, 1741–5

9. Coope, J., Thomson, J. M. and Pollan, L. (1975). Effects of 'natural estrogen' replacement therapy on menopausal symptoms and blood clotting. *Br. Med. J.*, **4**, 139–43

10. Haas, S., Walsh, B. and Evans, S. (1988). The effect of transdermal estrogen on hormone and metabolic dynamics over a six-week period. *Obstet. Gynecol.*, **71**, 671–6

11. Schiff, I., Tulchinsky, D. and Crand, D. (1980). Oral medroxyprogesterone in the treatment of postmenopausal symptoms. *J. Am. Med. Assoc.*, **244**, 1443–5

12. Clayden, J. R., Bell, J. W. and Pollard, P. (1974). Menopausal flushing, double-blind trial of non-hormonal medication. *Br. Med. J.*, **1**, 409–12

13. Bachman, G. A. (1994). Vulvovaginal complaints. In Lobo, R. A. (ed.) *Treatment of the Postmenopausal Woman: Basic and Clinical Aspects*, pp. 137–42. (New York: Raven Press)

14. Mettler, L. and Olson, P. G. (1991). Long-term treatment of atrophic vaginitis with low-dose estradiol vaginal tablets. *Maturitas*, **14**, 23–31

15. Sherwin, B. B. and Gelfand, M. M. (1985). Differential symptom response to parenteral estrogen and/or androgen administration in the surgical menopause. *Am. J. Obstet. Gynecol.*, **151**, 153–60

16. Bachman, G. A., Lieblum, S. R. and Gill, J. (1989). Brief sexual inquiry in a gynecologic practice. *Obstet. Gynecol.*, **73**, 1425–7

17. Bhatia, N. N., Bergman, A. and Karram, M. M. (1989). Effects of estrogen on urethral function in women with urinary function. *Am. J. Obstet. Gynecol.*, **160**, 176–81

18. Sherwin, B. B. and Gelfand, M. M. (1985). Sex steroids and affect in the surgical menopause: a double-blind, crossover study. *Psychoneuroendocrinology*, **10**, 325–35

19. Hammond, C. B. (1994). The climacteric. In Scott, J. R., DiSaia, P. J., Hammond, C. B. and Spellacy, W. N. (eds.) *Danforth's Obstetrics and Gynecology*, 7th edn, p. 777. (Philadelphia, PA: J. B. Lippincott)

20. Sherwin, B. B. (1996). Hormones, mood and cognitive function in postmenopausal women. *Obstet. Gynecol.*, **87**(Suppl. 2), 20s–6s

21. Hui, S. L., Slemenda, C. W. and Johnson, C. C. (1989). Baseline measurement of bone mass predicts fracture in white women. *Ann. Int. Med.*, **111**, 355–61

22. Lindsay, R. (1996). The menopause and osteoporosis. *Obstet. Gynecol.*, **87**(Suppl. 2), 16s–19s

23. Lindsay, R., Hart, D. M. and Clark, D. M. (1984). The minimum effective dose of estrogen for prevention of postmenopausal bone loss. *Obstet. Gynecol.*, **63**, 759–63

24. Riis, B. J., Thomsen, K., Strom, V. and Christiansen, C. (1987). The effect of percutaneous estradiol and natural progesterone on postmenopausal bone loss. *Am. J. Obstet. Gynecol.*, **157**, 61–5

25. Fleisch, H. (1993). New biophosphonates in osteoporosis. *Osteoporosis Int.*, **2**, 15–22

26. Kirk, J. K. and Spangler, J. G. (1996). Alendronate: a bisphosphonate for treatment of osteoporosis. *Am. Fam. Physician.*, **54**, 2053–60

27. Overgaard, K., Riis, B. J. and Christiansen, C. (1989). Nasal calcitonin for treatment of established osteoporosis. *Clin. Endocrinol. (Oxford)*, **30**, 435–42

28. Gorodeshi, G. I. and Utian, W. H. (1994). Epidemiology and risk factors of cardiovascular disease in postmenopausal women. In Lobo, R. A. (ed.) *Treatment of the Postmenopausal Woman: Basic and Clinical Aspects*, pp. 199–221. (New York: Raven Press)

29. Bush, T. L. (1990). The epidemiology of cardiovascular disease in postmenopausal women. *Ann. NY Acad. Sci.*, **592**, 263–71

30. Kalin, M. F. and Zumoff, B. (1990). Sex hormones and coronary disease. *Steroids,* **55**, 330–52

31. Ditkoff, E. C., Crary, W. G., Cristo, M. and Lobo, R. A. (1991). Estrogen improves psychological functioning in asymptomatic postmenopausal women. *Obstet. Gynecol.,* **78**, 991–5

32. Stampfer, M. J. and Brodstein, F. (1994). In Lobo, R. A. (ed.) *Treatment of the Postmenopausal Woman: Basic and Clinical Aspects,* p. 227. (New York: Raven Press)

33. Miller, V. T. (1990). Dyslipoprotenemia in women: special considerations. *Endocrinol. Metab. Clin. North Am.,* **19**, 381–98

34. Adams, M. R., Kaplan, J. R. and Clarkson, T. B. (1987). Effects of psychosocial stress, menopause and pregnancy on coronary artery atherosclerosis. In Eaker, E. D. (ed.) *Coronary Heart Disease in Women,* p. 151–7. (New York: Haymarket Doyman)

35. Lobo, R. A. and Speroff, L. (1994). International Consensus Conference on postmenopausal hormone therapy and the cardiovascular system. *Fertil. Steril.,* **62**(Suppl. 2), 176S–9S

36. Wild, R. A. (1996). Estrogen: effects on the cardiovascular tree. *Obstet. Gynecol.,* **87**(Suppl. 2), 27s–35s

37. Sullivan, J. M. and Foulkes, L. P. (1996). The clinical aspects of estrogen and the cardiovascular system. *Obstet. Gynecol.,* **87**(Suppl. 2), 36s–42s

38. McEwen, B. S. (1980). The brain as a target organ of endocrine hormones. In Kreiger, D. T. and Hughes, J. S. (eds.) *Neuroendocrinology.* (Sunderland: Sinauer Assoc)

39. Fillit, H., Weinreb, H. and Cholst, I. (1986). Observations in a preliminary open trial of estradiol therapy for senile dementia – Alzheimer's type. *Psychoneuroendocrinology,* **11**, 337–45

40. Paganini-Hill, A. and Henderson, V. W. (1994). Estrogen deficiency and risk of Alzheimer's disease in women. *Am. J. Epidemiol.,* **140**, 256–61

41. Speroff, L. (1996). Postmenopausal hormone therapy and breast cancer. *Obstet. Gynecol.,* **87**(Suppl. 2), 44s–54s

42. Wingo, P. A., Layde, P. M., Lee, N. C., Rubin, G. and Ory, H. W. (1987). The risk of breast cancer in postmenopausal women who have used estrogen replacement therapy. *J. Am. Med. Assoc.,* **257**, 209–15

43. Colditz, G. A., Stampfer, M. J. and Willett, W. C. (1992). Type of postmenopausal hormone use and risk of breast cancer. 12-year follow-up from the Nurses' Health Study. *Cancer Causes Control,* **3**, 433–9

44. Golditz, G. A., Hankinson, S. E. and Hunter, D. J. (1995). Use of estrogens and progestins and the risk of breast cancer in postmenopausal women. *N. Engl. J. Med.,* **332**, 1589–93

45. Spicer, D. V. and Pike, M. D. (1994). Epidemiology of breast cancer. In Lobo, R. A. (ed.) *Treatment of the Postmenopausal Woman: Basic and Clinical Aspects,* p. 318. (New York: Raven Press)

46. Armstrong, B. K. (1988). Oestrogen therapy after the menopause – boon or bane? *Med. J. Aust.,* **148**, 213–14

47. Bates, S. K. (1990). *J. Soc. Obstet. Gynecol. Can.,* **12**, 9

48. Dupont, W. D. and Page, D. L. (1991). Menopausal estrogen replacement therapy and breast cancer. *Arch. Intern. Med.,* **151**, 67–72

49. Sillero-Arenas, M., Delgado-Rodriguez, M., Rodrigues-Canteras, R., Bueno-Cavanillas, A. and Galvez-Vargas, R. (1992). Menopausal hormone replacement therapy and breast cancer. A meta-analysis. *Obstet. Gynecol.,* **79**, 286–94

50. Sternberg, K. K., Thacker, S. B. and Smith, S. J. (1991). A meta-analysis of the effect of estrogen replacement therapy on the risk of breast cancer. *J. Am. Med. Assoc.,* **265**, 1985–90

51. Colditz, G A., Egan, K. M. and Stampfer, M. J. (1993). Hormone replacement therapy and risk of breast cancer. Results from epidemiologic studies. *Am. J. Obstet. Gynecol.,* **168**, 1473–80

52. Nachtigall, M. J., Smilen, S. W., Nachtigall, R. A. D., Nachtigall, R. H. and Nachtigall, L. I. (1992). Incidence of breast cancer in a 22-year study of women receiving estrogen–progestin replacement therapy. *Obstet. Gynecol.,* **80**, 827–30

53. Gambrell, R. D. (1986). Prevention of endometrial cancer with progestogens. *Maturtitas,* **8**, 159–68

Hormone replacement therapy for all?　39

E. Barrett-Connor

Introduction

Should hormone replacement therapy (HRT) be the standard of care, i.e. prescribed for all postmenopausal women who have no known contraindication? In the United States, physicians' enthusiasm for HRT in healthy asymptomatic women varies by discipline. Saver and colleagues[1] performed a stratified random survey of gynecologists, internists and family physicians in Washington, Alaska, Montana and Idaho. Nearly all respondents believed in the value of HRT, but gynecologists ranked mammography first and HRT second on a list of eight preventive services, while the other physicians ranked smoking cessation first and HRT fourth ($p < 0.0001$).

Fewer than 20% of US postmenopausal women currently use HRT. This low rate worries physicians, but most women assign less importance to the menopause as a life event than do their doctors[2]. The healthy postmenopausal woman does not consider the menopause to be a disease, and dislikes the terms 'estrogen deficiency' and 'replacement therapy', which imply that she is defective. She is suspicious of the medicalization of a natural process and doubts that she needs therapy. In our society, medication is for treatment, not prevention. It is easier to treat the sick than to persuade a healthy person to take a medication to prevent a disease she may never get. In the United States, the average woman who survives to age 50 and does not take HRT will live to be almost 83 years old[3].

Treatment as standard of care

Treatment of the symptomatic woman is relatively non-controversial: HRT relieves symptoms and can be tapered off after a few years. Treatment to prevent disease in a healthy woman is quite another matter, probably requiring life-long therapy and involving some risks – but it is here where the greatest potential benefits also lie.

The cardiovascular protection observed in epidemiological studies conducted in the United States and Northern Europe is greater than the protection or risk of all other estrogen-associated conditions combined[3]. On these grounds, HRT as standard of care can be defended in a country like the United States – where heart disease is the leading cause of death in postmenopausal women, where it contributes significantly to female morbidity, and where breast-cancer rates are much lower than heart-disease rates. Based on a meta-analysis of studies, in which most women were treated with unopposed conjugated equine estrogen, HRT is associated with a 35% reduction in risk of coronary heart disease, and (on average) a healthy US woman at no particular risk for heart disease, osteoporosis or breast cancer would gain 1 year of life[3].

Two recent studies[4,5] found similar risk reductions in women taking estrogen plus a progestin, primarily medroxyprogesterone acetate, suggesting that this combination is similarly protective. These studies had relatively few events, however, and suffer from the selection biases that characterize all observational studies of HRT. It has been known for years that the addition of a progestin blunts the estrogen-induced increase in high-density lipoprotein (HDL) cholesterol[6]. The decreased dilatation of atherosclerotic coronary arteries when progestins, particularly medroxyprogesterone acetate, are added to estrogen, was the subject of nearly 20 presentations at the November 1996 meeting of the American Heart Association. In one analysis, compatible with the observed differences in HDL and blood flow, HRT would add only 0.3 years of life[3]. Obviously the uncertain effects of adding a progestin to the estrogen are critical to the risk–benefit ratio attributed to HRT.

Some US physicians think that there is sufficient evidence to recommend estrogen as standard of care for the postmenopausal woman, based on the consistent if circumstantial evidence from observational studies and the number of positive estrogen-effects on lipoproteins, coagulation factors, and coronary artery endothelium and smooth muscle. Others worry that the cardiovascular benefit is exaggerated because women who use estrogen are more educated and healthier than those who do not[7]. For example, a recent report from the Healthy Women's Study in Pennsylvania showed that women who took estrogen had better levels of heart disease risk factors even before the menopause[8]. If cardioprotection is exaggerated by various prevention, compliance and prescription biases, the true risk reduction may be 20% instead of 35%. Is that enough? Clearly that depends on the competing causes of morbidity and mortality in each country.

If the risk–benefit estimates based on United States data and United States life-expectancy showing 35% reduction in heart disease are real, this benefit would outweigh the increased risk of all other complications combined, including breast cancer[3]. Nevertheless, one in 10 women in the United States will develop breast cancer after age 50, in the absence of HRT, and the risk doubles if she has a mother or sister with breast cancer[3]. Breast cancer is a more common cause of death in US women under 60 years of age than cardiovascular disease; only later do heart disease death rates exceed breast-cancer death rates. Most peri- and early postmenopausal women have several friends their own age who have had breast cancer: at least one of them has

died of breast cancer. In contrast, women less than 65 years of age rarely have friends their age who have had a heart attack.

The statement that there is no consistent evidence that HRT promotes breast cancer is based on nearly 40 epidemiological studies of women who had *ever* used HRT, but most 'ever users' used estrogen for less than 5 years, typically for only a few months. In contrast, eight of 12 epidemiological studies of HRT for ≥ 9 to ≥ 20 years found a 50–80% increased risk of breast cancer[9]. The large prospective Nurse's Health Study reported a 50% increased risk of breast cancer with similar risks in women treated with estrogen alone or estrogen plus a progestin[10]. Recently, Cauley and associates[11] reported that one standard deviation increase in bone density predicted a 50% higher risk of breast cancer in postmenopausal women, adding to the circumstantial evidence for an estrogen–breast cancer association.

This uncertainty about the risk (breast cancer) and benefit (heart disease) has led to the initiation of clinical trials. One secondary prevention trial, the Heart Estrogen/Progestin Replacement Study (HERS), a 5-year trial, is now in its third year; 2673 women who have known coronary artery disease and an intact uterus have been randomly assigned to daily placebo or conjugated equine estrogen (0.625 mg) plus continuous medroxyprogesterone acetate (2.5 mg). The risk of another cardiovascular event in women who already have heart disease is much larger than the risk in women without heart disease, so the sample size and duration of the trial are smaller and shorter than for a primary prevention trial. Results are expected in 1998.

The Women's Health Initiative (WHI) is a primary prevention trial of mostly healthy women (although women with heart disease are not excluded). It will include 27 500 women assigned to estrogen plus progestin in the same regimen used in HERS, or unopposed estrogen for women who have had a hysterectomy. This study should complete recruitment in 1997 and continue for 9 more years.

In the meantime, some US physicians are recommending that their 45- to 55-year-old menopausal patients who have no immediate indications for HRT wait 10 years for the trial results before making an estrogen decision. They argue that these women would be unlikely to suffer a heart attack or hip fracture, since over 80% of these events occur after age 70. They also note recent studies suggesting that lower doses of estrogen may prevent heart disease[4] and bone loss[12] with fewer side-effects and better compliance in older women. Others, persuaded by the consistency and biological plausibility of the data, think that clinical trials are unnecessary, possibly even unethical[13].

Conclusion

It is unlikely that patients or physicians will agree to the need for, or compliance with, lifetime HRT until we have the results of clinical trials. The history of medicine is full of examples of treatments that looked very effective in the absence of a control group. Without clinical trial data, in another 15 years we will still be having these debates about HRT with each other and with our patients[14,15].

Acknowledgement

This research was partially supported by grant DK31801 from the National Institute of Diabetes, Digestive, and Kidney Disease.

References

1. Saver, B. G., Tayler, T. R., Woods, N. F. and Stevens, N. G. (1996). Physician policies on hormone replacement; a survey of four western states. Presented at the *North American Menopause Society (NAMS) Meetings,* Chicago, IL, September

2. Delorey, C. (1989). Women at midlife: women's perceptions, physician's perceptions. *J. Women Aging,* **1**, 57–69

3. Grady, D., Rubin, S. M., Petitti, D. B., *et al.* (1992). Hormone therapy to prevent disease and prolong life in postmenopausal women. *Ann. Intern. Med.,* **117**, 1016–37

4. Grodstein, F., Stampfer, M. J., Manson, J. E., *et al.* (1996). Post-menopausal estrogen and progestin use and the risk of cardiovascular disease. *N. Engl. J. Med.,* **335**, 453–61

5. Psaty, B. M., Heckbert, S. R., Atkins, D., *et al.* (1994). The risk of myocardial infarction associated with the combined use of estrogens and progestins in postmenopausal women. *Arch. Intern. Med.,* **154**, 1333–9

6. Tikkanen, M. J. (1993). Mechanisms of cardiovascular protection by postmenopausal hormone replacement therapy. *Cardiovasc. Risk Factors,* **3**, 138–43

7. Barrett-Connor, E. (1996). The menopause, hormone replacement, and cardiovascular disease: the epidemiologic evidence. *Maturitas,* **23**, 227–34

8. Matthews, K. A., Kuller, L. H., Wing, R. R., Meilahn, E. N. and Plantinga, P. (1996). Prior to use of estrogen replacement therapy, are users healthier than nonusers? *Am. J. Epidemiol.,* **143**, 971–8

9. Lindsay, R., Bush, T. L., Grady, D., Speroff, L. and Lobo, R. A. (1996). Therapeutic controversy: estrogen replacement in menopause. *J. Clin. Endocrinol. Metab.,* **81**, 3829–38

10. Colditz, G. A., Hankinson, S. E., Hunter, D. J., *et al.* (1995). The use of estrogens and progestins and the risk of breast cancer in postmenopausal women. *N. Engl. J. Med.,* **332**, 1589–93

11. Cauley, J. A., Lucas, F. L., Kuller, L., *et al.* for the Study of Osteoporotic Fractures Research Group (1996). Bone mineral density and risk of breast cancer in older women. *J. Am. Med. Assoc.,* **276**, 1404–8

12. Ettinger, B. (1993). Use of low-dosage 17β-estradiol for the prevention of osteoporosis. *Clin. Ther.,* **15**(6), 950–62

13. Bush, T. L. (1996). Clinical medicine and clinical trials: reflections on a shotgun marriage. *Presented at the 8th International Congress on the Menopause,* Sydney, Australia, November, Abstract A02

14. Toozs-Hobson, P. and Cardozo, L. (1996). Hormone replacement therapy for all? Universal prescription is desirable. *Br. Med. J.,* **313**, 350–1

15. Jacobs, H. S. (1996). Not for everybody. *Br. Med. J.,* **313**, 351–2

Does continuing medical education improve professional performance? 40

H. C. Visscher

Continuing Medical Education (CME) can improve professional performance. It is more likely to do so if certain principles are followed.

CME is the process of improving health-care outcomes through individual learning or through utilization of educational activities, products and services as provided by sponsors of CME. It is anticipated that this effort will maintain or enhance professional competence and performance and promote the effectiveness and efficiency of health-care organizations. Operating under the principle that CME can improve competence and perhaps patient care outcome, these factors are essential:

(1) The practicing obstetrician and gynecologist must be involved in the clear identification of the learning needs.

(2) The educational program must have clear goals and clinically oriented objectives.

(3) Learning activities must incorporate relevant methods with emphasis on learner participation.

(4) The central focus must be on improving patient care by changing physician behavior.

(5) The impact of the learning must be systematically evaluated in order to assist in planning future CME activity.

It is important to relate CME to the full spectrum of medical education. There is the continuous need for education throughout the approximate 45 years of a doctor's professional lifetime, including undergraduate, postgraduate and practicing years. Along this continuum, students, through gradual acquisition of knowledge, skills and experience, increasingly gain independence in their approach to learning and practice. They also acquire attitudes and habits that will help them assess continually their performance and professional needs. Faculty by precept and design eventually become facilitators and information brokers, rather than primarily instructors and content experts as they prepare students for independent, self-directed and lifelong learning. The individual practicing physician assumes primary control over identifying learning needs, setting goals and objectives, choosing learning approaches, selecting methods of evaluation, and applying acquired competence to clinical practice.

A compelling motivation for continual learning on the part of the obstetrician–gynecologist is the constant increase in medical knowledge and technology in the specialty and the pressures of the changing medical marketplace. It is important to recognize that CME programs are intended to be evidence-based educational aids to presenting recognized methods and techniques of clinical practice for consideration by obstetricians and gynecologists for incorporation into their practice. Programs should not be based solely on minimally acceptable modes or practice standards. Variations of practice that take into account the needs of the individual patient, resources, and limitations unique to the institution or type of practice, are appropriate.

The following are the basic essentials for any CME program that could be developed by any of the FIGO organizations[1]:

(1) The organization should develop a written statement of its educational mission and it

should be formally approved by the governing body. The statement should describe the goals of the overall medical education program, outline the characteristics of the potential participants, and describe in general terms the activities and services which the organization desires to provide. It must be demonstrated how the CME mission is congruent with, and supported by, the mission of the parent organization. For the organization to be successful, the intended participants must be truly represented in the organizational structure and be involved in the planning process.

(2) The organization must establish procedures for indentifying and analyzing the educational needs and interest of the prospective participants. The assessments of these needs should go beyond the perception of a few individuals or potential faculty. Educational needs should be identified by looking at practice outcome data, for example, by studying the benefits of risk analysis. Epidemiological and prevalence data that identify common causes of morbidity and mortality would be useful in this regard. Prevention, screening, and long-term cost containment data are also relevant.

(3) Based on the needs assessment analysis as identified by the organization, the next step would be the development of explicit objectives that the organization would like to accomplish in their medical education activities. They should state the educational needs which the individual educational activity will address, indicate the obstetrician/gynecologist for whom the activity is designed, and list any special background requirements of the prospective participants. They should highlight the instructional content and the expected learning outcomes in terms of knowledge, skills and attitudes.

(4) The organization should design and implement educational activities consistent in content and format with the stated objectives. These formats must be responsive to the characteristics of prospective participants such as their knowledge levels, professional experience, and preferred learning styles. The format chosen might be a self-assessment program, a course program, an educational publication or an information management program. The educational content and methods used for any CME program must be known to the prospective participants. The program should encourage and foster self-directed learning and the sense that individuals should be actively responsible for their own continuing medical education. Indeed, active pursuit of CME should become a matter of personal pride and duty.

(5) The organization must evaluate the effectiveness of any one of existing medical education programs as well as the overall effectiveness of the total CME activity, and use this information in CME planning for the future. This involves periodically reviewing the extent to which the CME mission is being achieved. Evaluations must assess the extent to which the educational objectives are being met and the overall quality of the instructional process, and listen to the participants' perception as to whether enhanced professional effectiveness is achieved. The focus must be on changing the individual's performance which can be evaluated through process or outcome data.

(6) The organization should decide who will manage the educational activity and where the necessary resources will come from to carry out the program effectively. An organizational structure would have to be identified, responsible individuals would have to be named, and a budget for the program would have to be developed. This would vary according to the structure of health provision in the countries concerned.

FIGO should organize workshops to assist its member organizations in developing high-quality CME programs which focus on improving the provision of health care for women and their newborn infants. Those who are developing their own programs could gain valuable advice and assistance by consulting members of FIGO who have well-established CME programs. It is hoped that external funding would become available at least for planning purposes, but for any organization's program to be successful there has to be significant input on the part of the organization itself, including seed money. This assumes that the participants of the intended program will also be very involved in organizing, planning and evaluating the CME program.

A recent review[2] has demonstrated that the probability of clinical guidelines being effective is high if the development strategy is an internal one, the strategy for dissemination of these guidelines use specific educational intervention, and the implementation involves specific reminders for managing individual patients at the time of consultation. The probability of this education being effective is low if development is external or national, dissemination is in journals, and is implemented only with general reminders. FIGO strategy should therefore be to facilitate the organization of workshops by its member societies on how to teach high-quality CME principles and methods to have the greatest impact. These workshops would automatically seek the appropriate level of expertise required for each country's needs, best suited for its professional body. At the same time, the important underlying principles to ensure success would apply. This would be the most useful way for FIGO to make a difference.

At the American College of Obstetricians and Gynecologists (ACOG), our most effective methods of changing practice behavior are based on a complex structure that involves:

(1) National ACOG committees which, with input from the epidemiological, academic, and practice perspectives, produce educational bulletins. These bulletins discuss areas of practice, committee opinions and practice guidelines which focus on a specific technology or treatment, and criteria sets which define minimal standards.

(2) These documents then serve as the tools to help our practicing members relate these facts to the local practice environment. They help institutional quality assessment committees to evaluate minimal acceptable practice, help departments to grant privileges, and help educational committees to identify the highest levels of clinically proven modes of practice. In our various medical marketplaces where product and technology promotion are so sophisticated, these documents help our members, institutions, and health care payers differentiate between what is experimental and what is clinically proven.

(3) The ACOG produces a series of patient education pamphlets which are co-ordinated with all of the above documents to enable our members to inform their patients better about the meaning of diagnosis, introduce them to new treatments and technologies, and discuss the risks and benefits of a particular intervention. This leads to better understanding and informed consent, better compliance, and better results.

(4) The ACOG also produces annual self-assessment programs and knowledge updates at 4-year intervals to aid individual practitioners and residents to evaluate their knowledge base; and enduring materials, such as programmed texts, audiotapes, videotapes and computer-assisted instructional materials, to help them improve their practice skills.

References

1. Accreditation Council for Continuing Medical Education (1997). *Essentials, Guidelines, and Standards for Accreditation of Sponsors of Continuing Medical Education.* (Chicago: ACCME)

2. Grimshaw, J. M. and Russell, I. T. (1993). Effect of clinical guidelines on medical practice: a systematic review of rigorous evaluations. *Lancet,* **342**, 1317–22

Further reading

Report of the Committee on Education in Obstetrics and Gynecology and Human Reproduction (1995). *Standards of education in obstetrics and gynecology. FIGO News/Int. J. Gynec. Obstet.,* **50**, 85–95

Visscher, H. C. (1991). Workshop on continuing medical education for obstetricians and gynecologists. Presented at the *CREOG/APGO Annual Meeting,* New Orleans, February

Does continuing medical education lead to improved performance? 41

A. D. Hewson

Vital importance of continuing medical education

The concept that lifelong learning is extremely important in our profession dates back to the time of Hypocrates when the great teacher reminded his listeners that 'life is short but the art is long'[1]. Sir William Osler in 1905 gave the same message to medical undergraduates and reminded them that they were beginning a life course in medical education[2]. In subsequent decades there were further references to the importance of lifetime learning for physicians, recently summarized by Manning[3].

In the second half of this century, this emphasis on continuing medical education has been supplemented by formalized approaches to linking continuing education with competence and performance, and as a corollary, linking these to continuing certification for medical practice, most notably in the formalized recertification protocols widely adopted in the United States under the umbrella of the American Board of Medical Specialties[4].

Opinion leaders have continued to stress the importance of continuing medical education: C. Everett Koop, former Surgeon General of the United States, in 1989 commented 'continuing medical education should be an inherent part of our belief system as physicians. The era in which we live makes it critical that we embrace the concept of continuous learning'[5].

Definitions

Definitions of the terms we use in this area are important. Continuing medical education consists of educational activities which serve to maintain, develop or increase the knowledge, skills, professional performance and relationships that a physician uses to provide services for patients, the public or the profession[6].

Competence is defined as 'the quality or state of being functionally adequate'[7], but for our purposes can be paraphrased into 'what one can do'. This is a theoretical construct, and is not really observable. Performance, on the other hand, is 'what one does do'. It therefore refers to behavior patterns which can be observed[8].

The objective of continuing medical education is to improve competence, with the anticipation that this will lead to improved performance and health-care outcomes. While this sequence is part of our 'belief system', there must be measures in place to demonstrate objectively that the sequence does occur.

Community, government and professional concerns

Such confirmation as described above has now become essential. In recent years the community has been taking an increasing interest in the standards of medical care provided by our profession. The community is concerned about increasing costs and the implications of increasing litigation as we are now part of a more questioning society. Governments are also concerned regarding competence, performance and standards of practice because of taxpayer funding of services and professionals[9].

Various statutory authorities concerned with licensure increasingly ask for guidance in measures of competence and dyscompetence. Further, the profession itself is increasingly aware of the rapid explosion of medical knowledge and the demonstrated incompetence of some professional 'outliers', and has to be seen to be protecting its own standards[10].

The outcome of all of the above is that we can no longer assume that the desirable sequence referred to always happens in practice: fortunately there are now many studies in the literature which address this issue.

Studies in the literature

Earlier studies in the literature which sought to evaluate the effect of traditional continuing medical education on subsequent practitioner competence failed to establish a cause and effect relationship. However, later reviews by Bertram and Brooks-Bertram, and Lloyd and Abrahamson, established methodological errors in these earlier papers[11,12]. Importantly, more recent studies by Steyn, and Raymond, demonstrated that particular forms of continuing education can and do produce measurable changes in practitioner behavior[13,14]. Beaudry carried out a quantitative synthesis of previous articles and also came to the same conclusion[15].

Most importantly, a definitive article by Davis and colleagues provided even more well-researched information on this topic[16]. The difficulty of obtaining objective data linking continuing medical education with competence and performance was demonstrated in their review. Davis and co-workers reviewed 777 continuing medical education studies and found only 50 which met their strict criteria, i.e. randomized controlled trials; specific educational programs, activities or other interventions; studies which included 50% or more physicians; follow-up assessment of at least 75% of study subjects; and objective assessments of either physician performance or health-care outcomes. Davis and associates divided medical interventions into predisposing, enabling or facilitating. They assessed physician performance outcomes and patient outcomes as either positive, negative or inconclusive. Of the final

50 studies meeting these criteria, 32 analyzed physician performance, seven evaluated patient outcomes and 11 examined both measures. The majority of the 43 studies of physician performance showed positive results in some important measures of resource utilization, counseling strategies and preventive medicine. Of the 18 studies of health-care outcomes, eight demonstrated positive changes in patient health-care outcomes.

Principles underlying effective continuing medical education

A review of the data in these papers establishes important principles. It is only possible to confirm that continuing medical education leads to improved competence provided that there is an educationally sound determination of the needs of the study group, and the attempt to meet these needs is in accordance with appropriate educational principles. These include recognition that practicing professionals use a wide variety of educational resources to update their knowledge, that the initiatives used utilize the principles of adult learning, that success rates improve if the initiative has a demonstrably close link to the practice of the individual, that there is appropriate reinforcement throughout the study time-frame and subsequently, that there is feedback and evaluation of the program, which give benefits to both the provider and the recipient.

Importance of opinion leaders

One of the papers reviewed by Davis and colleagues is of particular interest to obstetricians. This study by Lomas and co-workers was a randomized controlled trial of 76 physicians in 16 community hospitals which evaluated audit and feedback versus local opinion leaders as ways of encouraging compliance with guidelines for the management of women with a previous Cesarean section: it involved a study of the management of 3552 cases[17]. It demonstrated that the influence of a recognized opinion leader was very effective in altering the management of patients, and more effective than groups of physicians being involved in audit and feedback: the overall Cesarean-section rate was reduced, and the duration of hospital stay was lower in the opinion-leader groups, and the authors concluded that the use of opinion leaders significantly improved the quality of care[17].

The comparative failure of the audit feedback strategy via an administrative mechanism to influence performance in the desired direction is contrary to much of the evidence in the literature, and the poor effectiveness in the study of Lomas and associates, may be related to its multi-institutional focus, as opposed to the success of other studies in single units using the peer-review and audit approach.

However, there is an important principle in the Lomas study which is applicable to opinion leaders in our discipline world-wide. Respected leaders clearly continue to have great potential, by personal example and involvement, to produce improved performance and health-care outcomes, and it is comforting to have had this documented.

Problems of studies using volunteers

A possible criticism of even well-documented studies of randomized trials is that they involve volunteer physicians who may well be above the general standard of their peers in performance, and so are comfortable having their performance and patient health-status scrutinized. There are other possible sources of bias which are explored in the paper of Davis and colleagues. Therefore, because of the questions raised regarding studies which only use volunteers, many countries have moved towards obligatory involvement in continuing medical education as a major step in ensuring that all physicians become involved in the continuing medical education process, i.e. to ensure that those who may be most in need of education are obliged to become involved.

For example, the McAuley paper identified the high-risk group of the 'Geographically and professionally isolated practitioners' who usually stand apart from all continuing medical education and who were shown to have a poor standard of practice[10].

Links between continuing medical education and recertification programs

The obligatory recertification program of the American Board of Obstetrics and Gynecology in the USA is predicated on the view that a formal examination at 10-year intervals is an appropriate way to ensure that obstetricians in that country keep themselves up to date and can confirm that their knowledge base is appropriate for continuing practice[18]. While most would accept that this is a strategy which has some merit, and is certainly much better than no evaluation whatsoever, there remain concerns that just reviewing the knowledge base of a practitioner by itself may not ensure continuing competence and performance. For this reason, the obstetrics colleges in some other countries have developed other strategies aimed at ensuring competence: these programs demand involvement in medical education in various forms as well as assessment of competence and performance at the workface.

The Royal Australian College of Obstetricians and Gynaecologists (RACOG) was one of the pioneers in this field, and when that College was formed in 1979 it adopted the principle of time-limited certification dependent on documented involvement in continuing medical education activities specified by the College[9]. The RACOG program accepts that professionals utilize a wide range of educational activities for their continuing education, and therefore allocates educational credits (cognate points) to College-approved educational programs (needs-directed and continually evaluated). However, it also recognizes involvement in teaching, contributions to the literature, self-assessment tests of many types, and peer-review and quality-assurance programs in the workplace using guidelines from the College[19].

The program is obligatory and ensures that all Fellows of the College remain active participants throughout their practicing life in order to continue to have specialist certification in Australia. The acceptance of the program and its continuing evaluation has been described elsewhere, and its success has led to virtually all other specialist colleges in Australia introducing similar programs[20]. Similar systems have been developed in New Zealand[21] and the United Kingdom[1].

All of these programs, to varying degrees, ensure that all practitioners in the discipline are involved in specified continuing medical education initiatives: there is emphasis on the link with medical auditing, i.e. reviews at the workface with one's peers.

Canadian maintenance of competence program

The maintenance of competence of medical practitioners (MOCOMP) program now functioning in Canada also includes peer review of an individual's clinical practice, utilizing a continuous log of educational activities directed to learning objectives established by the individual practitioner. The data are then available to be compared with those of similarly placed colleagues. While the aims of this program are laudable, it remains open to the criticism that it is a voluntary program and that after some years only a minority of specialists in Canada are involved[22].

Difficulties in evaluating competence and performance

A review of the world literature clarifies the many difficulties in evaluating these interrelationships. Questions can be raised as to how competence and performance are assessed: there needs to be clarification of the standards set, particularly the impact of evidence-based medicine on current practice[23]. Also, studies to document the sequence are time-consuming and expensive. A significant advantage of the systems which are compulsory is that there is the opportunity to continually monitor the impact of education on outcomes covering the whole professional group, and this will become increasingly important in the future. However, over and above the competence and performance of health-care professionals, the outcomes of care are significantly influenced by a wide range of other factors.

Multiplicity of factors influencing outcomes

Individual obstetricians have their own beliefs, goals, attitudes, cultures and concerns regarding their patients and their practice. Moreover, the recipients of care also have their own beliefs, goals, attitudes, cultures and individual concerns. In addition, the way obstetricians interact with patients is further affected by our communication skills, the impact of their family and friends and society on their thinking, and the impact of our fellow health professionals on the health-care mix in which we work. There is also the significant impact of economic factors on patients; the physical framework in which we provide care; the ever-present impact of litigation on our relationships; and all of these have a continuing and significant impact on overall health-care outcomes[24]. Moreover, societal changes, including the increased questioning of all professionals by society, the misdeeds of some members of professional groups and an increased cynicism regarding the effectiveness of traditional medical care, have altered the whole intellectual and cultural framework in which we and our patients live. All these factors have an impact on our ability to influence health-care outcomes, and obstetricians need education in all of these areas if they are to be able to provide effective health-care in the future[25].

Turnberg has pointed out that patient satisfaction is also an outcome of health-care and, like any other outcome, requires measurement[26].

Impact of modern technology

The explosion of information and increasing access of obstetricians to data poses new challenges for us as we approach the next century.

277

The provision of enormous amounts of information on CD-ROM and computer disk, and the increased access to data via video links and telecommunication modalities, means that information is more rapidly and easily available than ever before. The decreasing costs of all these modalities means that in the future they will become increasingly available to all countries, even those with limited resources to spend on medical care.

However, the effectiveness of these new tools in the world of continuing medical education is still being evaluated, and we still do not have clear data regarding the extent to which there is transfer from the experience of multimedia simulation to the way professionals go about their work in real wards, surgeries or operating theatres[27].

The importance of recognized opinion leaders referred to above is important in this context: the views of world-recognized authorities via voice or image in our discipline are now widely available, and so can provide continuing encouragement to practitioners to update their knowledge and improve their competence and performance.

Medical-records accessibility and privacy issues

The rapidly expanding computerization of medical records, which facilitates easier review of charts and hospital records for audit purposes, clearly makes these avenues more accessible and less time-consuming.

The increasing availability of a direct print-out of the spoken word via the new software programs also increases the privacy of confidential information, so that its dissemination is limited to the recorder and receivers of the confidential information, instead of being potentially available to the unauthorized.

The computerization of records on a national scale again makes interhospital, interpractice and interpractitioner review progressively more available. Properly utilized, and with privacy safeguards, this provides yet another avenue for continuing education and feedback along the lines of the MOCOMP program.

Conclusion

In summary, the now established guidelines for effective continuing medical education can be much more readily implemented than ever before: it should be possible to progressively improve the prospects of continuing education for achieving desired outcomes.

Many of the time-tested methods should continue and these should be utilized in the educational framework and principles of adult learning. Our influence on health-care outcomes will be affected by our ability to recognize the changes occurring in society and the health-care environment in which we work: continuing education in this area will become progressively more important as we face the challenges of the new century.

References

1. Purdie, D. W. (1994). Continuing medical education. *Br. J. Obstet. Gynaecol.*, **101**, 101–281
2. Osler, W. (1905). The student life: farewell address to American and Canadian medical students. *NY Med. News.*
3. Manning, P. R. (1987). In Manning, R. R. and DeBakey, L. (eds.) *Medicine – Preserving the Passion*, pp. 26–7. (New York: Springer-Verlag)
4. Langsley, D. G. (1989). American Board of Medical Specialist Board Recertification: current status and requirements 1989. In *ABMS Annual Report and Reference Handbook,* Oklahoma City, OK C3104
5. Koop, C. E. (1990). Why CME? Address to the Third International Conference on Continuing Medical Education, Annenberg Centre, 1989. *J. Contin. Educ. Health Prof.*, **10**, 103

6. Maitland, F. M. (1992). Accreditation of sponsors and certification of credit. In Primer, A., Rosof, A. B. and Felsch, W. C. (eds.) *Continuing Medical Education*, p. 15. (New York: Praeger)

7. Pease, R. W. Jnr. (ed.) (1986). *Webster's Medical Desk Dictionary*, p. 136. (Springfield, MA: Merrian-Webster Inc.)

8. Mast, T. and Davis, D. (1994). Concepts of competence. In Davis, D. R. and Fox, R. D. (eds.) *The Physician as Learner*, p. 141. (Chicago, IL: American Medical Association)

9. Hewson, A. D. (1989). The development of the obligatory education and certification programme of the RACOG: a practical response to the increasing challenges of a modern society. *Med. Teacher*, **11**, 27–37

10. McAuley, R. G. (1984). Results of Peer Assessment Program of the College of Physicians and Surgeons of Ontario. *Can. Med. Assoc. J.*, **131**, 557–60

11. Bertram, D. A. and Brooks-Bertram, P. A. (1977). The evaluation of continuing medical education: a literature review. *Health Educ. Monogr.* **5**, 330–62

12. Lloyd, J. S. and Abrahamson, S. (1979). Effectiveness of continuing medical education: a review of the evidence. *Eval. Health Prof.* **2**, 251–80

13. Steyn, L. S. (1981). The effectiveness of continuing medical education: 8 research reports. *J. Med. Educ.*, **56**, 103–10

14. Raymond, M. R. (1986). The effectiveness of continuing education in the health professions: a re-analysis of the literature. Presented at *Annual Convention of the American Medical Research Association*, San Francisco, CA, April

15. Beaudry, J. S. (1989). The effectiveness of continuing medical education: a quantitative synthesis. *J. Contin. Educ. Health Prof.*, **9**, 285

16. Davis, D. A., Thomson, M. A., Oxman, A. D. and Haynes, B. (1992). Evidence of the effectiveness of CME. A review of 50 randomized controlled trials. *J. Am. Med. Assoc.*, **268**, 1111–17

17. Lomas, J., Enkin, M., Anderson, G. M., Hannah, W. J., Vayda, E. and Singer, J. (1991). Opinion leaders vs. audit and feedback to implement practice guidelines – delivery after previous Cesarean section. *J. Am. Med. Assoc.*, **265**, 2202–7

18. Langsley, D. G. (1991). Recredentialing. *J. Am. Med. Assoc.*, **265**, 772

19. Gabb, R. and Hewson, A. D. (eds.) (1987). *A Guide to Quality Assurance in Obstetrics and Gynaecology.* (Melbourne, Australia: Royal Australian College of Obstetricians and Gynaecologists)

20. Hewson, A. D. (1996). CME and recertification in Australia 1995. *Postgrad. Med. J.*, **72**(Suppl. 1), S43

21. Fiddes, T. M. (1989). Guidelines for the development of continuing medical education and continuing certification in the RNZCOG. *Workshop Proceedings.* (Auckland: Royal New Zealand College of Obstetricians and Gynaecologists)

22. Council of the Royal College of Physicians and Surgeons of Canada (1990). *Maintenance of Competence System (MOCOMP).* (Ottawa, Canada: RCPS)

23. Enkin, M., Kierse, M. J. N. C. and Chalmers, I. (1990). *A Guide to Effective Care in Pregnancy and Childbirth.* (Oxford: Oxford University Press)

24. Watts, M. S. M. (1990). A third component to continuing education in health professions. *J. Contin. Educ. Health Prof.*, **10**. 377–8

25. Hewson, A. D. (1991). Continuing medical education in obstetrics and gynaecology: the challenge of the 90s. *Aust. NZ J. Obstet. Gynaecol.*, **31**, 249–53

26. Turnberg, L. M. (1993). In Fitzpatrick, R. and Hopkins, A. (eds.) *Measurement of Patient Satisfaction with their Care*, p. iii. (London: Royal College of Physicians)

27. Atkins, M. J. and O'Halloran, C. (1995). AMEE Medical Education Guide No. 6: evaluating multimedia applications for medical education. *Med. Teacher*, **17**, 149–59

Factor V Leiden: a beginning of an explanation for venous thrombosis risk with oral contraceptives

42

K. W. M. Bloemenkamp, F. R. Rosendaal, F. M. Helmerhorst and J. P. Vandenbroucke

Oral contraceptives and venous thrombosis

From the early days of use of combined oral contraceptives, reports have emerged on an association between the use of oral contraceptives (OCs) and the development of venous thromboembolism. After the report of Jordan[1], numerous case–control and cohort studies followed. The estimated relative risk of developing thromboembolism during OC use was reported to be between 2 and 11; the most recent studies[2,3] in which mainly low-dose OCs are used still report a relative risk of 4.

Inherited clotting defects and venous thrombosis

The overall annual incidence of venous thrombosis is estimated to be 1 in 1000. Individuals with clotting factor gene abnormalities are at higher risk to develop venous thrombosis in comparison with individuals without these abnormalities. Antithrombin, protein-C and protein-S deficiency are examples of already long-known inherited clotting defects. From case–control and cohort studies it can be concluded that they are present in 0.02–0.5% of healthy individuals, in 1–3% of consecutive patients with a first deep-vein thrombosis and in 0.5–13% of thrombophilic patients[4]. In 1994, the single point mutation in the factor V gene was identified as the genetic defect causing the phenotype of activated protein-C (APC) resistance[5]. It involves a G→A transition of nucleotide 1691 in exon 10, which predicts the synthe-sis of variant factor V molecule (factor V Arg506 to Gln or factor V Leiden). Thus, factor V Leiden leads to resistance to APC and is commonly found among patients with venous thrombosis. The mechanism by which the mutation leads to the phenotype of APC resistance is not yet clear, but replacement of Arg506 by Gln will prevent cleavage of factor V(a) at this site by APC, and by that delay the inactivation of factor V(a). To date, factor V Leiden has been the only genetic defect identified in APC-resistant families. The frequency of occurrence of factor V Leiden is 3–6% in healthy individuals, 20% in consecutive patients with a first deep-vein thrombosis and up to 52% (APC resistance) in thrombophilic patients[4]. In the Caucasian population higher frequencies were found than in Japanese and other Eastern populations[6,7].

Inherited thrombophilia acknowledges the presence of an inherited factor that by itself predisposes towards thrombosis, but due to the episodic nature of thrombosis, requires interaction with other components (inherited or acquired) before onset of the clinical disorder (Table 1).

Interaction between factor V Leiden and oral contraceptives

A new insight into the relation between OC use and thromboembolism was reported in 1994[8]. In a population-based case–control study on the causes of venous thrombosis (the Leiden thrombophilia study), 155 consecutive pre-menopausal women, aged 15–49, who had developed an objectively diagnosed first deep-vein thrombosis in the absence of other underlying diseases, were compared with 169 population controls. Factor V Leiden mutation displayed a strong interaction with use of OCs. In non-carriers who used OCs the risk of venous thrombosis was increased fourfold and in carrier non-users the risk was increased eightfold, but the risk rose 30-fold in users of OCs who also carried the factor V Leiden mutation. Recalculation of population incidences from these relative risks showed that the absolute risk of venous thrombosis in young women who use OCs is much larger when they carry the factor V Leiden mutation (Figure 1). Also, for the other inherited clotting factors which are themselves risk factors of venous thrombosis, namely protein-C, protein-S and antithrombin deficiency, OC use appeared to synergistically lead to an excess risk for development of venous thrombosis[9].

Venous thrombosis during first year of oral contraceptive use

Recent studies showed that the risk for venous thrombosis is highest during initial OC use[10–12]. We investigated whether women with inherited clotting defects who use OCs develop their venous thrombosis at an earlier stage compared with women without known inherited clotting defects. Therefore, we analyzed the data of the Leiden thrombophilia study with regard to OC use and duration of OC use. Women were termed deficient when they proved to have protein-C, protein-S or antithrombin deficiency, or factor V Leiden. In the total group the risk of developing deep-vein thrombosis was greatest in the first half-year of use. Of the 109 OC-using cases, 35 women were deficient, and of the deficient women, 25.7% (9/35) had their venous thrombosis during the first year of use, in comparison with 4.1% (3/74) of the non-deficients ($p < 0.05$). The risk of developing deep-vein thrombosis during the first year of OC use was eightfold increased (OR 8.2, 95% CI 2.1–32.6) for a woman with a deficiency. We conclude that inherited clotting defects lead to development of deep-vein thrombosis in OC users at an earlier stage, compared with women without inherited clotting defects who also developed their deep-vein thrombosis during OC use. It should be a warning signal for the clinician when a woman develops venous thrombosis during the first year of OC use, because this could be an indication that she has an inherited clotting defect.

Table 1 Risk factors for deep-vein thrombosis

Acquired
Surgery
Malignancies
Trauma
Immobilization
Pregnancy, puerperium
Use of oral contraceptives

Inherited
Antithrombin deficiency
Protein-C deficiency
Protein-S deficiency
APC resistance/factor V Leiden mutation
Dysfibrinogenemia
(Hyperhomocystenemia?)

APC, activated protein C

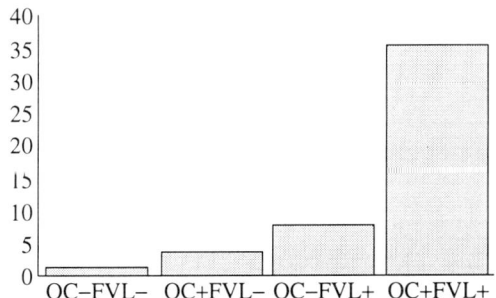

Figure 1 Deep-vein thrombosis per year per 10 000 women. OC, oral contraceptive; FVL, factor V Leiden

Third-generation oral contraceptives

In the Leiden thrombophilia study, we also compared the risk of developing deep-vein thrombosis during use of the newest OCs, containing a third-generation progestogen, with the risk during use of 'older' OCs containing other progestogens. In this analysis we also investigated the influence of family history of thrombosis, previous pregnancy, age and the thrombogenic factor V Leiden mutation upon these risks[10].

We selected 126 women with deep venous thrombosis and 159 control women who were aged 15–49 (mean age 34.9 years) and pre-menopausal, and found, compared with non-users, the highest age-adjusted relative risks for an OC containing desogestrel and 30 µg ethinylestradiol (OR 8.7, 95% CI 3.9–19.3). In contrast, we found lower relative risks for use of all other types of OC, ranging from 2.2 to 3.8. In a direct comparison, users of the desogestrel-containing OC had a 2.5-fold higher risk of developing deep-vein thrombosis (95% CI 1.2–5.2) than users of all other OC types combined.

The relative risk for the desogestrel-containing OC was similar among women with and without a family history of deep-vein thrombosis, i.e. preferential prescription because of family history cannot explain our findings. The excess risk could also not be explained by women having ever been pregnant or not, and was highest in the youngest age categories where we would expect most new users. The age-adjusted odds ratio for the desogestrel-containing contraceptive was 9.2 (95% CI 3.9–21.4) among non-carriers of the factor V Leiden mutation and 6.0 (95% CI 1.9–19.0) among carriers of the mutation. This latter risk was then superimposed on the eightfold increased risk of venous thrombosis for carriers of the factor V Leiden mutation. The risk of carriers using the desogestrel-containing OC compared with non-carrier non-users would, therefore, be almost 50-fold increased.

Low-dose OCs with a third-generation progestogen have a higher risk of deep venous thrombosis associated with them than the previous generation of OCs. The absolute risk of deep venous thrombosis associated with these OCs appears to be particularly high among carriers of the factor V Leiden mutation and

among women with a family history of thrombosis. However, the higher risk associated with oral contraception containing a third-generation progestogen compared with that containing previous generations was also present in women without factor V Leiden and without a positive family history.

The increasing mortality of young women due to venous thrombosis, in The Netherlands and the United Kingdom, supports this excess in risk associated with the more often used third-generation OCs[13].

Oral contraceptives, factor V Leiden and activated protein-C resistance

Recently, several studies reported that OC use leads to an increase in APC resistance[14–17], and it has also been described that women without factor V Leiden mutation show APC resistance[18]. One problem when comparing these studies is that different types of assay to measure APC resistance were used and they seem different in their sensitivity to sex-steroids. Also, other variables, such as lupus anticoagulants and platelets, can interfere with the results of the assay. We found that women who developed deep-vein thrombosis during OC use and from whom blood was collected more than 6 months after their event showed more APC resistance than their control subjects, irrespective of OC use during time of blood collection.

Biological explanation

One objection to the findings of excess risk of venous thrombosis by use of third-generation OCs was that there was no biological mechanism that could explain these unexpected findings. However, to date, the mechanism by which OCs cause venous thrombosis has never been understood. Very recently, Rosing and colleagues showed that healthy women using third-generation OCs have twofold increased plasma levels of APC resistance when compared with healthy women using the older second-generation OCs[19]. The degree of the acquired resistance to APC (by the use of third-generation OCs) is close to that of asymptomatic non-OC-using women who carry factor V Leiden. These data are in agreement with the estimates (OR of 8 for factor V Leiden carrier and OR of 8 for use of third-generation OCs) found in epidemiological studies[8,10].

Screening

It is questionable whether routine screening for genetic clotting disorders before starting OCs is useful or feasible. When there is a family history of inherited thrombophilia in a first-degree relative, how useful it really is to screen for genetic disorders, even in patients with thrombosis, is not yet agreed. A major problem is that venous thrombosis is a rather frequent disease when viewed over the course of a lifetime, so many people will have a positive history without having a genetic defect[20]. We calculated that, when estimating the death rate from pulmonary embolism at 5.7 per 100 000 a year, 20 000 women positive for factor V Leiden should be denied the use of OCs during 1 year to prevent one death. At an estimated population-prevalence of factor V Leiden of 1 in 20, 400 000 women would need to be screened to find them[21].

Recurrence

An answer to the extremely relevant, clinical question on the recurrence rate when continuing OCs after a first thrombosis is still lacking. Therefore, it remains a question whether OCs should be continued after a woman has developed her venous thrombosis during OC use. Probably, in some countries, legal problems can be expected if a woman develops a recurrent venous thrombosis after a clinician has advised her to continue OCs after her first thrombotic event. However, in our opinion, when a woman is an asymptomatic homozygote carrier of the factor V Leiden mutation, is asymptomatic but a carrier of a combination of inherited clotting defects or is a heterozygote carrier and has had a venous thrombosis, OCs should not be prescribed or should be discontinued. Asymptomatic carriers of factor V Leiden can be prescribed OCs after counseling about the effect of the interaction between factor V Leiden and OC use and discussing all disadvantages and possible benefits of other types of contraception. If a woman chooses to use OCs this should be a second-generation OC, because there is an excess in risk for use of the third-generation OCs, especially in combination with factor V Leiden.

References

1. Jordan, W. M. (1961). Pulmonary embolism. *Lancet*, **2**, 1146–7
2. Hannaford, P. C. (1996). Combined oral contraceptive use and venous thromboembolism. *Gynecol. Endocrinol.*, **10**(Suppl. 2), 13–18
3. Bloemenkamp, K. W. M., Rosendaal, F. R., Helmerhorst, F. M. and Vandenbroucke, J. P. (1996). Evidence that currently available pills are associated with cardiovascular disease: venous disease. In Hannaford, P. C. and Webb, A. M. C. (eds.) *Evidence-Guided Prescribing of the Pill*, pp. 61–76. (Carnforth, UK: Parthenon Publishing)
4. Lane, D. A., Mannucci, P. M., Bauer, K. A., Bertina, R. M., Bochkov, N. P., Boulyjenkov, V., Chandy, M., Dahlback, B., Ginter, E. K., Miletich, J. P. *et al.* (1996). Inherited thrombophilia 1. *Thromb. Haemost.*, **76**, 651–62
5. Bertina, R. M., Koeleman, B. P., Koster, T., Rosendaal, F. R., Dirven, R. J., de Ronde, H., van der Velden, P. A. and Reitsma, P. H. (1994). Mutation in blood coagulation factor V associated with resistance to activated protein C. *Nature (London)*, **369** , 64–7
6. Rees, D. C., Cox, M. and Clegg, J. B. (1995). World distribution of factor V Leiden. *Lancet*, **346**, 1133–4

7. Ridker, P. M., Hennekens, C. H., Lindpainter, K., Stampfer, M. J., Eisenberg, P. R. and Miletich, J. P. (1995). Mutation in the gene coding for coagulation factor V and the risk of myocardial infarction, stroke, and venous thrombosis in apparently healthy men. *N. Engl. J. Med.*, **332**, 912–7

8. Vandenbroucke, J. P., Koster, T., Briet, E., Reitsma, P. H., Bertina, R. M. and Rosendaal, F. R. (1994). Increased risk of venous thrombosis in oral-contraceptive users who are carriers of factor V Leiden mutation. *Lancet*, **344**, 1453–7

9. Pabinger, I. and Schneider, B. (1994). Thrombotic risk of women with hereditary antithrombin III-, protein C- and protein S-deficiency taking oral contraceptive medication. The GTH Study Group on Natural Inhibitors. *Thromb. Haemost.*, **71**, 548–52

10. Bloemenkamp, K. W. M., Rosendaal, F. R., Helmerhorst, F. M., Buller, H. R. and Vandenbroucke, J. P. (1995). Enhancement by factor V Leiden mutation of risk of deep-vein thrombosis associated with oral contraceptives containing third-generation progestagen. *Lancet*, **346**, 1593–6

11. Poulter, N. R., Farley, T. M. M., Chang, C. L., Marmot, M. G. and Meirik, O. (1996). Authors' reply: safety of combined oral contraceptive pills. *Lancet*, **347**, 547

12. Spitzer, W. O., Lewis, M. A., Heinemann, L. A. J., Thorogood, M. and MacRae K. D. (1996). Third generation oral contraceptives and risk of venous thromboembolic disorders: an international case–control study. *Br. Med. J.*, **312**, 83–8

13. Vandenbroucke, J. P., Bloemenkamp, K. W. M., Helmerhorst, F. M. and Rosendaal, F. R. (1996). Mortality from venous thromboembolism and myocardial infarction in young women in The Netherlands. *Lancet*, **348**, 401–2

14. Bokarewa, M. I., Falk, G., Sten-Linder, M., Egberg, N., Blomback, M. and Bremme, K. (1995). Thrombotic risk factors and oral contraception. *J. Lab. Clin. Med.*, **126**, 294–8

15. Henkens, C. M. A., Bom, V. J. J., Seinen, A. J. and van der Meer, J. (1995). Sensitivity to activated protein C; influence of oral contraceptives and sex. *Thromb. Haemost*, **73**, 402–4

16. Østerud, B., Robertsen, R., Åsvang, G. B. and Thijssen, F. (1994). Resistance to activated protein C is reduced in women using oral contraceptives. *Blood Coagul. Fibrinolysis*, **5**, 853–4

17. Bokarewa, M. I., Falk, G., Sten-Linder, M., Egberg, N., Blomback, M. and Bremme, K. (1995). Thrombotic risk factors and oral contraception. *J. Lab. Clin. Med.*, **126**, 294–8

18. Olivieri, O., Friso, S., Manzato, F., Guella, A., Bernardi, F., Lunghi, B. *et al.* (1995). Resistance to activated protein C in healthy women taking oral contraceptives. *Br. J. Haematol.*, **91**, 465–70

19. Rosing, J., Tans, G., Nicolaes, G. A. F. *et al.* (1997). Oral contraceptives and venous thrombosis; different sensitivities to activated protein C in women using second- and third-generation oral contraceptives. *Br. J. Haematol.*, **97**, 233–8

20. Briët, E., van der Meer, F. J., Rosendaal, F. R., Houwing-Duistermaat, J. J. and van Houwelingen, H. C. (1994). The family history and inherited thrombophilia. *Br. J. Haematol.*, **87**, 348–52

21. Vandenbroucke, J. P., van der Meer, F. J. M., Helmerhorst, F. M. and Rosendaal, F. R. (1996). Factor V Leiden: should we screen oral contraceptive users and pregnant women? *Br. Med. J.*, **313**, 1127–30

Venous thrombosis and oral contraceptives: point of view of an epidemiologist

43

L. A. J. Heinemann and E. Garbe

Introduction

Recently, a number of observational epidemiological studies were published pointing at a slightly increased risk of venous thromboembolism (VTE) associated with the use of third-generation vs. second-generation oral contraceptives (OCs)[1-7]. The controversial discussion continues whether this is due to residual confounding factors and bias associated with the studies, or if this is a clinically relevant result.

However, this reopened methodological discussion about the strengths and limitations of epidemiology, especially if the outcome of interest is rare or the diagnostic procedure is weak such as in mild cases of venous thrombosis. Before coming to a critical assessment of the epidemiological study results and their clinical implications, some considerations about the clinical entity 'venous thrombosis' are needed.

Venous thrombosis

It is known that clinical symptoms of a deep venous thrombosis vary a great deal and are often not impressive, i.e. might neither attract the attention of the patients nor the doctor. Clear symptoms that initiate further diagnostic measures were estimated to range between 2 and 50%[8,9], i.e over 50% of VTE may not be detected, unless there are reasons for better surveillance (such as risk factors for VTE, or OC use). Moreover, the misclassification rate of VTE is also high, i.e. in the order of 30–50%[10-13]. In other words, VTEs are often not detected because neither the affected person nor the consulted doctor find the mild or non-specific symptoms worth following up, unless there are reasons to search for such an event (unmasking bias).

The risk of suffering from a VTE is very low. The risk estimates range between 0.4 and about 2 cases per 10 000 women-years, and the case fatality was estimated from vital statistics to be about 1% (i.e. one fatal case in about one million women). The problem is that these estimates are derived not from population-based registers, which are unavailable, but from various 'cohort-like studies', e.g. very often selected-patient cohorts. Thus, these estimates comprise very weak data, and are obviously affected by the above-mentioned diagnostic procedure and very much subject to an 'unmasking bias' if the patient or the treating doctor has good reasons to search for this diagnosis. The real incidence rates might well be higher in the population if women are screened according to defined diagnostic criteria, i.e. taking into account cases with clinically mild symptoms and also considering misclassification (false-positive or false-negative diagnosis).

It has been well established for some decades that the risk for idiopathic VTE is associated with the use of OCs, and depends on the dose of estrogens. Only the recent studies[1-7] established the suspicion that the newer progestins (so-called third-generation progestins) might also increase the relative risk compared with that for non-users, leading to an impaired safety of these drugs.

285

Safety and risk

Safety of a drug is not just the opposite of its risk. Risk is no clear-cut term, but rather a perceived value. Risk is primarily the probability of an outcome and secondarily the value of this outcome for the person perceiving this risk. Obviously, the perceived risk of a very rare cancer can be higher than that of a frequent allergy: it is a personal or social judgement.

Everything in life is associated with some risk. There is only a degree of safety. Two problems are derived from this: measurement of the absolute risk (usually done with epidemiological methods) and judgement of the acceptability of this risk at the individual and social level. This is not easy to communicate to the public, neither to patients nor to their physicians. The misperception by the public persists that drugs should be without any risk at all.

The issue can be more focused on the individual decision: can I accept the risk of an effective drug, or do I accept the problems, complaints and symptoms of the disease instead? In this respect some diseases create more fear and emotion than others, e.g AIDS, cancer and cardiovascular events. Moreover, an adverse effect in the future is usually considered less serious than the same event today, and a benefit today is better than one in the future. This is also very relevant for OC utilization patterns.

The confusion about risk is also a confusion about terms used to describe it:

(1) The *absolute risk* is the incidence of events in a population;

(2) The difference in incidence for the exposed and non-exposed group is called *absolute attributable risk*, but also *excess risk*;

(3) *Relative risk* is the ratio of the incidence in the exposed group divided by the incidence in the non-exposed group, under certain circumstances called the *odds ratio*.

The relative risk (odds ratio) gives an answer for questions of causation e.g. is there an association between OC use and the risk of thromboembolism, and if so, what is the magnitude? The excess risk, i.e. the absolute difference between exposed and non-exposed is useful to answer public health questions, i.e. what is the impact of a two-fold increased relative risk? If, for instance, the absolute risk is very low, even a four-fold relative risk would still be low.

If one assumes an absolute risk for fatal VTE events of one case per one million women, this compares with other fatal lifestyle risks such as[14]: fatal accidents in the household 1 : 33 000; football 1 : 25 000; pregnancy and delivery in the UK 1 : 10 000 or in Ecuador 1 : 476; fatal accidents of pedestrians 1 : 17 000; car accidents 1 : 6000; parachuting 1 : 500.

The risk of cardiovascular disease associated with OC use was carefully monitored over more than two decades. It became clear that the benefits of OC use in healthy women by far outweigh any risks.

Risk of third-generation OC use

Venous thromboembolism

Although VTEs are rare events in young women, the relative VTE risk for OC users is increased about four-fold compared with non-users in all studies, i.e. still very rare. Newer progestins (third-generation) were reported to have 1.5- to more than twofold higher relative risk estimates[1-7]; however, the latest study[7] found no significantly increased VTE risk associated with third-generation pills.

The relative risk for VTE associated with OC use reported in the literature has not stabilized over time: starting with an eight- to 11-fold risk for OC users compared with non-users in the early 1970s, this estimate went down to three- to fourfold increased odds ratio in the late 1980s to early 1990s. Each pill generation began with high risk estimates after its introduction onto the market with a declining trend thereafter, and then again an increase, at a slightly lower level, with introduction of a new generation. The reason for this is that women who have problems with older pills usually switch to the newer types. In other words, when we compare the risk of VTE of a new drug with that of an old product, we are likely to be comparing a group of individuals at the peak risk level with a group with reduced risk, namely a group from which susceptibles (those at high risk) have been removed because they had already incurred that risk. This has been called the 'healthy user effect' in publications of the Transnational Study Team[15].

The problem is that none of the case–control studies were specifically designed for a head-to-head comparison of third- and second-generation OCs, and therefore data for some of the essential variables – at least for venous thromboembolism – were not collected[16].

One could say that an unbiased odds ratio of less than two is not meaningful[17], if dealing with clinically relatively important but uncommon events such as VTE, because the absolute rates are so low. But in the case of the VTE risk there is evidence that bias and residual confounding factors may explain much, if not all, of the calculated relative risk. Biases to be considered in this context are prescription and diagnostic behavior as well as the 'healthy user' phenomenon. Newer preparations (e.g. third-generation pills), thought to be safer, were preferentially given to women at higher risk of VTE (prescribing bias)[18–22], who were then preferentially referred for further diagnosis (diagnostic or referral bias)[18–23], which led to higher diagnostic confirmation of VTE in third-generation OC users (unmasking bias) and therefore higher inclusion of women with clinically mild VTE not usually diagnosed (selection bias)[23]. Evidence was found for all of these biases, but not in the study data, because of insufficient design for detecting the biases[16].

On these and other grounds, the European Drug Committee (CPMP)[24] could not agree on firm actions against third-generation pills. In their Position Statement of January 1997 they underlined that VTEs are rare, difficult to study and that incidence estimates are not precise. The committee made efforts to reanalyze the studies 'seeking for additional control of bias and confounders'. But 'this has not been fully possible since all relevant information was not available'. Thus 'the impact of biases and confounding [factors] . . . cannot be fully evaluated'. The CPMP Working Group Assessment Report[25] came to similar conclusions.

A final point is that of insufficient biological plausibility of a differential VTE risk between third- and second-generation pills. However, some evidence is available that the risk of arterial events (myocardial infarction) associated with third-generation pills might be lower due to better effects on high-density lipoprotein (HDL), insulin level, insulin resistance and blood pressure because of higher estrogenicity of third-generation progestins[26,27]. Factors that influence venous thrombosis formation include those activating the hemostatic system (e.g. fibrinogen, factor VII, antithrombin, protein C) and factors relating to fibrinolysis (e.g. plasminogen activator inhibitor-1). Recently, one study found higher factor VII activity with third-generation OCs, but many studies in the past did not find this result. Some reviews were published that could not find enough evidence to show that hemostatic factors can explain a higher VTE risk with third- vs. second-generation OCs[28,29].

Another study was published by a group in Maastricht pointing to a higher acquired activated protein C (APC) resistance associated with third-generation OCs[30]; this study was performed using some patients of general practitioners. But our group could not find any differences regarding APC resistance between different types of OC user in an unselected population-based survey[31]. The discussion about biological mechanisms of the VTE risk will continue and new studies are about to be launched.

Other cardiovascular events

Myocardial infarction   The highest case fatality is associated with myocardial infarction (MI) in women under age 45, i.e. 30–40% case fatality, mainly before hospital admission. But it is a very rare event: the absolute risk ranges between 0.4 and 0.6 cases per 10 000 women under 45.

The relative risk for MI of any OC use compared to non-use is increased about twofold[32–35]. First-generation OCs exhibited the highest risk, followed by the second and third generations. All studies already published or on their way to being published show an even lower risk estimate for newer progestins (third-generation) than for older types. It cannot be ruled out that fewer acute MIs occur with use of third-generation OCs, but this needs to be confirmed. Cautious interpretation is currently recommended: there were only a few studies of MI cases that used third-generation OCs; only one study published so far shows statistically significant results; many studies are not yet published and details are not known to the scientific community; bias and confounding factors cannot be fully excluded; and biological plausibility – although available – needs further elaboration. The message to women and physicians seems to be clear: there is no increased risk of myocardial infarction for healthy young women using modern OCs, but cardiovascular risk factors need to be checked prior to prescribing the pill, and monitored thereafter.

Thromboembolic stroke The absolute risk of ischemic stroke is between 0.8 and 1.6 cases per 10 000 women under age 45, but the case fatality is also high (10–20%).

Two recent studies (World Health Organization, Transnational)[36,37] have reported relative risk of stroke for users of second- or third-generation pills: both studies found that the relative risk compared with that for non-users was increased 2.9-fold (conditional logistic regression). There was no significantly increased relative risk for third- vs. second-generation OCs. The risk was found to be lower in non-smokers that have their blood pressure controlled, indicating that cardiovascular risk factors should be checked before prescribing OCs. Similar results were reported from a Danish study[38].

Observational research and drug safety

Randomized clinical trials are the standard to test the efficacy of a drug, and to control for unknown and unmeasurable confounders (by means of random allocation of the drug). But this design is most expensive, artificial and logistically most difficult to implement. Thus, randomized clinical trials are rarely useful for safety–risk consideration, whereas observational studies are most relevant and feasible.

Findings of observational studies, however, should be discussed in the light of a critical review of methodological limits of epidemiology that was recently published in *Science*[17]. Epidemiologists expressed in this article their opinion that relative risk estimates below three- to four-fold should be ignored in view of practical considerations if there is lack of biological plausibility or if the risks are brand new. Therefore, it is a great challenge for every critical clinician or epidemiologist to give priority to thorough contemplation and careful consideration without being persuaded by the attraction of quick, additional statistical analyses. The results of sophisticated statistical approaches often lead to an alleged safety that should be replaced by a more critical view of interpretation[23].

Conclusion

Oral contraceptives are the most widely used and carefully investigated drug and have many well-established benefits, but also some rare side-effects. There is not enough evidence yet that any one of the modern oral contraceptive formulations is safer than any of the others. The balance of a small risk and overwhelming benefits should lead to an informed consent at the individual level, i.e. between the woman and her doctor.

References

1. World Health Organization Collaborative Study of Cardiovascular Disease and Steroid Hormone Contraception (1995). Effect of different progestagens in low estrogen oral contraceptives on venous thromboembolic disease. *Lancet*, **346**, 1582–8

2. Spitzer, W. O., Lewis, M. A., Heinemann, L. A. J., Thorogood, M. and McRae, K. D. (1996). Third-generation oral contraceptives and risk of venous thromboembolic disorder: an international case–control study. *Br. Med. J.*, **312**, 83–8

3. Jick, H., Jick, S. S., Gurevich, V., Myers, M. W. and Vasilakis, C. (1995). Risk of idiopathic cardiovascular death and nonfatal venous thromboembolism in women using oral contraceptives with differing progestagen components. *Lancet*, **346**, 1589–93

4. Bloemenkamp, K. W, M., Rosendaal, F. R., Helmerhorst, F. M., Büller, H. R. and Vandenbrouke, J. P. (1995). Enhancement by factor V Leiden mutation of risk of deep vein thrombosis associated with oral contraceptives containing a third-generation progestagen. *Lancet*, **346**, 1593–6

5. Farmer, R. D. T. and Preston, T. D. (1995). The risk of venous thromboembolism associated with low oestrogen oral contraceptives. *J. Obstet. Gynaecol.*, **1**, 13–20

6. Farmer, R. D. T. (1996). Letter to the editor. Results of AAH Meditel Study. *Lancet*, **347**, 259

7. Farmer, R. D. T., Lawrenson, R. A., Kenned, J. G. and Hambleton, I. R. (1997). Populations-based study of risk of venous thromboembolism associated with various oral contraceptives. *Lancet*, **349**, 83–8

8. Fobbe, F. and Koppenhagen, K. (1995). Diagnostik der symptomatischen und asymptomatischen venösen Thrombose. *Hämostaseologie*, **15**, 148–55

9. Geerts, W. H., Karen, K. I. and Jay, R. M. (1994). A prospective study of venous thromboembolism after major trauma. *N. Engl. J. Med.*, **331**, 1601–6

10. Großmann, K. (1979). Die Diagnostik venöser Erkrankung der Extremitäten mit apparativen Methoden. *Z. Ärztl. Fortbild. Jena*, **73**, 13–17

11. Heinemann, L. and Heine, H. (1981). *Angiologie in der Ärztlichen Praxis*, p. 235. (Jena: Fischer Verlag)

12. Bergquist, D. and Bergentz, S. E. (1990). Diagnosis of deep vein thrombosis. *World J. Surg.*, **14**, 679–87

13. Nielsen, H. K., Fasting, H. and Husted, S. E. (1990). Venous thromboembolism. 'The emperor's new clothes' or 'a silent menance'? *Nord-Med.*, **105**, 139–43

14. Neumann, H. G. (1985). Zur Bewertung von Mitteilungen über Nebenwirkungen hormonaler Kontrazeptiva. *Z. Ärztl. Fortbild.*, **79**, 1033–6

15. Lewis, M. A., Heinemann, L. A. J., McRae, K. D., Bruppacher, R. and Spitzer, W. O. Transnational Research Group on Oral Contraception and the Heath of Young Women (1996). The increased risk of venous thromboembolism and the use of third-generation progestagens: role of bias in observational research. *Contraception*, **54**, 5–13

16. Heinemann, L. A. J. (1997). Möglichkeiten und Grenzen der Epidemiologie. Steroidhormone und venöse Thrombosen? *Gynäkologie*, **30**, 296–304

17. Mann, C. C. and Taubes, G. (1995). Epidemiology faces its limits. *Science*, **269**, 164–9

18. Heinemann, L. A. J., Lewis, M. A., Assmann, A., Gravens, L. and Guggenmoos-Holzmann, I. (1996). Could preferential prescribing and referral behaviour of physicians explain the elevated thrombosis risk found to be associated with third-generation oral contraceptives? *Pharmacoepidemiol. Drug Safety*, **5**, 285–94

19. Farmer, R. D., Lawrenson, R. A. and Hambleton, I. R. (1996). Oral contraceptive switching patterns in the United Kingdom: an important potential confounding variable of venous thromboembolism. *Eur. J. Contracept. Reprod. Health Care*, **1**, 31–7

20. Farmer, D. T. and Lawrenson, R. (1996). Utilization patterns of oral contraceptives in UK general practice. *Contraception*, **53**, 211–5

21. Van Lunsen, H. W. (1996). Recent oral contraceptive use patterns in four European countries: evidence for selective prescribing of oral contraceptives containing third-generation progestogens. *Eur. J. Contracept. Reprod Health Care*, **1**, 39–45

22. Creatsas, G. Pitsavos, C., Amy, J. J., Aubeny, E., Bartfai, G., Coll, C., Elstein, M., Eskes, T, Kovacs, L., Lazdane, G., Lidegaard, O., Winkler, U. H. and Unzeitig, V. (1996). A multicenter European survey of the attitudes to contraception in women at high risk or with established cardiovascular diseases. *Eur. J. Contracept. Reprod. Health Care*, **1**, 267–73

23. Heinemann, L. A. J. (1996). Background to epidemiology of the recent pill scare. In Cohen, J. (ed.) *Oral Contraceptives and Cardiovascular Disease*, pp. 19–32. (Carnforth, UK: Parthenon Publishing)

24. CPMP (1997). Position Statement of the CPMP on oral contraceptives containing desogestrel or gestodene. London, 22 January, CPMP/073/97 Rev.2.

25. Wilholm, B. E. (1996). CPMP Working Group Assessment Report. Third-generation oral contraceptives. *Draft Pharmacovigilance Assessment Report.* (Unpublished document), 20 December

26. Godsland, I. F. (1997). Risk markers and risk factors: metabolism and the pill with reference to arterial and venous risk. Presented at *European Congress on Pediatric and Adolescent Gynecology*, Vienna, March

27. Collins, J. A. (1995). Progestins and lipoproteins: the implications for clinical practice. *J. Soc. Obstet. Gynecol. Can.*, **17** (Suppl.), 12–18

28. Speroff, L. and De Chemey, A. (1993). The advisory board for the new progestins. Evaluation of a new generation of oral contraceptives. *Obstet. Gynecol.*, **81**, 1034–47

29. Winkler, U. H. (1996). Role of screening for vascular diseases in pill users: the hemostatic system evidence on acute long-term effects. In Hannaford, P. C. and Webb, A. M. C. (eds.) *Evidence-Guided Prescribing of the Pill*, pp. 109–20. (Carnforth, UK: Parthenon Publishing)

30. Rosing, J., Tans, G., Nicolaes, G. A. F., Thomassen, P., van Oerle, R., van der Ploeg, P. M. E. N., Hejnen, P., Hamalyak, K. and Hemker, H. C. (1997). Oral contraceptives and venous thrombosis: different sensitivities to activated protein C in women using second- and third-generation oral contraceptives. *Br. J. Haematol.*, **97**, 23–38

31. Schramm, W. and Heinemann, L. A. J. (1997). First results of the Bavarian Thromboembolic Risk Study. *Br. J. Haematol.*, in press

32. Lewis, M. A., Spitzer, W. O., Heinemann, L. A. J., McRae, K. D., Bruppacher, R. and Thorogood, M. Transnational Research Group on Oral Contraception and Health of Young Women (1996). Third-generation oral contraceptives and risk of myocardial infarction: an international case–control study. *Br. Med. J.*, **312**, 88—90

33. Lewis, M. A., Spitzer, W. O., Heinemann, L. A. J., McRae, K. D., Thorogood, M. and Bruppacher, R. (1997). Third-generation oral contraceptives and risk of myocardial infarction: final results of an international case–control study. *Br. Med. J.*, in press

34. Jick, H., Jick, S. S., Myers, M. W. and Vasilakis, C. (1996). Risk of acute myocardial infarction and low-dose combined oral contraceptives (letter). *Lancet*, **347**, 627

35. WHO Collaborative Study of Cardiovascular Disease and Steroid Hormone Contraception (1997). Acute myocardial infarction and combined oral contraceptives: results of an international, multicentre, case–control study. *Lancet*, **348**, 505–10

36. WHO Collaborative Study of Cardiovascular Disease and Steroid Hormone Contraception (1996). Ischaemic stroke and combined oral contraceptives: results of an international, multicentre, case–control study. *Lancet*, **348**, 498–505

37. Heinemann, L. A. J., Lewis, M. A., Thorogood, M., Spitzer, W. O., Guggenmoos-Holzmann, I., Bruppacher, R. (1997). Oral contraceptives and risk of thromboembolic stroke. Results from the Transnational Study on oral contraceptives and health of young women. *Br. Med. J.*, in press

38. Lidegaard, O. (1993). Oral contraceptives and the risk of a cerebral thromboembolic attack: results of a case–control study. *Br. Med. J.*, **306**, 956–63

Venous thrombosis with oral contraceptives: the reaction of a clinician

S. O. Skouby

44

Introduction

Since the introduction of oral contraceptives (OCs) in the 1960s, clinicians have received several official warnings on cardiovascular risks, issued by regulating agencies. In 1969, the use of OCs containing more than 50 μg estrogen was banned by the UK Committee on Safety of Drugs (CSN, now CSM) because a consensus was reached following investigations in the UK and Sweden which pointed to a dose-dependent risk of venous thromboembolism. As a consequence, the principle of prescribing the lowest feasible dose of hormones was accepted. In addition, the importance of other risk factors, in particular, smoking, was established by the use of mortality data on cardiovascular disease, also including stroke and myocardial infarction, from the Royal College of General Practitioners (RCPG) and Oxford Family Planning Association (FPA) cohort studies[1,2]. The so-called third-generation progestins, desogestrel, gestodene and norgestimate, were introduced in the late 1970s in an attempt to further reduce and refine the hormonal content in combined OCs. Pharmaceutical companies have invested enormous resources into the development of these products and research activities have been based, at least partly, on advice from the medical profession regarding relevant safety studies on risk of cardiovascular disease. Clearly, such studies have been directed towards those risk indicators considered to have causal links with cardiovascular disease, and not on clinical end-points. Despite these efforts, the CSM felt it necessary in October 1995 to warn physicians and pharmacists about third-generation OCs because

investigators from the World Health Organization Collaborative Study of Cardiovascular Disease and Steroid Hormone Contraception unexpectedly had found an increased risk of deep venous thrombosis in user of third-generation OCs containing desogestrel or gestodene compared with second-generation type OCs[3]. This finding was supported by unpublished data from two other studies, the Transnational Study on Oral Contraception and the Health of Young Women[4] and data from the UK General Practice Research Database (GPRD)[5].

Epidemiology

The data from the three case–control studies on third-generation OCs, one of them nested in a cohort study, were published in December 1995 and January 1996, together with data from the Leiden thrombophilia case–control study[6]. Altogether, the studies reported a statistically significant increase in the adjusted odds ratio of deep venous thrombosis in users of third- rather than second-generation OCs.

In the multinational hospital-based World Health Organization study carried out in 21 centers in Africa, Europe, Asia, and Latin America, use of OCs was associated with a three–four-fold increased risk of venous thromboembolism. The risk estimates for deep venous thrombosis were generally higher compared to pulmonary embolism. In a subanalysis, the odds ratio value associated with the use of OCs containing a third-generation progestin was 2.6 (95% confidence interval (CI): 1.4–2.6) compared to second-generation products containing levonorgestrel. The values were 2.2 (95% CI: 1.2–4.1) and 3.0 (95% CI: 1.6–5.8) for desogestrel and gestodene, respectively, after adjustment for differences in body mass index[3].

In the transnational matched case–control study performed in ten centers in Germany and the UK, the odds ratio value for deep venous thrombosis with any kind of OC was 4.0 (95% CI: 3.2–5.3). The odds ratio for third-generation products vs. no use was 4.8 (95% CI: 3.4–6.7), and for third-generation products vs. second-generation products it was 1.5 (95% CI: 1.1–2.2).

In the data obtained from the UK GPRD, healthy women exposed to OCs with either levonorgestrel, gestodene or desogestrel were compared with regard to cardiovascular events. Compared with levonorgestrel users, the adjusted relative risk estimates for gestodene users were 1.9 (95% CI: 1.1–3.2) and 1.8 (95% CI: 1.0–3.2) for desogestrel. In a nested, case–control study, relative risk estimates for desogestrel and gestodene users were 2.2 (95% CI: 1.1–4.4) and 2.1 (95% CI: 1.0–4.4), respectively, compared with levonorgestrel users.

In the population-based Leiden thrombophilia case–control study, the highest age-adjusted risk for deep venous thrombosis among OC users was found in users of the third-generation desogestrel product (the only third-generation product included in the study) with a relative risk of 8.7 (95% CI: 3.9–19.3) compared to non-users. In a direct comparison, users of desogestrel products had 2.5-fold higher risk (95% CI: 1.2–5.2) compared to users of all other OC types combined. The magnitude of the added risk was not influenced by a family history of deep venous thrombosis, but was found to be significantly higher in women who had never been pregnant or were carriers of the factor V Leiden mutation.

The interpretation of the results from these primary studies on third-generation OCs and deep venous thrombosis raised a number of issues. Despite their different designs and different populations, these observational studies showed similar magnitude and direction of effect; important issues when a causal relationship is determined from epidemiological data. In contrast, it may be argued that a consistent finding in the same direction may suggest presence of the same confounding factors, study limitations and potential biases in all studies. In fact, the non-randomized design of all OC studies makes them sensitive to diagnostic and referral bias, prescribing bias and the phenomenon of attrition of susceptibles as well as recency of market introduction.

Detection and referral bias take their origin in the well-known fact that diagnosis of deep venous thrombosis is difficult. If phlebography or ultrasound is not performed, the risk of a false-positive diagnosis may be as high as 50%. Referral bias occurs if only individuals considered to be at high risk, for example, third-generation users, are preferentially hospitalized. Consequently, therefore, these women are more likely to enter a hospital-based case–control study. Prescribing bias will appear if physicians consider the use of third-generation products to be 'safer' compared to more traditional compounds, and thus prescribe to individuals whom they perceive to be at some risk, or to women who have experienced OC problems in the past, or to first-time users. The term 'attrition of susceptibles' or recency refers to the possibility that women newly started on OCs may be at the greatest risk for the development of deep venous thrombosis and women who have taken an OC for a longer period without development of deep venous thrombosis may be at relatively low risk of doing so in the future. Data from the UK MediPlus study, published early 1997[7], emphasizes the significance of confounders and bias. The MediPlus database is similar to the GRPD, but with no overlap of practices. In common with the GRPD, the cohort analysis estimated and compared the incidence of venous thromboembolism in users of main OC preparations, and a nested case–control study compared the odds ratio of deep venous thrombosis associated with use of different types of OC, but in contrast to the GRPD, diagnosis was not based on hospital submission. Adjustments were made for confounding factors such as age, duration of use, body mass index and previous pregnancy. When these adjustments were performed, the odds ratio for second-generation products was 3.10 (95% CI: 2.08–4.45) and for third-generation products 4.96 (95% CI: 3.73–6.47). No significant difference between second- and third-generation products could be demonstrated (odds ratio 1.34; 95% CI: 0.74–2.39). In addition, and in accordance with these findings, re-analysis of the Transnational Study have failed to substantiate the original findings[8]. Thus, among epidemiologists there is no consensus about the causality between increased risks of deep venous thrombosis and the use of third-generation OCs after the strengths and weaknesses of the primary studies have been analyzed.

Another important factor for the clinician to consider is not only relative risk, but also absolute figures. Deep venous thrombosis is a rare event with a prevalence of 1–2 cases per 10 000 women per year who are not using OCs. In OC users, the rate is 3–4 per 10 000 women per year, but during pregnancy 6–7 events will take place in 10 000 women per year. Only 1–2% of deep venous thrombosis in OC users will be fatal, whereas mortality from myocardial infarction and ischemic stroke may be as high as 40–50%. It is, therefore, of interest that the most recent epidemiological data indicate that the resulting mortality from all thrombotic events is lower in users of the third-generation products compared to users of the second-generation products[9]. The statistical power of the analysis on association of third-generation OCs with myocardial infarction and stroke is, however, strongly impacted by the small number of exposed cases. In contrast, the potential biases associated with the studies on deep venous thrombosis will be reduced due to a lower risk of diagnostic bias.

Biological plausibility

The biochemical and cellular composition of a venous thrombus consists mainly of fibrin and few platelets, whereas the arterial thrombus consists of less fibrin and more platelets (white and red thrombus). This difference in thrombus composition, therefore, makes the discussion of changes in the hemostatic balance more relevant compared with inflammatory changes or cholesterol plaque formation which are highly important when discussing the impact of OCs on an arterial lesion. The hemostatic balance determines the amount of fibrin formed by the generation and dissolving processes in the coagulation and fibrinolytic system. Any deviation from this delicate balance may be of clinical significance, resulting in a tendency towards thrombosis or bleeding. The balance is characterized by its capacity or degree of activation and molecular markers reflecting activation of coagulation and fibrinolysis are currently available. It is, therefore, possible to measure not only the zymogen, but also the enzyme and the activation peptides; within coagulation, for example, prothrombin, thrombin and prothrombin fragment 1 + 2 and the thrombin–antithrombin complexes. The ability to determine such specific activation peptides and degradation inhibition products has increased our knowledge of the dynamics of the thrombotic process and the predictive diagnosis of thrombosis.

A substantial number of studies have been performed comparing second- and third-generation OCs using these different hemostatic variables of predictive value for the occurrence of thrombosis. The overall results from such studies found no difference between second- and third- generation compounds, apart from the influence on the level of factor VIIc[10]. When the changes of factor VIIc, however, are put into a clinical perspective, based on population studies, it appears that, although the association to vascular disease is clear and significant, the risk is solely associated to arterial and not venous disease. Moreover, there is a clear association between the intake of fat, the concentration of triglycerides and levels of factor VIIc. Changes in factor VIIc levels are, therefore, considered to be irrelevant for the occurrence of venous thromboembolism during OC intake[11].

Another aspect affecting the hemostatic balance is the possibility of OC-induced presence of resistance towards protein C. Activated protein C (via the thrombomodulin/thrombin complex) and the co-factor protein S inactivate blood coagulation factors VIII and V, respectively. It is via this mechanism that activated protein C prolongs the clotting time when added to plasma *in vitro*. In some individuals, this expected prolongation of the clotting time does not take place and these individuals are defined as activated protein C-resistant. Ultimately, this resistance may lead to increased thrombin generation when the carrier of this defect are exposed to thrombosis triggers[12]. In one study released early in 1997, it was demonstrated that women who used third-generation monophasic OCs were significantly less sensitive to activated protein C than those using second-generation contraceptives[13]. A follow-up commentary in *The Lancet* referred to this study as the 'end of the line for third-generation pill controversy'[14]. There are, however, some design and methodological problems with this study as also recognized by the authors. The volunteers are not randomized to the different OC regimens and blood samples are collected at different times throughout the treatment cycles. The specific activated protein C assay used is influenced from other OC-induced changes in the coagulation system and the results are not in accordance with the more commonly used activated partial thromboplastin time-based assay for activated protein C. One should, therefore, be very cautious with the clinical interpretation of a study before the reproducibility of the assay and the clinical relevance in OC users have been further validated.

Concluding remarks on clinical relevance

In a global perspective, the oral contraceptive is one of the most effective methods of birth control, with non-contraceptive benefits such as a protective effect on the development of ovarian cancer, endometrial cancer and pelvic inflammatory disease. Beneficial effects may also be obtained in the presence of specific gynecological conditions such as dysmenorrhea and bleeding disturbances. The widespread usage and the non-contraceptive benefits, however, do not mean universal acceptance of oral contraceptives or absence of clinical hazards. The recent epidemiological data link third-generation oral contraceptive use to an increased risk of deep venous thrombosis, but proper adjustment for confounding factors and bias has not been possible and the biological plausibility is not convincing. It is a matter of concern if the supposed risk only exists due to special genetic or environmental conditions and is, therefore, irrelevant in 'normal' users or in women who have been using the pill for more than 1 year without any side-effects. Thus, there is no apparent medical basis for switching current users to other products. From a morbidity and mortality point of view, arterial thrombotic events are much more serious than venous thrombosis and the most recent data indicate an overall lower risk of thrombosis with third-generation oral contraceptives. However, a proactive discussion with oral contraceptive users is still warranted in order to provide adequate information for making a well-informed choice, together with the women seeking contraceptive guidance. Information on absolute risk figures may increase compliance and counteract media reports which focus on high relative risk. Particular emphasis should be placed on the social and medical problems associated with the risk of unintended conception if a less effective method is used. Determination of inherited or environmental risk factors are clinical hazards that should be addressed, first and foremost, by a carefully recorded anamnesis, although, clearly, more research is needed to clarify the cost benefits of biochemical tests on imbalances in the hemostatic system during oral contraceptive use. Clinicians, together with regulatory authorities, should promulgate not only evidence-based guidelines for oral contraceptive prescription, but also communication strategies, before positions are made public.

References

1. Inman, W. H. W., Vessey, M. P. and Westerholm, B. (1970). Thromboembolic disease and the steroid content of oral contraceptives. A report to the Committee on Safety of Drugs. *Br. Med. J.*, **2**, 203–9

2. Royal College of General Practitioners (1967). Oral contraception and thromboembolic disease. *J. R. Coll. Gen. Pract.*, **13**, 267–79

3. World Health Organization Collaborative Study of Cardiovascular Disease and Steroid Hormone Contraception (1995). Effect of different progestagens in low oestrogen oral contraceptives on venous thromboembolic disease. *Lancet*, **346**, 1582–8

4. Spitzer, W O., Lewis, M. A., Heinemann, L. A. J., Thorogood, M. and MacRae, K. D. (1996). Third generation oral contraceptives and risk of venous thromboembolic disorders; an international multicenter case–control study. *Br. Med. J.*, **312**, 83–8

5. Jick H, Jick, S. S., Gurewich, V., Myers, M. W. and Vasilakis, C. (1995). Risk of idiopathic cardiovascular death and non-fatal venous thromboembolism in women using oral contraceptives with differing progestagen components. *Lancet*, **346**, 1589–93

6. Bloemenkamp, K. W. M., Rosendaal, F. R., Helmerhorst, F. M., Büller, H. R. and Vandenbroucke, J. P. (1995). Enhancement by factor V Leiden mutation of risk of deep-vein thrombosis associated with oral contraceptives containing a third generation progestagen. *Lancet*, **346**, 1593–6

7. Farmer, R. T. D., Lawrenson, R. A., Thomson, C. R., Kennedy, J. G. and Hambleton, I. R. (1997). Population-based study of risk of venous thromboembolism associated with various oral contraceptives. *Lancet*, **349**, 83–8

8. Suissa, S., Blais, L., Spitzer, W. O., Cusson, J., Lewis, M. and Heinemann, L. (1997). First-time use of newer oral contraceptives and the risk of venous thromboembolism. *Contraception*, **56**, 141–6

9. Lidegaard, Ø. and Edström, B. (1997). Myocardial infarction, cerebral thrombosis and oral contraceptives. Two case–control studies. *Acta Obstet. Gynecol. Scand.*, **76**, 53

10. Kluft, C. and Lansink, M. (1997). Effects of oral contraceptives on haemostasis variables. *Thomb. Haemost.*, **78**, 315–26

11. Koster, T., Rosendal, F. R., Reitsma, P. H., Van der Velden, P. A., Briët, E. and Vandenbroucke, J. P. (1994). Factor VII and fibrinogen levels as risk factors for venous thrombosis. A case–control study of plasma levels and DNA polymorphisms. Leiden Thrombophilia Study. *Thromb. Haemost.*, **71**, 719–22

12. Jespersen, J. (1996). Plasma resistance to activated protein C: an important link between venous thromboembolism and combined oral contraceptives – a short review. *Eur. J. Contracep. Reprod. Health Care*, **1**, 3–11

13. Rosing, J., Tans, G., Nicolaes, A. E., Thomassen, M. C. L. G. D., *et al.* (1997). Oral contraceptives and venous thrombosis: different sensitivities to activated protein C in women using second- and third-generation oral contraceptives. *Br. J. Haematol.*, **97**, 233–8

14. Vandenbroucke, J. P. and Rosendaal, F. R. (1997). End of the line 'third generation pill' controversy? *Lancet*, **349**, 1113–4

Early diagnosis of breast cancer by dynamic angiothermography

45

G. C. Montruccoli, D. Montruccoli-Salmi and D. Barnabé

Introduction

The most useful resource that we have at our disposal in the fight against breast cancer can be said to be early diagnosis. Much work has been done to improve and expand the possibilities of those instrumental techniques that aim to 'see' the tumor at the earliest possible stage. Nevertheless, this approach will never be capable of permitting organ-specific secondary prevention, as however small the tumor may be when we manage to catch it, it is still already a cancer. Furthermore, various factors but especially desmoplasia and the histological type make it difficult for us to 'see' the tumor.

In this light, we believe that it is worthwhile to consider the diagnostic possibilities afforded by aspects of turmoral biology, such as angiogenesis or genetic alterations like loss of heterozygosity (LOH), that are either indispensible to the birth of a cancer (as in the case of angiogenesis)[1] or else often precede its appearance (as with LOH)[2,3]. A method that is providing increasingly interesting results in the detection of tumoral angiogenesis and of pretumoral lesions, most often associated with LOH, is dynamic angiothermography (DATG), which is also the subject of this chapter.

Biological premises for dynamic angiothermographic detection

Any state, whether physiological, inflammatory, preneoplastic or cancerous necessitates a blood supply, whose intensity must vary depending on the requirements of the particular condition. On anatomical grounds, in the case of the breast, blood is mainly supplied from the external and internal mammary arteries, which progressively branch off into a microcirculatory network that irrigates the entire organ. In particular, this network, comprising countless tiny vessels, passes through the connective tissue stroma to concentrate at a capillary level around the lobules, where it forms a basket-like structure. It is highly probable that due to the intense physiological requirements expressed by the mammary gland (such as in lactation), the blood supply system to its functional units, i.e. the lobules, must be highly developed with respect to the rest of the breast.

It is now widely accepted that malignant breast pathology generally originates from the morphological structure known as the terminal ductal–lobular unit (TDLU)[4–6]. At a later stage, its histology may become definitively ductal or lobular in nature, but its birthplace is in the TDLU, with its highly developed blood supply system.

Ottinetti and Sapino[7] have demonstrated that, in the presence of hyperplastic alterations (with or without atypia) of lobular or ductal epithelium, there is an increment in blood-vessel dilatation with respect to normal tissue. This implies that an elevated quantity of blood will be able to reach these lesions. It is not surprising, therefore, that we should also be able to find a localized rise in heat caused by a localized increase in the blood supply when one or more lobules have become hyperplastic, which can be distinguished from that of the surrounding healthy tissue with its normal circulation. It is even less surprising if greater heat-pattern modifications can be detected after the angiogenic switch in cancerous lesions of the TDLU where progressive neovascularization is already under way.

Specific studies would be required to confirm this explanation of DATG's ability to reveal surprisingly small pathological changes, including lobular carcinoma *in situ* (LCIS) and lobular/ductal precancerous lesions. Nevertheless, we think that the considerations outlined above can be said to form a valid working hypothesis.

Novel strategy in fight against breast cancer

We believe that a diagnostic tool capable of identifying breast cancer in its earliest stage (the so-called precancerous lesions or the smallest *in situ* lesions) could be of great importance in the fight against the disease. This is the strategy that has been successfully applied, for example, in the cervix[8]. Unfortunately, the breast, unlike the cervix (or other organs such as the bowel), is not accessible to endoscopic or external exploration. However, we have found that very reliable indications of tiny precancerous or neoplastic lesions can be obtained with the DATG method[9,10].

Over the last 25 years, we have used this approach with almost 6000 self-referred women in the gynecology department of our clinic. Our work with DATG has had three main aims:

(1) To successfully diagnose and remove the whole range of neoplastic breast lesions, even the very small *in situ* lesions measuring just a few millimeters;

(2) To remove the so-called precancerous lesions, which have been traditionally referred to as hyperplastic lesions with or without atypia;

(3) To provide regular monitoring for our clients, so that they can be reassured that they are cancer free.

Characteristics of dynamic angiothermography

Table 1 shows the histological results of the breast biopsies we have performed in the last 11 years. A straightforward wide excisional biopsy was used to remove a large number of preneoplastic lesions as well as 46 very small LCIS, all undetected at X-ray mammography.

An important characteristic of DATG is that it is completely pattern-based: no quantitative measurements, such as thermal gradients, are attempted. To spotlight individual patterns, DATG requires plates that are highly sensitive to detail.

Dynamic angiothermography patterns are composed of peduncular branch-like formations in correspondence with the four major arteries: (1) the external mammary, which represents the principle peduncle; (2) the internal mammary, which is often the second strongest; (3) the acromial; (4) the subscapular, which is comparatively rare. Although each of the peduncles tends to have its own general characteristics, individual patterns are always different, like fingerprints. In our experience, even identical twins have similar overall patterns, which differ in their details.

Another characteristic of DATG patterns is that, in the absence of pathology, the outlines of the branches remain constant, even over the course of decades. The pattern can grow, as for example during pregnancy and lactation, or sometimes with use of the pill. After menopause,

Table 1 Histological findings of 596 excisional breast biopsies performed at Toniolo Clinic, Bologna, Italy on indication of dynamic angiothermography (DATG) between 1 January 1986 and 31 December 1996

Finding	n
Ductal infiltrating carcinoma	98 (16.4%)
Lobular infiltrating carcinoma	28 (4.7%)
DCIS	21 (3.5%)
LCIS	46 (7.7%)
Atypical ductal hyperplasia	35 (5.9%)
Atypical lobular hyperplasia	63 (10.6%)
Severe hyperplasia (lobular/ductal)	146 (24.5%)
Phyllodes tumor	3 (0.5%)
Other (mild–moderate hyperplasia, sclerosing adenosis, ductal ectasia, adenoma)	156 (26.2%)

DCIS, ductal carcinoma *in situ*; LCIS, lobular carcinoma *in situ*

the pattern retracts. But in the absence of pathology, the visible detail remains constant, again like a fingerprint.

We have found that certain alterations to the pattern (in particular to the terminations of the branches, and the capitation of branches) are suspicious and require clinical interpretation. It should be underlined that, in DATG, the thermographic interpretation is always done strictly in accordance with the age and clinical circumstances of the patient. This is why we have avoided making classification schemes for DATG patterns. Instead, we have identified a series of objective, abnormal pattern features (ball or spatula branch terminations, benign and malignant varieties of hotspot, malignant stars and rings, etc.) which require accurate interpretation in the light of the age and clinical conditions of the patient.

A DATG breast atlas illustrating signs and their correct interpretation in differing clinical contexts will soon become available. A clearly formulated interpretational system is fundamental for the reproducibility of any diagnostic tool. Problems of interpersonal discrepancy are encountered in every imaging technique, including X-ray mammography[11], and DATG lays no claim to be an exception. Nevertheless, the atlas should illustrate how DATG is based on impersonal, objective interpretative principles that can be clearly formulated and applied by others, rather than on the subjective value judgements commonly attributed to thermography.

Functional blood supply and tumoral angiogenesis

How do we explain these peduncular patterns? In the early days, we thought that the peduncles corresponded to anatomical blood vessels. But mapping of the main vessels at biopsy showed that this was not the case. So, we now think that the most plausible explanation is that the peduncles trace the flow lines of the functional blood supply as it is delivered to the mammary gland through countless vessels, especially in the microcirculation, as outlined above: hence

the term 'dynamic angiothermography'. As regards the notion that tumoral cell proliferation can generate enough heat to create thermographic abnormalities[12], we agree with Sterns and colleagues[13] that this is unlikely, at least in small lesions.

Neoplastic breast lesions also have functional blood supply requirements. Since we started applying DATG, Judah Folkman in particular has patiently demonstrated how neoplastic lesions require their own special blood supply for their growth[1,14–17]. This supply is satisfied by a process of angiogenesis and neovascularization around the tumor. Without the switch to angiogenesis, a tumor cannot expand. The earliest stage in the process seems to be vessel dilatation in correspondence with hyperplastic lesions[7], followed by capillary sprouting when an angiogenic clone is present in neoplastic lobules[1,17] and, finally, neovascularization.

Possibility of organ-specific secondary prevention by dynamic angiothermography

The women regularly followed by us with DATG have not gone on to develop breast cancer. This suggests the possibility of organ-specific secondary prevention of breast cancer by DATG[10,18]. This hypothesis is supported by recent molecular biology studies of precancerous lesions using the polymerase chain reaction (PCR). These studies have demonstrated that a percentage of so-called hyperplasias (with or without atypia) express LOH and, therefore, are already monoclonal[2,3]. In other words, these lesions already comprise neoplastic cell populations. It is interesting to note that these findings seem to provide biological support[19] for a proposal made by Juan Rosai in 1991[20] to reclassify precancerous breast lesions along the lines of the cervical intra-epithelial neoplasia, or CIN, classification system (this would also permit the clinically unfortunate term LCIS[21] to be dropped, perhaps in favor of 'mammary intra-epithelial neoplasia', or MIN). We think that the diagnostic possibilities of DATG could provide a clinical argument in favor of such a change.

The PCR method has been performed by Cavazzana and colleagues in Rome on a number of the preneoplastic lesions removed by us on indication of DATG. They found that about 70–75% of these so-called hyperplasias expressed LOH and, therefore, were already, strictly speaking, neoplastic (personal communication, January 1997). We think that this finding may help to explain the preventive potential of DATG.

In this context, it is also interesting to note that, whereas most biopsies performed on indication of X-ray mammography are done in postmenopausal women, the majority of those carried out by us with DATG were in premenopausal women (Figure 1). This was also true for the positive biopsies, including those that revealed pretumoral lesions.

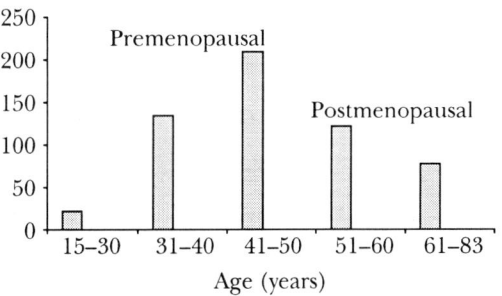

Figure 1 Number of biopsies performed with respect to different age groups on indication of dynamic angiothermography (DATG) between 1 January 1986 and 31 December 1996 ($n = 596$)

Dynamic angiothermography and breast cancer screening

Regarding the possibility of employing DATG for mass breast cancer screening, it must be underlined that, although we have a very large series of several thousand patients, these were all self-referred clients in a major gynecological practice. Our series, therefore, is not comparable with a screening population or a screening situation. Nevertheless, we think that DATG could prove to be suitable for screening. Equipment costs are low, and the examination is rapid, completely uninvasive and easily repeatable. Photographic records of the DATG images would be easily producible for reference at future screening check-ups.

At present, breast cancer screening is generally only performed with X-ray mammography. Its rationale is that it allows tumors to be caught at an earlier, more favorable stage in asymptomatic women over the age of 50 years from the general population, with a corresponding decrease in breast cancer mortality. By contrast, the rationale for breast cancer screening with DATG could also be a preventive one. Furthermore, DATG screening would not present a 'minimum age' problem, as it could, in theory,

be applied at any age. If DATG were to be employed in this way in mass screening, interpretative guidelines for the physicians involved would have to be prepared very carefully to avoid the pitfall of an unacceptable number of biopsies. Contemporary clinical check-ups of the women receiving screening would be mandatory for the DATG interpretation.

Conclusion

Today, advances in molecular biology are opening up new diagnostic, therapeutic and preventive possibilities in all sectors of the oncological field. In recent years, loss of heterozygosity has been shown to represent an important step in the carcinogenic process in many organs. Likewise, angiogenesis is now known to play a decisive role in the birth, growth and metastasis of malignant tumors[4]. Regarding the possible clinical applications of the phenomenon[22], studies are ongoing to test the ability of antiangiogenic agents to arrest tumoral development and extend dormancy of micrometastases in human cancer[23].

Dynamic angiothermography can be seen within this context. In the mammary gland, some epithelial cells either with loss of heterozygosity or the angiogenic phenotype (or both) have greater blood supply requirements than normal cells. Dynamic angiothermographic pattern analysis seems capable of evidencing corresponding localized blood supply increases and, thus, of indirectly revealing two important moments of initial mammary carcinogenesis. We think that the diagnostic and preventive potentials that the detection of these phenomena could offer should justify further and more widespread studies of dynamic angiothermography.

References

1. Folkman, J. (1994). Angiogenesis and breast cancer. *J. Clin. Oncol.*, **12**, 441–3
2. Lakhani, S. R., Collins, N., Stratton, M. R. and Sloane, J. P. (1995). Atypical ductal hyperplasia of the breast: clonal proliferation with loss of heterozygosity on chromosomes 16q and 17p. *J. Clin. Pathol.*, **48**, 611–5
3. Lakhani, S. R., Slack, D. N., Hamoudi, R. A., Collins, N., Stratton, M. R. and Sloane, J. P. (1996). Detection of allelic imbalance indicates that a proportion of mammary hyperplasia of usual type are clonal, neoplastic proliferations. *Lab. Invest.*, **74**, 129–35
4. Rosen, P. P. (1996). *Rosen's Breast Pathology*, pp. 507–44. (New York: Lipincott-Raven)
5. Wellings, S. R. (1980). A hypothesis of the origin of human breast cancer from the terminal ductal lobular unit. *Pathol. Res. Pract.*, **166**, 515–35
6. Wellings, S. R., Jensen, H. M. and Marcum, R. G. (1975). An atlas of sub-gross pathology of the human breast with special reference to possible precancerous lesions. *J. Natl. Cancer Inst.*, **55**, 231–73
7. Ottinetti, A. and Sapinio, A. (1988). Morphometric evaluation of microvessels surrounding hyperplastic and neoplastic mammary lesions. *Breast Cancer Res. Treat.*, **11**, 241–8
8. Anderson, C. M. and Thornton, J. G. (1994). Screening for cervical cancer. *Br. Med. J.*, **309**, 953–4
9. Montruccoli, G. C. (1994). Diagnosing breast diseases: selecting and integrating instrumental procedures. In Popkin, D. R. and Peddle, L. J. (eds.) *Women's Health Today: Perspectives on Current Research and Clinical Practice*, pp. 331–6. (Carnforth, UK: Parthenon Publishing)
10. Montruccoli, G. C. and Montruccoli-Salmi, D. (1997). Timely diagnosis by means of angiothermography. In Montruccoli, G. C. (ed.) *The Female Breast: Gynecological Considerations*, pp. 29–35. (Bologna: Edizioni Balesl)
11. Boyd, N. F., O'Sullivan, B., Fishell, E., Simor, I. and Cooke, G. (1984). Mammographic patterns and breast cancer risk: methodologic standards and contradictory results. *J. Natl. Cancer Inst.*, **72**, 1253–9

12. Head, J. F. and Elliott, R. L. (1997). Thermography: its relation to pathologic characteristics, vascularity, proliferation rate and survival of patients with invasive ductal carcinoma of the breast. *Cancer*, **79**, 186–8
13. Sterns, E. E., Zee, B., SenGupta, S. and Saunders, F. W. (1996). Thermography: its relation to pathologic characteristics, vascularity, proliferation rate, and survival of patients with invasive ductal carcinoma of the breast. *Cancer*, **77**, 1324–8
14. Folkman, J. (1993). Tumor angiogenesis. In Holland, J. F., Frei, E., Bast, R. C., *et al.*, (eds.) Cancer Medicine, 3rd edn., pp. 153–70. (Philadelphia: Lea & Febriger)
15. Folkman, J. (1990). What is the evidence that tumors are angiogenesis dependent? *J. Natl. Cancer Inst.*, **82**, 4–6
16. Folkman, J., Watson, K., Ingber, D. and Hanahan, D. (1989). Induction of angiogenesis during the transition from hyperplasia to neoplasia. *Nature (London)*, **339**, 58–61
17. Hanahan, D. and Folkman, J. (1996). Patterns and emerging mechanisms of the angiogenic switch during tumorigenesis. *Cell*, **86**, 353–64
18. Montruccoli, G. C., Montruccoli, D. S., D'Errico, A. and Grigioni, W. F. (1994). Angiothermography in an integrated diagnosis for secondary prevention of breast cancer. In Fox, R. (ed.) *Lancet Conference – The Challenge of Breast Cancer*, p. 49 (London: The Lancet)
19. Sloane, J. P., Lakhani, S. R. and Stratton, M. R. (1996). Terminology for carcinoma-in-situ of the breast (Letter). *Lancet*, **347**, 1259–60
20. Rosai, J. (1991). Borderline epithelial lesions of the breast. *Am. J. Surg. Pathol.*, **15**, 209–21
21. Baum, M. (1996). Terminology for carcinoma-in-situ of the breast (Letter). *Lancet*, **347**, 1260
22. Folkman, J. (1995). Clinical applications of research on angiogenesis. *N. Engl. J. Med.*, **333**, 1757–63
23. Holmgren, L., O'Reilly, M. S. and Folkman, J. (1995). Dormancy of micrometastases: Balanced proliferation and apoptosis in the presence of angiogenesis suppression. *Nature Med.*, **1**, 149–53

Prediction of outcome of assisted reproduction in the female patient

46

S. Daya

Introduction

The availability of assisted reproductive techniques has provided the infertile couple with a wide array of options to achieve pregnancy. However, despite gradual improvements that have occurred in the probability of pregnancy with such therapy, the overall success rate is still relatively low. Although there are several reasons for the less than desirable pregnancy rates being achieved, it is well known that, in some couples, success rates are quite high whereas, in others, despite numerous attempts, pregnancies are unlikely to occur. Based on this observation, it becomes important to identify the constellation of factors that is associated with good outcome so that couples can be given therapy in an efficient manner. Couples who fall into poor prognosis group can be appropriately counseled to be realistic in their expectations so that they can consider other options. Such categorization into the prognostic risk groups can also allow improvements in technology to occur more rapidly and direct researchers to focus their attention on identifying reasons for the poor outcome in the poor prognosis group.

Several methods of identifying predictors of success have been established and require consistent recording of data on variables that may be associated with the outcome of interest. Statistical methods are then used to analyze the data. This paper will use several examples to illustrate the different analytical tools that are available.

Meta-analysis: the effect of hydrosalpinges on *in vitro* fertilization outcome

In vitro fertilization (IVF), originally introduced for couples with infertility resulting from tubal damage, is now available for most categories of infertility. Several reports have appeared in the last few years associating the hydrosalpinx with a lower probability of success with IVF, whereas other reports have suggested otherwise. One method of resolving this state of equipoise is to conduct a prospective study, after stratifying the patients into groups of increasing hydrosalpinx severity, and comparing their outcome with a control group with normal tubes. This process is time-consuming and involves exposing women in a potentially poor prognosis category to possibly inappropriate therapy. Another option is to review the literature to determine whether there is enough evidence to resolve this issue.

A literature review was initiated to try to answer the question of whether the presence of hydrosalpinges affected the pregnancy success rate and outcome of the pregnancy in patients undergoing treatment with IVF. The search period extended from 1994 to 1997 and included access to electronic databases such as Medline and Embase, and manual searching of journals in the areas of infertility and obstetrics and gynecology. The bibliography of relevant articles and abstracts from scientific meetings were also scanned to identify other articles. Studies were selected if the outcome of IVF was compared in women having hydrosalpinx with those having other categories of infertility. Data from cases with male factor infertility were excluded. The search yielded 35 studies in which controls were available for comparison. The vast majority of controls were patients with non-hydrosalpinx tubal disease (27/35 studies). Other controls included non-tubal disease (five studies), previous tubal ligation (two studies) and bilateral salpingectomy (two studies, one of which also included women with previous tubal ligation).

The studies ranged in size from 75 to 1766 cycles and provided data from a total of 16 523 cycles of treatment. The data from each study were extracted and expressed as odds ratios (ORs) with their 95% confidence intervals (CIs) (Figure 1). The point estimate for all except two studies indicated that the presence of hydro-salpinx was associated with a reduction in the odds of clinical pregnancy (the results were statistically significant in 13/33 of these studies). There was no significant statistical heterogeneity ($\chi^2 = 43.5$, $p = 0.127$) among the individual estimates when compared with the overall pooled estimate.

The pooled odds ratio was 0.56 (95% CI, 0.51–0.62) demonstrating a significant reduction in the probability of pregnancy in the presence of hydrosalpinx. A subgroup analysis of the data, separated into the various control groups, showed a similar effect (Table 1).

The effect of hydrosalpinx on the outcome of the pregnancy was also evaluated, and demonstrated a significant increase in the rates of spontaneous abortion (OR = 1.83; 95% CI, 1.39–2.42) and ectopic pregnancy (OR = 3.44; 95% CI, 2.06–5.75). The data displayed in 2×2 tables from each trial that used tubal infertility controls were then crudely aggregated to obtain summary results (Figure 2). Compared with the overall pregnancy rate per cycle of 27.3%, there was an absolute reduction in rate of 9.4% (representing a relative reduction of 34%). The absolute increase in spontaneous abortion and ectopic pregnancy rates were 9.2% and 5.8% respectively, which represented relative

Table 1 Odds ratios for clinical pregnancy per cycle in the presence of hydrosalpinges compared to various controls

	Clinical pregnancy per cycle	
Controls used	Odds ratio	95% confidence interval
All controls	0.56	0.51–0.62
Tubal disease	0.58	0.52–0.65
Non-tubal disease	0.44	0.33–0.60
Tubal ligation or salpingectomy	0.52	0.36–0.74

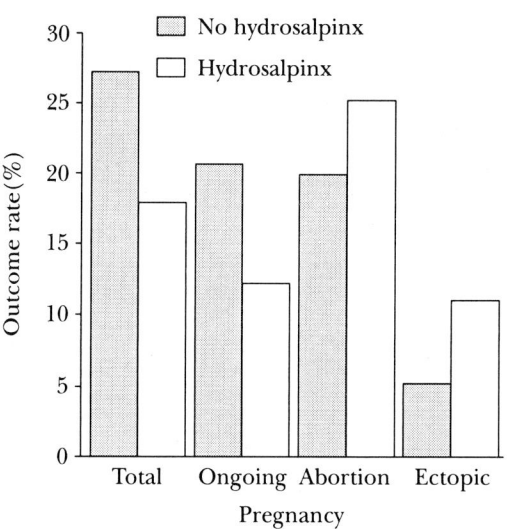

Figure 2 Effect of hydrosalpinges on the probability and outcome of pregnancy

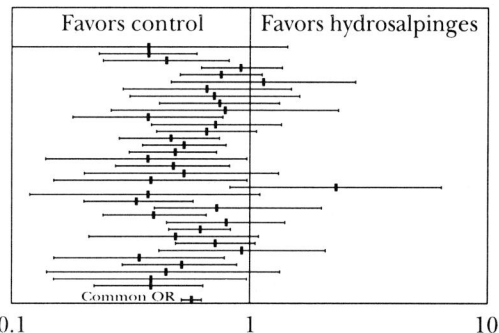

Figure 1 Odds ratios (OR) for clinical pregnancy per cycle in the presence of hydrosalpinges

increases of 26% and 111%, respectively. Consequently, the ongoing pregnancy rate was reduced by 8.6% (a relative reduction of 42%).

The cycle performance characteristics in patients with tubal infertility were then evaluated. There were no significant differences in the mean number of oocytes retrieved (9.3 without hydrosalpinx versus 9.8 with hydrosalpinx), number of embryos obtained (6.1 versus 6.9), number of embryos transferred (3.2 versus 3.3), and fertilization rate (77.7% versus 74.2%). However the implantation rate was significantly lower (10.7% versus 6.9%, $p = 0.003$).

Although many theories have been advanced to explain the mechanism of implantation failure in the presence of hydrosalpinges, the mechanical displacement by fluid leaking from the hydrosalpinx into the uterine cavity seems the most plausible. Much work remains to be done to elucidate the exact mechanism of reproductive failure so that corrective measures can be suggested. The options of tubal ligation, salpingostomy, aspiration of hydrosalpinx fluid and salpingectomy await evaluation by controlled trials, some of which are currently under way.

Logistic regression analysis: predictors of pregnancy with donor insemination

The switch from fresh to cyropreserved sperm for donor insemination became necessary to reduce the risk of transmitting the human immunodeficiency virus. The consequence of this decision was a lower pregnancy rate per cycle, resulting in the need for a higher number of cycles of treatment to achieve the same cumulative pregnancy rate obtained with fresh sperm insemination. It becomes necessary, therefore, to identify the factors that are able to optimize the pregnancy rate.

We conducted a prospective cohort study in 87 women who underwent 220 cycles of treatment with intrauterine insemination with thawed cryopreserved donor sperm. One insemination was performed in each cycle on the morning after the luteinizing hormone (LH)

surge was detected using a urine LH kit. There were 35 pregnancies in this study (15.9% per cycle and 40% per patient) with a cumulative pregnancy rate of 60% after five cycles.

Logistic regression analysis was used to identify which of several variables examined entered the final model that predicted pregnancy. Once total motile sperm (TMS) concentration in the inseminated sample (after undergoing preparation in the laboratory using a swim-up procedure) entered the model, no other variables were able to significantly improve the model. The variables that had no effect included female age, number of insemination cycles, endometrial thickness, total motile sperm concentration in the pre-swim-up sample, degree of male factor infertility and history of previous pregnancy. A discriminatory threshold of TMS = 8 million was observed when the pregnancy rate was displayed as a function of the total motile sperm concentration in the insemination cycle. The odds ratio for pregnancy using this cut-off level was 1.61 (95% confidence interval, 1.11–2.34) and translated into a clinical pregnancy rate per cycle of 23.2% for a TMS above this level versus 10.4% for a TMS below this threshold level. The respective cumulative pregnancy rate curves are shown in Figure 3, in which it can be seen that, after five cycles of treatment, a cumulative pregnancy rate of 80% was observed with the higher TMS compared to 38% with the lower TMS.

This type of analysis is useful in identifying predictors of outcome so that optimal care can be provided. It is clear from this analysis that more attention should be paid to the concentration of motile sperm used in the insemination sample.

Receiver operator characteristic curve analysis: motile sperm concentration for natural cycle IVF

The costs and morbidity associated with IVF cycles, in which ovarian stimulation is used, have led to increasing interest in the option of using a natural cycle, in which no fertility drugs are administered. However, there are many disadvantages with the latter option including a higher cancellation rate from premature LH surge, failure to retrieve the oocyte from the single follicle, failure of fertilization of the single oocyte and lack of cleavage of the fertilized oocyte. Although the double bore aspiration needle and flushing technique has resulted in a higher likelihood of successful retrieval[1], the problem of fertilization failure persists despite normal semen quality in the male partner.

The objective of this study was to identify a discriminatory level of motile sperm concentration that is associated with a higher likelihood of fertilization in a natural cycle so that patients being considered for this treatment could be better selected. Infertile women less than 38 years in age with regular (25–35-day) cycles, with evidence of fertilization in a previous stimulated cycle and with follicle-stimulating hormone (FSH) level < 15 IU/l on day 3, were selected for the study. To be included in the study, the male partner had to have a total motile sperm concentration of > 5 million. Follicle development was monitored with daily transvaginal ultrasound examination until the follicle was ≥ 16 mm in diameter, at which time 10 000 IU human chorionic gonadotropin (hCG) was

given intramuscularly. Transvaginal oocyte retrieval was performed 34–36 h later provided no LH surge had occurred in the interim. Embryo transfer was performed 48–52 h after oocyte retrieval and the luteal phase was supported with intravaginal natural progesterone at a dose of 50 mg twice daily.

The cycle was canceled (on day 3 of the cycle) if ovarian cyst(s) were observed, the endometrial thickness was > 5 mm or the estradiol level was > 300 nmol/l. The semen sample was prepared using a standard sperm wash procedure. Each oocyte was inseminated with 50 000 spermatozoa 6 h after retrieval. Fertilization was assessed 18 h later. Receiver operator characteristic (ROC) curve analysis was performed to identify a discriminatory threshold for sperm concentration that would provide optimal sensitivity and specificity.

There were 84 cycle cancellations out of 240 that were initiated. Successful oocyte retrieval occurred in 129 and fertilization was observed in 104 (81%) cases. Significant differences were observed in the sperm concentration (both before and after sperm wash) in the group that achieved fertilization compared with the group that did not. The ROC analysis identified a discriminatory threshold of 45 million motile sperm/ml in the pre-wash analysis producing a likelihood ratio for a positive test of 2.60 (Table 2) and a fertilization rate of 89% versus 62% for values below this threshold. Similarly, in the post-wash analysis, the discriminatory threshold was 5 million motile sperm/ml producing a likelihood ratio for a positive test of 3.58 and a fertilization rate of 90% versus 53% for values below this threshold. By combining the two

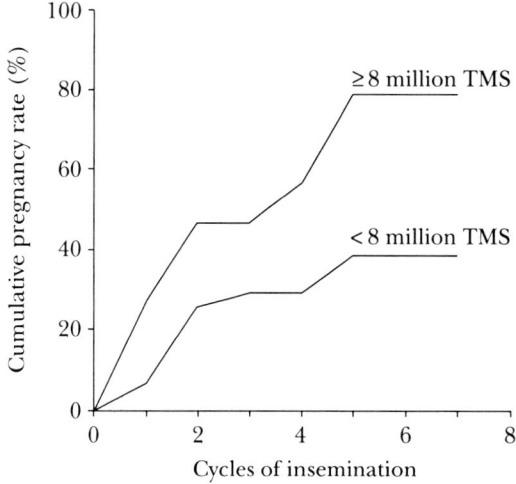

TMS, total motile sperm

Figure 3 Cumulative pregnancy rates according to total motile sperm count

Table 2 Motile sperm concentration and likelihood of fertilization in natural cycles. Likelihood ratio for positive test = 2.6; likelihood ratio for negative test = 0.52

Motile sperm concentration (million/ml)	Fertilization		
	No	Yes	Total
< 45	15	24	39
≥ 45	10	80	90
Total	25	104	129

Table 3 Fertilization rate with motile sperm concentration before and after sperm preparation

Motile sperm concentration (million/ml)		Fertilization rate (%)
Before preparation	After preparation	
< 45	< 5	46
≥ 45	< 5	70
< 45	≥ 5	92
≥ 45	≥ 5	91

tests, better discrimination was obtained as shown in Table 3. Thus, the sperm of male partners of couples considering natural-cycle IVF should be subjected to pre- and post- swim-up analysis to identify those who have a high likelihood of achieving fertilization so that the probability of pregnancy can be increased.

Summary

There are many methods of analyzing data to identify predictors of outcome of assisted reproduction in the female patient. In this paper, the different methods illustrated include meta-analysis, logistic regression analysis and receiver operator characteristic curve analysis. Through techniques such as these, factors associated with a higher probability of pregnancy can be ascertained so that therapeutic interventions can be directed appropriately.

Reference

1. Daya, S., Gunby, J., Hughes, E. G., Collins, J. A., Sagle, M. A. and Younglai, E. V. (1995). Natural cycles for *in vitro* fertilization – cost effectiveness analysis and factors influencing outcome. *Hum. Reprod.*, **10**, 1719–24

Prevention of eclampsia

47

J. M. Belizán, E. Bergel and F. Althabe

Introduction

Many requirements must be met for the prevention of a disease. One of them is to have an accurate method for the early detection of patients at a higher risk of developing the disease in order to apply diagnostic tools and preventive measures. These preventive measures should ideally be applied to the patients who have a greater likelihood of developing the disease. Furthermore, when the disease has become established, treatments are required which can be applied during the mild stage to prevent the development of the severe stage. This is the case for eclampsia which threatens maternal and fetal life.

This article will try to answer a number of questions that arise from the above ideas, based on the available scientific evidence.

Do we have any methods that can accurately predict eclampsia early?

We have reviewed the literature dealing with the use of testing for the prediction of pre-eclampsia[1]. To be included in the review, the reports had to yield the necessary information to construct a 2×2 table in order to calculate the sensitivity, specificity, predictive value and relative risk. In addition, the subjects under study were not to have had any therapeutic intervention induced as a result of testing. There is no overall accepted definition of what a 'good' test is. The ideal predictive test for pre-eclampsia should be simple, innocuous, rapid, inexpensive and easy to perform early in pregnancy as well as reproducible and non-invasive, with both a high sensitivity and positive predictive value.

A summary of all included studies is given in Table 1. It can be seen that the angiotensin II sensitivity test showed the highest median of

sensitivity (75–78%) whereas hematocrit and platelet count had the lowest (33%). The remainder of the tests had medians of sensitivity that ranged between 42 and 70%. The ranges of sensitivity for all these tests were wide.

The vast majority of tests showed medians of specificity above 80% (Table 1). Isometric exercise and angiotensin II sensitivity tests showed the highest values of relative risk (14.3 and 10.1 respectively), with wide confidence intervals. The 95% lower limit of typical relative risk of these two tests was greater than the 95% upper limit of the typical relative risks of mean arterial pressure, roll-over, serum uric acid level, hematocrit, fibronectin, platelet count and Doppler ultrasonography testing methods.

We concluded that at present there is no test for the prediction of pre-eclampsia that is simple, innocuous, rapid, inexpensive and easy to perform early in pregnancy as well as reproducible and non-invasive, with both a high sensitivity and positive predictive value. Currently, plasma levels of ED1 + cellular fibronectin, platelet angiotensin II receptors and urinary kallikrein, and the increase in the sensitivity of platelet calcium to arginine vasopressin are new test methods proposed. Although these tests are promising as predictors of pre-eclampsia, additional evaluation is required to establish their effectiveness before their implementation in clinical practice.

Do we have any preventive interventions for the development of pre-eclampsia?

Over the past few years, two interventions for the prevention of pre-eclampsia have aroused great interest among obstetricians. These are the

Table 1 Evaluation of methods used in prediction of pre-eclampsia[1]

Test	Number of studies	Number of women studied	Sensitivity (%)		Specificity (%)		Positive predictive value		Typical relative risk (95% confidence interval)
			Median	Range	Median	Range	Median	Range	
Roll-over	22	2 502	61.5	0–88	84.5	35–100	40	0–100	3.1 (2.7–3.6)
Mean arterial pressure in second trimester									
cut-off point 90 mmHg	9	40 508	63	8–93	87	62–95	24	6–78	3.5 (3.1–3.8)
cut-off point 85 mmHg	5	—	67	60–88	79	48–88	22	6–47	4.9 (4.1–5.8)
Angiotensin II sensitivity									
<8 ng kg^{-1} min^{-1}	5	350	75	20–90	87	39–99	67	7–90	10.1 (5.9–17.3)
<10 ng kg^{-1} min^{-1}	4	395	78	67–92	83	30–86	47	11–53	9.5 (5.4–16.7)
Isometric exercise	2	300	61.5	54–81	97	96–98	80	79–81	14.3 (8.1–25.4)
Urinary calcium excretion	3	632	70	33–88	84	78–95	32	5–64	5.4 (2.9–10.2)
Serum uric acid	2	536	42	27–56	81	77–85	17	4–29	2.2 (1.0–4.7)
Fibronectin	3	374	57	30–97	94	75–94	67	39–86	2.9 (2.1–3.9)
Doppler ultrasonography	6	1 543	58	29–100	73	64–93	38	9–70	4.0 (3.2–5.0)
Microalbuminuria	1	88	50	—	82	—	26	—	3.6 (1.2–11.3)
Hematocrit	1	445	33	—	83	—	6	—	2.1 (1.3–3.5)
Platelet count	1	445	33	—	72	—	4	—	1.3 (0.8–2.1)

early intake of a low dose of aspirin and calcium supplementation. Unfortunately, the careful evaluation of these interventions through randomized trials showed that the preliminary satisfactory results are not so clinically important.

Low-dose aspirin

There have been 19[2-4] trials assessing the effect of a low dose of antiplatelet agents on the development of pre-eclampsia, involving a total of 18 606 women randomized to either aspirin or placebo. The meta-analysis that includes all the trials shows an overall reduction of 18% in the incidence of pre-eclampsia with aspirin supplementation (confidence interval 24–9%) (Figure 1a). Considering the great expectations created at the end of the last decade, it is a surprisingly modest clinical effect. If we observe the results of the trials included we can see they are heterogeneous (homogeneity test, $p = 0.003$). Including only the large trials, the relative risk reduction on the development of pre-eclampsia with the use of aspirin is 14% (typical relative risk 0.86, confidence interval 0.78–0.95). By contrast, the meta-analysis that includes only the smaller trials shows a 79% reduction (confidence interval 64–88%). The effect size (relative risks) of the smaller trials is distributed asymmetrically among those of the largest trials, with an excess of strong-positive results among the smallest studies.

There are several possible explanations for these discrepancies. The first is the possibility of publication bias; perhaps some small trials with unpromising results have not been published because they were less remarkable. This possibility is consistent with the less extreme results observed in the largest trial[5].

An alternative explanation is that the benefit of antiplatelet agents could be confined to special categories of women at risk included only in the smaller trials. A recently published trial[4] designed to explore the effect of aspirin in high-risk women does not support this hypothesis. This large trial funded by the National Institutes of Health randomized 471 women with

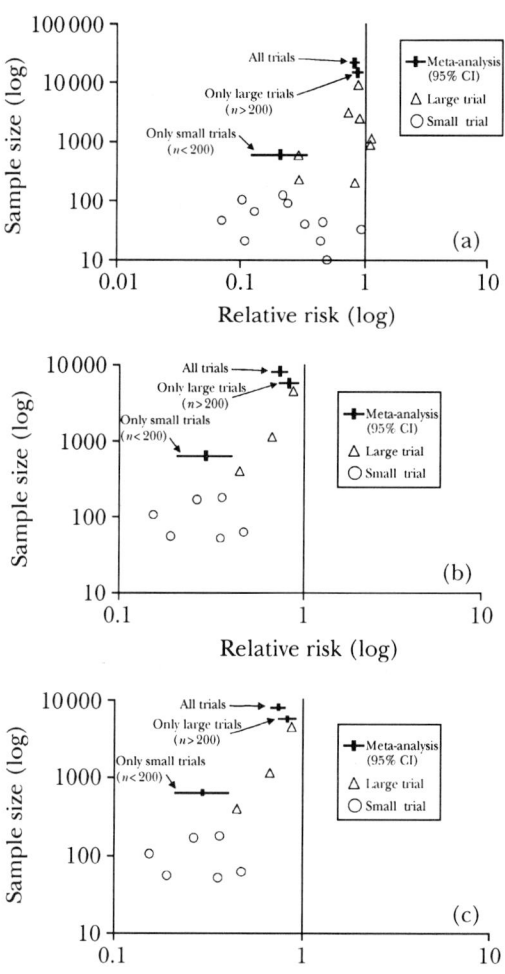

Figure 1 Meta-analysis of effect of (a) aspirin on proteinuric pre-eclampsia (19 trials), (b) calcium supplementation on proteinuric pre-eclampsia (nine trials) and (c) calcium supplementation on pregnancy-induced hypertension (nine trials). In each case, results of smaller trials cluster asymmetrically around those of larger trials; there is much larger treatment effect in small trials than in larger ones

insulin-dependent diabetes, 774 with chronic hypertension, 688 with multifetal gestations and 606 with pre-eclampsia in previous pregnancies. The study concludes that aspirin does not reduce the incidence of pre-eclampsia in the aggregate group (relative risk reduction 9%, 95% confidence interval 13 to –6%) or in any of the individual risk groups. Only in the multifetal gestation group is the treatment effect large enough to be of clinical significance (relative risk reduction 27%, 95% confidence interval 50 to −7%) although it is not statistically significant. The idea that low-dose aspirin may be a general prophylactic agent has been discarded[6], and its effect in high-risk groups is not obvious.

In a *post hoc* analysis of the Collaborative Low Dose Aspirin Study in Pregnancy (CLASP) data it has been shown that there was a protective effect on women developing pre-eclampsia at early gestational ages[5]. If we consider that early-onset pre-eclampsia has the most serious implications for the neonate, this observation needs corroboration. Another *post hoc* analysis of data from the same study showed that if there is any benefit it may be prophylactic rather than therapeutic; there is a protective effect that increases as the gestational age at entry decreases[6]. These data are in contradiction with the results of the trials of Wallenburg and colleagues[7] and McParland and co-workers[8] that showed a significant reduction in the incidence of pre-eclampsia in women treated after 28 and 24 weeks of gestation, respectively. But there is agreement with the results of Bowler and associates[9], a trial that was part of the CLASP study but women-inclusion criteria included the presence of an abnormal uterine-artery Doppler flow-velocity waveform at 18–22 weeks of gestation. There was a non-significant reduction in the incidence of pre-eclampsia with the use of aspirin, although the authors pointed out a protective effect in the incidence of severe pre-eclampsia. This finding does not agree with the fact that there was no reduction in perinatal mortality in any of the subgroups of the CLASP trial[5]. This may be due to lack of power, but we cannot reject the hypothesis that aspirin may have simply prevented maternal manifestations without any effect on the uteroplancental circulation[6].

Some of these hypotheses are being tested in ongoing trials. A multicenter study is being conducted in Spain and Latin America to test the early administration of aspirin (between 12 and 16 weeks of gestation) in the prevention of pre-eclampsia.

In summary, in the light of the current evidence, there is no place for general prophylaxis of pre-eclampsia with low-dose aspirin.

Calcium supplementation

There have been nine randomized controlled trials, including 7232 women, with a treatment regimen containing calcium supplementation during pregnancy and outcome data on pre-eclampsia[10–18]. A meta-analysis including all trials shows a statistically significant difference (relative risk reduction 24%, 95% confidence interval 37–10%) (Figure 1b), but only one trial had enough sample size to detect a clinically significant difference in pre-eclampsia[18]. This methodologically sound study by the National Institutes of Health (NIH) randomized 4589 nulliparous women to either 2 g supplemental calcium daily or placebo. Supplementation began at 12 to 21 completed weeks of gestation and continued until the termination of pregnancy. In this trial, 6.9% of women in the calcium group and 7.3% of women in the placebo group developed pre-eclampsia (relative risk reduction 6%, 95% confidence interval 24 to −16%). This difference between treatment groups is not clinically or statistically significant.

A recent, thorough meta-analysis including all randomized trials with the exception of the NIH trial concludes that calcium supplementation during pregnancy leads to an important reduction in systolic and diastolic blood pressure and pre-eclampsia[19]. The discrepancy between the results of the largest trial and the meta-analysis deserves a detailed analysis that is outside the scope of this paper, although we will try to sum up the possible explanations. Six of the randomized trials were small, with fewer than 200 study subjects. Small trials are more likely to be submitted and accepted for publication if they suggest a beneficial effect of the treatment, a concept usually referred to as publication bias. Figure 1b shows that there is a much larger treatment effect in the small trials than in the large trials suggesting that publication bias might be present. If we include only large trials in the meta-analysis, the summary measure is in agreement with the result of the NIH trial (relative risk reduction 11%, 95% confidence interval 27 to −1%).

Differences in baseline characteristics of the study subjects can also partly explain the discrepancy between large and small trials, causing calcium supplementation to be more effective in certain groups of patients. The incidence of pre-eclampsia in the control group, or baseline risk, varies considerably among trials, from 7.3% in the NIH trial to 44.1% in one of the smallest trials, showing that the smallest trials included a population at a higher risk to develop pre-eclampsia. The NIH trial[20] is the only large trial conducted in a patient population where the median daily calcium intake (approximately 1000 mg with prenatal vitamins) approaches the recommended level of 1200 mg[21], raising the issue of a possible stronger effect of the intervention in populations where calcium intake is lower.

A meta-analysis of the effect of calcium supplementation on pregnancy-associated hypertension (Figure 1c) including all randomized trials (relative risk reduction 25%, 95% confidence interval 33–16%), or only the largest trials (relative risk reduction 18%, 95% confidence interval 27–8%) shows a statistically significant effect. These results might indicate that calcium supplementation does reduce blood pressure, an observation supported by studies in non-pregnant subjects[22] and in animal models[23].

From this evidence one can conclude that calcium supplementation during pregnancy does not reduce the incidence of pre-eclampsia in a well-nourished, low-risk population. The question remains unanswered for high-risk and low dietary-calcium intake populations, like those of developing countries.

Another concern is the long-term effect of calcium supplementation during pregnancy on the offspring. Much attention has been paid to the potential implications that modifications to the fetal environment might have on the development of the fetus, and their amplification throughout childhood and adult life[24–26].

The results of the follow-up of a cohort of children from the second largest trial of calcium supplementation during pregnancy up to 7 years of age show that the intervention does not have any remarkable long-term deleterious effect on the offspring[27]. This study was designed to test the hypothesis that calcium supplementation during pregnancy is associated with lower blood pressure in children. In this cohort the proportion of children with high systolic blood pressure was lower in the calcium group (11.4%) than in the placebo group (19.3%) (relative risk reduction 41%, 95% confidence interval 61–10%). If these findings are confirmed by further studies, calcium supplementation during pregnancy will have a substantial impact on the prevention of adult hypertension since high blood pressure in childhood is a strong predictor of hypertension in adult life[28].

In conclusion, although the importance of an adequate intake of calcium during pregnancy is well known, the routine use of calcium supplementation during pregnancy for the prevention of pre-eclampsia is not justified by the current evidence. More research is needed to explore the effect of calcium supplementation on the offspring.

Do we have any preventive measures for development of eclampsia in women with severe pre-eclampsia?

Many treatments have been used in women with severe pre-eclampsia in order to avoid the development of convulsions and consequently the development of eclampsia. But a search of the literature to select studies that assessed treatments through randomized trials found only a very small number. In relation to the treatment of eclampsia, a recent multicenter randomized trial performed in developing countries showed conclusive results favoring magnesium sulfate in comparison with phenytoin or diazepam[29].

We performed a search for reports of randomized clinical trials that compared different treatments in women with pre-eclampsia, showing the development of convulsions as outcome. The search was performed through the MEDLINE, manual search and the Cochrane

Table 2 Characteristics of clinical trials comparing different treatments on women with pre-eclampsia for prevention of eclampsia

Authors	Method	Participants	Interventions
Moodey and Moodey[30]	consecutively numbered sealed opaque envelopes	228 women with severe pre-eclampsia: DBP at least 110 mmHg for 4–6 h, proteinuria + and delivery imminent. Excluded if prior anticonvulsant (except phenobarbitone) or antihypertensive	MgSO$_4$, 4 g iv over 20 min and 10 g im (5 g into each buttock), then 5 g 4-hourly for 24 h. Control, no anticonvulsant
Chen et al.[31]	randomized (no other information)	64 women with BP 150/100 mmHg or above, plus at least one of 11 listed features of severe pre-eclampsia. Excluded if intrauterine death, chronic hypertension or eclampsia	MgSO$_4$, 4 g iv over 10 min, then 1 g/h until 24 h after delivery. Control, no anticonvulsant
Ramsay et al.[32]	alternate days	59 women of at least 26 weeks' gestation, with DBP 90 mmHg or more and proteinuria. Excluded if seizures in this pregnancy, any anticonvulsant drugs or history of epilepsy	Diazepam, 10 mg orally, followed by 5 mg 8-hourly. Control, no anticonvulsant
Lucas et al.[33]	numbered opaque envelopes, no other information	2138 women with BP 140/90 mmHg or above. Excluded if postpartum or delivery imminent, epilepsy or eclampsia	MgSO$_4$, 10 g (50% solution) im (5 g in each buttock), then 5 g im every 4 h. If severe pre-eclampsia, additional 4 g iv (20% solution) before first im dose. Phenytoin, 1000 mg iv over 1 h. 10 h later, 500 mg orally. If eclampsia developed, all women received MgSO$_4$
Friedman et al.[34]	sealed opaque envelopes, sequence generated from random number table	103 women with BP 140/90 mmHg (or above), or rise in SBP of 30 mmHg (or more), or rise in DBP of 15 mmHg (or more), plus either proteinuria + (or more), or significant edema or eclampsia. Also, two women with eclampsia (data not included in this review). Excluded if MgSO$_4$ before admission, history of seizure disorder, cardiac arrhythmia, phenytoin sensitivity or myasthenia gravis	MgSO$_4$, 6 g iv, then infusion of 2 g/h. Mg levels every 6 h. Phenytoin, 1000, 1250 or 1500 mg, depending on weight. Serum levels 1–2 h later to determine next dose (0–500 mg), once stable checked every 12 h. Both regimens continued for 24 h after delivery
Walls Rodriguez and Levario[35]	numbered opaque envelopes, no other information	38 women over 28 weeks' gestation with SBP 150 mmHg or above, DBP 110 mmHg or above, proteinuria 2+, no previous treatment, at least one symptom (of headache, blurred vision, epigastric pain) and no epilepsy	MgSO$_4$, 4 g iv over 15 min, then 1 g/h infusion. Diazepam, 30 mg in 500 ml 5% glucose iv at 60 µg/h. If convulsions, bolus of 10 mg iv
Adeeb and Ho[36]	consecutive sealed envelopes, no other information	28 women with pre-eclampsia (DBP at least 110 mgHg and proteinuria) plus 11 women with eclampsia (data not included in this review)	MgSO$_4$, 'Pritchard's regimen', no other information. Diazepam, not stated

DBP, diastolic blood pressure; iv, intravenously; im, intramuscularly; BP, blood pressure; SBP, systolic blood pressure

311

Data Base. The reports obtained are given in Table 2. As can be seen, there are only three studies comparing an anticonvulsant with a placebo[30–32]. Two studies comprising a total of 292 women compare magnesium sulfate with a placebo[30,31] and one study comprising 59 women compares diazepam with a placebo. Three other studies deal with the comparison between two anticonvulsants. Two studies comprising a total of 2241 women compare magnesium sulfate with phenytoin[33,34] and two studies with a total of 66 women compare magnesium sulfate with diazepam[35,36].

The results of these studies are given in Table 3. As previously mentioned, the sample size of the studies is small, a fact that precludes the statement of conclusions. However, in the comparison of magnesium sulfate and phenytoin, magnesium sulfate appears to be a better preventive measure for the development of convulsions.

It is remarkable to see that for a disease of the relevance of pre-eclampsia, with its well-known consequences, only a small number of well-designed studies is available to support evidence-based treatment.

Our conclusion is that it is desirable to have more information through randomized clinical trials about the best treatment for women with pre-eclampsia and that the performance of large, collaborative trials is warranted. Magnesium sulfate appears to be the most promising treatment and consequently studies should test this treatment. From the available information there is no evidence of magnesium sulfate as a preventive measure for the development of eclampsia and the test of this treatment versus a placebo is warranted. This study should have close supervision from a data-monitoring committee to examine whether the treatment shows clear benefits that would imply the discontinuation of the trial, and further testing of this treatment versus other commonly used treatments.

Final remarks

Eclampsia and pre-eclampsia remain important causes of maternal and perinatal morbidity and mortality world-wide. This condition is even more serious in developing countries. From this review it is concluded that we still have no effective approach to deal with this disease.

There is no simple and accurate test available to predict those women having a greater possibility of developing the disease, women that could benefit from better follow-up and preventive measures. Furthermore, there appear to be no effective preventive measures, and the initial enthusiasm raised by the possibility of using aspirin and calcium supplements seems to be inconclusive. Finally, treatments to prevent the development of eclampsia in women with severe pre-eclampsia have not been evaluated well

Table 3 Randomized trials of anticonvulsants for women with severe pre-eclampsia in development of convulsions

Authors	Year	Comparison	Experimental		Control		Risk ratio (95% confidence interval)
			Observed (n)	Total (n)	Observed (n)	Total (n)	
Moodly and Moodly[30]	1994	MgSO₄ vs. no anticonvulsant	1	112	0	116	3.11 (0.13–75.46)
Chen et al.[31]	1995	MgSO₄ vs. no anticonvulsant	0	34	0	30	not estimable
Ramsay et al.[32]	1994	Diazepam vs. no anticonvulsant	1	32	2	27	0.42 (0.04–4.40)
Lucas et al.[33]	1995	MgSO₄ vs. phenytoin	0	1049	10	1089	0.05 (0.00–0.84)
Friedman et al.[34]	1993	MgSO₄ vs. phenytoin	0	60	0	43	not estimable
Walls Rodriguez and Levario[35]	1992	MgSO₄ vs. diazepam	1	19	0	19	3.00 (0.13–69.32)
Adeeb and Ho[36]	1994	MgSO₄ vs. diazepam	0	10	0	18	not estimable

enough through effective experimental design. The design and performance of studies to reply to the three issues raised in this paper are fully warranted, and clinicians and clinical researchers should be encouraged to perform such studies.

References

1. Conde-Agudelo, A., Lede, R. and Belizán, J. M. (1994). Evaluation of methods used in the prediction of hypertensive disorders of pregnancy. *Obstet. Gynecol. Survey*, **49**, 210–21
2. Collins, R. (1994). Antiplatelet agents for IUGR and pre-eclampsia. In Enkin, M., Keise, M. J., Renfrew, M. and Neilson, J. P. (eds.) *Pregnancy and Childbirth Module*, Review Number 04000. (Oxford: Cochrane Database of Systematic Reviews)
3. ECPPA Collaborative Group (1996). ECPPA: a randomized trial of low dose aspirin for the prevention of maternal and fetal complications in high risk asymptomatic pregnancies. *Br. J. Obstet. Gynaecol.*, **103**, 39–47
4. Caritis, S. N. The National Institute of Child Health and Human Development Network (1997). Low dose aspirin does not prevent preeclampsia in high risk women. *Am. J. Obstet. Gynecol.*, **176**, S6
5. Collaborative Low Dose Aspirin Study in Pregnancy Collaborative Group (1994). CLASP: a randomized trial of low-dose aspirin for the prevention and treatment of pre-eclampsia among 9364 pregnant women. *Lancet*, **343**, 619–29
6. Pipkin, F. B., Crowther, C. *et al.* (1996). Where next for prophylaxis against pre-eclampsia? *Br. J. Obstet. Gynaecol.*, **103**, 603–7
7. Wallenburg, H. C. S., Dekker, G. A., Makovitz, J. W. and Rotmans, P. (1986). Low dose aspirin prevents pregnancy induced hypertension and pre-eclampsia in angiotensin-sensitive primigravidae. *Lancet*, **1**, 1–3
8. McParland, P., Pearce, J. M. and Chamberlain, G. V. P. (1990). Doppler ultrasound and aspirin in recognition and prevention of pregnancy-induced hypertension. *Lancet*, **335**, 1552–5
9. Bowler, S. J., Harrington, K. E., Schuchter, K., McGirr, C. and Campbell, S. (1996). Prediction of pre-eclampsia by abnormal uterine Doppler ultrasound and modification by aspirin. *Br. J. Obstet. Gynaecol.*, **103**, 625–9
10. Marya, R. K., Rathee, S. and Manrow, M. (1987). Effect of calcium and vitamin D supplementation on toxemia of pregnancy. *Gynecol. Obstet. Invest.*, **24**, 38–42
11. Montanaro, D., Boscutti, G., Antonucci, F., Messa, P., Messa, M., Adonati, M., Chopuzzo, M., Mioni, G., Driul, P. and Tosolini, G. (1986). Prevention of pregnancy-induced hypertension (PIH) and preeclampsia (PE) by oral calcium supplementation: preliminary results. *Miner. Metab. Res. Italy*, **7**, 121–4
12. Lopez-Jaramillo, P., Narvaez, M., Weigel, R. M. and Yepez, R. (1989). Calcium supplementation reduces the risk of pregnancy-induced hypertension in an Andes population. *Br. J. Obstet. Gynaecol.*, **96**, 648–55
13. Lopez-Jaramillo, P., Narvaez, M., Felix, C. and Lopez, A. (1990). Dietary calcium supplementation and prevention of pregnancy hypertension. *Lancet*, **335**, 293
14. Villar, J. and Repke, J. T. (1990). Calcium supplementation during pregnancy may reduce preterm delivery in high-risk populations. *Am. J. Obstet. Gynecol.*, **163**, 1124–31
15. Villar, J., Repke, J., Belizán, J. M. and Pareja, G. (1987). Calcium supplementation reduces blood pressure during pregnancy: results of a randomized controlled clinical trial. *Obstet. Gynecol.*, **70**, 317–22
16. Belizán, J. M., Villar, J., Gonzalez, L., Campodónico, L. and Bergel, E. (1991). Calcium supplementation to prevent hypertensive disorders of pregnancy. *N. Engl. J. Med.*, **325**, 1399–405
17. Sanchez-Ramos, L., Briones, D. K., Kaunitz, A. M., Del Valle, G. O., Gaudier, F. L. and Walker, C. D. (1994). Prevention of pregnancy-induced hypertension by calcium supplementation in angiotensin II-sensitive patients. *Obstet. Gynecol.*, **84**, 349–53
18. Levine, R. J. The CPEP Study Group (1997). Calcium for preeclampsia prevention (CPEP): a double blind, placebo-controlled trial in healthy nulliparas. *Am. J. Obstet. Gynecol.*, **176**, S2
19. Butcher, H. C., Guyatt, G. H., Richard, J. C. *et al.* (1996). Effect of calcium supplementation on pregnancy induced hypertension and preeclampsia. *J. Am. Med. Assoc.*, **275**, 1113–17
20. Levine, R. J., Esterlitz, J. R. *et al.* (1996). Trial of calcium for preeclampsia prevention (CPEP):

rationale, design, and methods. *Controlled Clin. Trials*, **17**, 442–169

21. National Research Council (US), Subcommittee on the Tenth Edition of the RDAs: *Recommended Dietary Allowances* (1989). Committee on Dietary Allowances, Food and Nutrition Board, Division of Biological Sciences. Assembly of Life Sciences. 10th Rev. edn. (Washington, DC: National Academy Press)

22. Butcher, H. C., Cook, R. J., Guyatt, G. H. *et al.* (1996). Effects of dietary calcium supplementation on blood pressure: a meta-analysis of randomized controlled trials. *J. Am. Med. Assoc.*, **275**, 1116–22

23. Belizán, J. M. Pineda, O. *et al.* (1981). Rise of blood pressure in calcium-deprived pregnant rats. *Am. J. Obstet. Gynecol.*, **141**, 163–9

24. Godfrey, K. M., Forrester, T., Barker, D. J. P., Jackson, A. A., Landman, J. P., Hall, J. S., Cot, V. and Osmond, C. (1994). Maternal nutritional status in pregnancy and blood pressure in childhood. *Br. J. Obstet. Gynaecol.*, **101**, 398–403

25. Campbell, D. M., Hall, M. H., Barker, D. J. P., Cross, J., Shiell, A. W. and Godfrey, K. M. (1996). Diet in pregnancy and the offspring's blood pressure 40 years later. *Br. J. Obstet. Gynaecol.*, **103**, 273–80

26. Law, C. M., de Swiet, M., Osmond, C., Fayers, P., Barker, D. P. J. and Cruddas, A. M. (1993). Initiation of hypertension *in utero* and its amplification throughout life. *Br. Med. J.*, **306**, 24–7

27. Belizán, J. M., Villar, J., Bergel, E. F., Del Pino, A., Di Fulvio, S., Galliano, S. and Kattan, S. (1997). The long-term effect of calcium supplementation during pregnancy on the blood pressure of the offspring: follow-up of a randomised controlled trial. *Br. Med. J.*, in press

28. Lever, A. and Harrap, S. (1992). Essential hypertension: a disorder of growth with origins in childhood. *J. Hyperten.*, **10**, 101–20

29. The Eclampsia Trial Collaborative Group (1995). Which anticonvulsant for women with eclampsia? Evidence from the Collaborative Eclampsia Trial. *Lancet*, **345**, 1455–63

30. Moodly, J. and Moodly, J. (1994). Prophlyactic anticonvulsant therapy in hypertensive crises of pregnancy – the need for a large randomised trial. *Hyperten. Pref.*, **13**, 245, 252

31. Chen, F. P., Chang, S. D. and Chu, K. K. (1995). Expectant management in severe preeclampsia: does magnesium sulfate prevent the development of eclampsia? *Acta Obstet. Gynecol. Scand.*, **74**, 181–5

32. Ramsay, M. M., Rimoy, G. H. and Rubin, P. C. (1994). Are anticonvulsants necessary to prevent eclampsia? *Lancet*, **343**, 540–1

33. Lucas, M. J., Leveno, K. J. and Cunningham, M. D. (1995). A comparison of magnesium sulfate with phenytoin for the prevention of eclampsia. *N. Engl. J. Med.*, **333**, 201–5

34. Friedman, S. A., Lim, K. H., Baker, C. and Repke, J. T. (1993). Phenytoin vs. magnesium sulfate in preeclampsia: a pilot study. *Am. J. Perinatol.*, **10**, 233–8

35. Walls Rodriguez, R. J. and Lavario, A. R. (1992). Anticonvulsant treatment of severe pre-eclampsia. Comparison of diazepam and magnesium sulfate. *Ginecol. Obstet. Mex.*, **60**, 331–5

36. Adeeb, N. and Ho, C. M. (1994). Comparing magnesium sulfate versus diazepam in the management of severe pre-eclampsia and eclampsia. *9th International Congress of the International Society for the Study of Hypertension in Pregnancy*, March, abstr. 38

Lipids and lipid peroxidation in pregnancy-induced hypertension

48

M. M. Anceschi, F. Pierucci, V. Brancato, E. Marchiani and E. V. Cosmi

Pre-eclampsia has been, for the last 40 years, the leading cause of maternal morbidity and mortality in the Western world. The pathogenesis of the disease remains unclear, although endothelial cell injury appears to play a key role in the genesis of the multisystem damage seen in pre-eclampsia. Rodgers and colleagues[1] reported that pre-eclamptic sera contain 'cytotoxic factors' that damage endothelial cells. The identity of these cytotoxic factors is unknown, but, currently, the attention has focused on potential endothelial activators as lipid peroxides and cytokines. It has been proposed that the origin of these factors is the placenta, poorly perfused because of the defective invasion of the maternal vessels observed in pre-eclampsia[2].

In pre-eclampsia a marked perturbation in lipid and lipoprotein metabolism has also been reported that may play a role in the pathogenesis of the disorder. Van den Elzen and colleagues[3] reported a significant association between serum total cholesterol levels in the first trimester of pregnancy and the risk of pre-eclampsia, with the adjusted relative risk exceeding 5 for women with serum total cholesterol levels above 6 mmol/l. Uslu and co-workers[4] found a significant increase in serum levels of apolipoprotein(a) and lipoprotein(a) in pregnancy-induced hypertension, but no significant correlation could be demonstrated for other lipoproteins.

In normal pregnant women, the total serum lipid concentration is significantly higher than that found in non-pregnant women and the concentration of each lipid component (triglyceride, cholesterol and phospholipids) is also higher in normal pregnant women when compared with non-pregnant women[5]. In pre-eclampsia, there is a significant increase in triglyceride concentration with respect to normal pregnancies. This may be explained by an increased flux of free fatty acid that occurs over and above that seen in normal pregnancies[6].

In normal pregnancies, in the late second trimester, the flux of free fatty acid is increased because of the stimulation of hormone-sensitive lipase by human placental lactogen[7] and the relative resistance to insulin, that normally suppresses the free fatty acid release from adipose tissue[8]. Normally, free fatty acid entering the liver has two routes of metabolism, being subjected to beta-oxidation or esterified and secreted as triglyceride in very low density lipoproteins (VLDL). Late pregnancy is associated with an increased flux of free fatty acid and impaired free fatty acid beta-oxidation, with increased triglyceride synthesis, compensated for by increased secretion of VLDL[9].

In pre-eclampsia, the flux of free fatty acid is further enhanced (and this phenomenon is observed long before the onset of clinical disease)[10] by the placental cytokines and the liver further increases the VLDL secretion, and particularly the secretion of large, triglyceride-rich VLDL. The elevation in plasma triglyceride levels leads to an associated increase in small, dense low density lipoproteins (LDL) that are more susceptible to oxidation than large LDL[11]. Large VLDL and small LDL (particularly when oxidized), both have the capacity to induce endothelial damage[12]. Oxidized LDL (ox-LDL) promotes rapid adhesion of neutrophils to the endothelium[13], inhibits endothelial prostacyclin synthesis, increases endothelin production and release and inactivates endothelium-derived relaxing factor (EDRF) (nitric oxide)[12].

Ox-LDL is also immunogenic and can elicit autoantibody formation. Branch and colleagues[14] observed significant higher titers of auto-antibodies to an epitope of ox-LDL in pre-eclamptic patients when compared to normal pregnant women.

The placenta is a source of lipid peroxides in pre-eclampsia. Lipid peroxides are formed when polyunsaturated fatty acids interact with free radicals. Several studies have demonstrated that maternal levels of lipid peroxides are increased in normal pregnancy as compared with non-pregnant women, and are significantly elevated in pre-eclampsia as compared to normal pregnancy. In contrast, the antioxidant activity of maternal blood is significantly decreased in pre-eclampsia as compared to normal pregnancy[15,16]. Antioxidants are derived from endogenous sources or from the diet. They may be classified into preventive antioxidants that act to inhibit the initiation of the peroxidation process, and chain-breaking antioxidants that act to trap or decompose radicals or peroxides already present in the system[17]. The most important chain-breaking antioxidants are α-tocopherol, ascorbic acid, carotenoids, glutathione and uric acid. The most important antioxidative enzymes are superoxide dismutase, catalase, glutathione peroxidase, glutathione-S-transferase and glucose-6-phosphate dehydrogenase.

Lipid peroxides secreted by the placenta have a relatively short half-life. However, some lipid peroxides, such as the oxidized polyunsaturated fatty acid in ox-LDL, have a half-life of about 3 h and are stable enough to function as circulating compounds[18].

We have investigated the susceptibility of isolated plasmatic LDL to copper-mediated oxidation as an indication of enhanced lipid (and particularly LDL) oxidation in pre-eclampsia[19]. We have observed a significant increase in LDL oxidation in pre-eclampsia, demonstrated by a reduction in lag time of oxidation and an increase in oxidation rate in isolated LDL, obtained from pre-eclamptic pregnant women as compared to normal pregnant women. We have also found a significant negative correlation

between serum levels of uric acid and lag time of oxidation in isolated LDL (unpublished data) (Figure 1).

Many and colleagues have proposed a correlation between oxidative stress and hyperuricemia through the xanthine oxidase activity[20]. Xanthine dehydrogenase/oxidase is present as two isoforms *in vivo*. Several factors, as hypoxia/reperfusion, cytokines and increased substrate availability (xanthine and hypoxanthine) may increase the conversion of xanthine dehydrogenase/oxidase to its oxidase form. When the enzyme is in its oxidase form, uric acid production is coupled with the formation of reactive oxygen species. The presence of a relatively hypoxic maternal–fetal interface, the increased turnover of trophoblastic tissue which can result in higher xanthine and hypoxanthine concentration and the increased levels of circulating cytokines in pre-eclampsia, may act to stimulate the conversion of the enzyme in its oxidase isoform, explaining the correlation between oxidative stress and uric acid levels.

The increased production of lipid peroxides may explain the increase in thromboxane synthesis observed in pre-eclampsia. Walsh and co-workers postulated that peroxides could increase the synthesis of thromboxane by

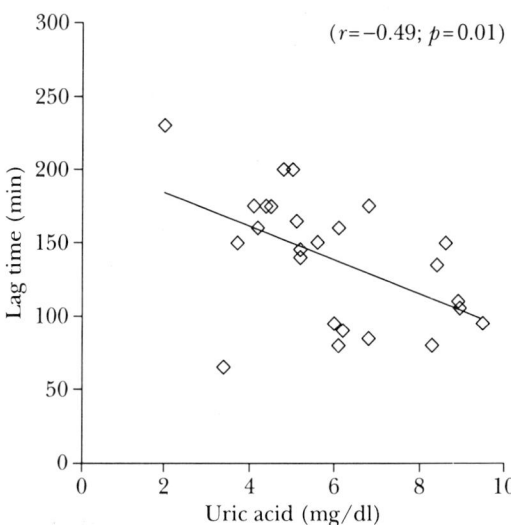

Figure 1 Linear regression between lag time and uric acid values

stimulating the activity of the PGH-synthase enzyme, particularly of the cyclooxygenase component that converts arachidonic acid in PGG_2[21]. The peroxidase component of PGH-synthase then converts the PGG_2 in PGH_2, with production of superoxide radicals. PGH_2 is converted in thromboxane by thromboxane synthase. Thromboxane is a potent vasoconstrictor and the perfusion of the placenta with peroxides could result in vasoconstriction (a common feature in pre-eclampsia). Walsh and colleagues[21] have also observed significantly lower levels of glutathione peroxidase activity in placentas obtained from women with pre-eclampsia than from those in normal pregnancies. Glutathione peroxidase is one of the most important antioxidants in tissues; a decrease in the activity of this enzyme in pre-eclamptic placentas could explain the increase in peroxide production and that of thromboxane synthesis.

Lipid peroxides may also contribute to vasoconstriction, leading to maternal hypertension, through their ability to inactivate nitric oxide. Pamarthi and co-workers reported an increased synthesis of nitric oxide in rat peritoneal macrophages after incubation with native VLDL and LDL and oxidized VLDL[22].

Finally, lipid peroxides may contribute to coagulation abnormalities associated with pre-eclampsia; indeed they increase thrombin generation and decrease antithrombin III levels, triggering thrombus formation, as observed in disseminated intravascular coagulation[23]. Moreover, oxidized LDL and high density lipoprotein (HDL) may cause platelet aggregation and activation, through changes in platelet membrane fluidity[24].

Altered cell membrane fluidity in pre-eclampsia has been described. In our previous study, we reported an increased cholesterol/phospholipids ratio in the erythrocyte plasma membrane of pre-eclamptic pregnant women as compared to normal pregnant women[25]. Similar abnormalities have been reported in the plasma membrane of platelets[26] and trophoblastic cells[27]. The increase in cholesterol/phospholipids ratio is associated with a reduction of cell membrane fluidity that alters cellular function. Lipid peroxides increase the incorporation of cholesterol into cell membranes, influencing their function. It is also likely that the composition, and then the function, of endothelial cells, is altered in pre-eclampsia.

In conclusion, the increased production of lipid peroxides may explain most of the clinical findings of pre-eclampsia, although it is not enough completely to understand the pathogenesis of this pregnancy-related disease.

References

1. Rodgers, G. M., Taylor, R. N. and Roberts, J. M. (1988). Preeclampsia is associated with a serum factor cytotoxic to human endothelial cells. *Am. J. Obstet. Gynecol.*, **159**, 908–14
2. Roberts, J. M. and Redman, C. W. G. (1993). Preeclampsia: more than pregnancy induced hypertension. *Lancet*, **341**, 1447–51
3. Van den Elzen, H. J., Wladimiroff, J. W., Cohen-Overbeek, T. E., de Bruijn, A. J. and Grobbee, D. E. (1996). Serum lipids in early pregnancy and risk of preeclampsia. *Br. J. Obstet. Gynaecol.*, **103**, 117–22
4. Uslu, A., Uslu, T., Bingol, F. and Aydin, S. (1996). Lipoprotein levels in patients with pregnancy induced hypertension. *Arch. Gynecol. Obstet.*, **258**, 21–4
5. Maseki, M., Nishigaki, I., Hagihara, M., Tomoda, Y. and Yagi, K. (1981). Lipid peroxide levels and lipid content of serum lipoprotein fractions of pregnant subjects with or without preeclampsia. *Clin. Chim. Acta*, **115**, 155–61
6. Sattar, N., Gaw, A., Packard, C. J. and Greer, I. A. (1996). Potential pathogenic roles of aberrant lipoprotein and fatty acid metabolism in pre-eclampsia. *Br. J. Obstet. Gynaecol.*, **103**, 614–20
7. Martin-Hidalgo, A., Hom, C., Belfrage, M., Schotz, M. C. and Herrera, E. (1994). Lipoprotein lipase and hormone-sensitive lipase activity and mRNA in rat adipose tissue during pregnancy. *Am. J. Physiol.*, **266**, 930–5
8. Silliman, K., Shore, V. and Forte, T. (1994). Hypertriglyceridaemia during late pregnancy is

associated with the formation of small, dense low density lipoprotein and the presence of large buoyant high density lipoproteins. *Metabolism*, **43**, 1035–41

9. Wasfi, I., Weinstein, I. and Heimberg, M. (1980). Increased formation of triglyceride from oleate in perfused livers from pregnant rats. *Endocrinology*, **107**, 584–90

10. Lorentzen, B., Endersen, M. J., Clausen, T. and Henriksen, T. (1994). Fasting serum free fatty acids and triglycerides are increased before 20 weeks of gestation in women who later develop preeclampsia. *Hypertens. Pregnancy*, **13**, 103–9

11. deGraaf, J., Hak-Lemmers, H. L. and Hectors, M. P. C. (1991). Enhanced susceptibility to *in vitro* oxidation of the dense low density lipoprotein subfraction in healthy subjects. *Arterioscler. Thromb.*, **11**, 298–306

12. Stewart, D. J. and Monge, J. C. (1993). Hyperlipidaemia and endothelial dysfunction. *Curr. Opin. Lipidol.*, **4**, 319–24

13. Lehr, H. A., Krombach, F., Munzing, S. *et al.* (1995). *In vitro* effects of oxidised low density lipoprotein on CD11b/CD18 and L-selectin presentation on neutrophils and monocytes with relevance for the *in vivo* situation. *Am. J. Pathol.*, **146**, 218–27

14. Branch, D. W., Mitchell, M. D., Miller, E., Palinski, W. and Witzum, J. L. (1994). Pre-eclampsia and serum antibodies to oxidise low-density lipoprotein. *Lancet*, **343**, 645–6

15. Ishihara, M. (1978). Studies on lipoperoxide of normal pregnant women and of patients with toxemia of pregnancy. *Clin. Chim. Acta*, **84**, 1–9

16. Uotila, J. T., Tuimala, R. J., Aarnio, T. M., Pyykko, K. A. and Ahotupa, M. O. (1993). Findings on lipid peroxidation and antioxidant function in hypertensive complications of pregnancy. *Br. J. Obstet. Gynaecol.*, **100**, 270–6

17. Poranen, A. K., Ekblad, U., Uotila, P. and Ahotupa, M. (1996). Lipid peroxidation and antioxidants in normal and pre-eclamptic pregnancies. *Placenta*, **17**, 401–5

18. Gorog, P. (1991). Activation of human blood monocytes by oxidized polyunsaturated fatty acids: a possible mechanism for the generation of lipid peroxides in the circulation. *Int. J. Exp. Pathol.*, **72**, 227–37

19. Pierucci, F., Piazze Garnica, J. J., Cosmi, E. V. and Anceschi, M. M. (1996). Oxidability of low density lipoproteins in pregnancy-induced hypertension. *Br. J. Obstet. Gynaecol.*, **103**, 1159–61

20. Many, A., Hubel, C. A. and Roberts, J. M. (1996). Hyperuricemia and xanthine oxidase in pre-eclampsia, revisited. *Am. J. Obstet. Gynecol.*, **174**, 288–91

21. Walsh, S. W. and Wang. Y. (1993). Deficient glutathione peroxidase activity in preeclampsia is associated with increased placental production of thromboxane and lipid peroxides. *Am. J. Obstet. Gynecol.*, **169**, 1456–61

22. Pamarthi, E. M. and Durisala, D. (1994). Very low density and low density lipoproteins induce nitric oxide synthesis in macrophages. *Biochem. Biophys. Res. Commun.*, **204**, 1047–53

23. Barrowcliffe, T. W., Gray, E., Kerry, P. J. and Gutteridge, J. M. C. (1984). Triglyceride-rich lipoproteins are responsible for thrombin generation induced by lipid peroxides. *Thromb. Haemost.*, **52**, 7–10

24. Ardlie, N. G., Selley, M. L. and Simons, L. A. (1989). Platelet activation by oxidatively modified low density lipoproteins. *Atherosclerosis*, **76**, 117–24

25. Piazze Garnica, J. J., Pierucci, F., Vozzi, G., Cosmi, E. V. and Anceschi, M. M. (1994). The cholesterol to phospholipids ratio (C/PL) of the erythrocyte membrane in normotensive, hypertensive pregnant and in cord blood as assessed by a simple enzymatic method. *Scand. J. Clin. Lab. Invest.*, **54**, 631–5

26. Coata, G., Frusca, T., Baranzelli, D., Cosmi, E. V., Di Renzo, G. C. and Anceschi, M. M. (1992). Abnormal platelet lipid membrane composition in pregnancy induced hypertension. *J. Perinat. Med.*, **20**, 123–7

27. Cester, N., Mazzanti, L., Benedetti, G., Cugini, A. M., Rabini, R. A., Tranquilli, A. L. and Valenzise, H. (1988). Pregnancy induced hypertension: observations on chemical–physical properties of syncytiotrophoblast plasma membranes from human placenta. *Clin. Exp. Hypertens. [B] Hypertens. Preg.*, **B7**, 57–66

Index